Springer Theses

Recognizing Outstanding Ph.D. Research

Aims and Scope

The series "Springer Theses" brings together a selection of the very best Ph.D. theses from around the world and across the physical sciences. Each volume has been selected for its scientific excellence by an internationally renowned institute or department. For greater accessibility to non-specialists, the published versions include an extended introduction, as well as a foreword by the student's supervisor explaining the special relevance of the work for the field. The series as a whole provides a valuable resource both for newcomers to the research fields, and for other scientists seeking detailed background information on special questions. Finally, it serves as an accredited documentation of the valuable contributions made by today's younger generation of scientists.

How to Apply

Theses prepared at internationally leading universities and institutes may be nominated for publication by supervisors with the endorsement of the head of department. Each such department is entitled to nominate one thesis per year. Enquiries and requests for a nomination form should be sent, together with the thesis, to Ms. Nathalie Berg (see link on right).

Eligibility Criteria

To qualify for consideration, theses should fulfil the following criteria:

- They must be written in good English.
- The topic should fall within the confines of Chemistry, Physics, Earth Sciences, Engineering and related interdisciplinary fields such as Materials, Nanoscience, Chemical Engineering, Complex Systems and Biophysics.
- The work reported in the thesis must represent a significant scientific advance.
- A maximum of 30% of the text may be a verbatim reproduction from the author's previous publications.
- They must have been examined and passed during the 12 months prior to nomination.
- The theses should have a clearly defined structure including an introduction accessible to new PhD students and scientists not expert in the relevant field.
- After acceptance, theses should be supplemented by a "Supervisor's Foreword" outlining the wider scientific relevance of the work.

Indexed by zbMATH.

Mihai Dragusanu

Design of Soft–Rigid Devices for Rehabilitative and Assistive Robotics

Doctoral Theses accepted by
University of Siena, Siena, Italy

Springer

Author
Dr. Mihai Dragusanu
Department of Information Engineering
and Mathematics
University of Siena
Siena, Italy

Supervisor
Prof. Monica Malvezzi
Department of Information Engineering
and Mathematics
University of Siena
Siena, Italy

ISSN 2190-5053 ISSN 2190-5061 (electronic)
Springer Theses
ISBN 978-3-031-84822-3 ISBN 978-3-031-84823-0 (eBook)
https://doi.org/10.1007/978-3-031-84823-0

This Springer imprint is published by the registered company Springer Nature Switzerland AG
The registered company address is: Gewerbestrasse 11, 6330 Cham, Switzerland

To my family, for their unconditional love and support, and to my beloved Serena.

Supervisor's Foreword

It is my great pleasure to introduce Dr. Mihai Dragusanu's thesis work, which has been accepted for publication within Springer Theses Book Series and recognized with an award for outstanding original work.

I have been the supervisor of his Master and Ph.D. Theses and I currently collaborate with him in several research projects, in which he is involved as a post-doctoral researcher. I can assure Dr. Mihai Dragusanu has a very strong background across various fields of robotics, including robotic grasping and manipulation, human-robot interaction, haptics, wearable robots, exoskeletons, and robotic augmentation. While his engineering expertise is impressive, his interdisciplinary approach, by means of working with neuroscientists, surgeons, psychologists, and educators, further strengthens the quality of his research.

The Ph.D. thesis in particular focuses on Mihai's journey in haptics, rehabilitation, and assistive robotics. It details the innovative devices he designed and developed, their practical applications, and the tests conducted. The development of robotic devices aimed at assisting individuals with impairments or disabilities in their daily lives is an exceptionally challenging area of research with significant potential for social impact

Wearable robotic devices as exoskeletons can support people in autonomously performing physiotherapy exercises, increasing their efficiency, providing supplementary information about results and progress, reducing physiotherapists' efforts and the need of their physical presence during exercise sessions, and encouraging autonomy and independence in people with disabilities. Robotic devices can be a fundamental support for people with impairments in their everyday activities, as for instance grasping objects, making bimanual operations, dressing, etc. Wearable haptics devices are becoming an important tool to enhance experiences in virtual or augmented reality and for human/human interactions.

Nevertheless, assistive and supportive technologies developed without the inputs and feedback of the end-user throughout the design process are less likely to be adopted for their intended purpose and use case.

Mihai's thesis presents the main results of a research in which different devices for rehabilitation, assistance, and haptic applications are designed and developed. The fil-rouge of the thesis is the user-centered perspective that has been employed in all the design and development phases, and the exploitation of soft robotics solutions, one of the most recent and challenging robotics branches, that in this context is mandatory for a safe and comfortable interaction with the user.

Siena, Italy
January 2025

Prof. Monica Malvezzi

Parts of this thesis have been published in the following articles

International Journal Articles

1. **M. Dragusanu**, S. Marullo, M. Malvezzi, G. M. Achilli, M. C. Valigi, D. Prattichizzo and G. Salvietti. The dressgripper: A collaborative gripper with electromagnetic fingertips for dressing assistance. *IEEE Robotics and Automation Letters*, 7(3), 7479–7486, 2022, doi: 10.1109/LRA.2022.3183756.
2. **M. Dragusanu**, Z. Iqbal, T. Lisini Baldi, D. Prattichizzo and M. Malvezzi. Design, Development, and Control of a Hand/Wrist Exoskeleton for Rehabilitation and Training. *IEEE Transactions on Robotics*, vol. 38, no. 3, pp. 1472–1488, 2022, doi: 10.1109/TRO.2022.3172510.
3. **M. Dragusanu**, D. Troisi, A. Villani, D. Prattichizzo and M. Malvezzi. Design and prototyping of an underactuated hand exoskeleton with fingers coupled by a gear-based differential. *Frontiers in Robotics and AI, section Biomedical Robotics*, p. 69, 2022, doi: 10.3389/frobt.2022.862340.
4. **M. Dragusanu**, A. Villani, D. Prattichizzo and M. Malvezzi. Design of a Wearable Haptic Device for Hand Palm Cutaneous Feedback. *Frontiers in Robotics and AI, section Haptics*, p. 254, 2021, doi: 10.3389/frobt.2021.706627.

International Conferences

1. A. Villani, **M. Dragusanu**, D. Prattichizzo and M. Malvezzi. Validation and Usability Assessment of The HapticPalm, a Wearable Device for Hand Palm Force Feedback. *2024 IEEE Haptics Symposium (HAPTICS), Long Beach*, CA, USA, 2024, pp. 372–378, doi: 10.1109/HAPTICS59260.2024.10520842.
2. **M. Dragusanu**, D. Troisi, D. Prattichizzo and M. Malvezzi. Compliant Finger Joint with Controlled Variable Stiffness based on Twisted Strings Actuation. *2023 IEEE International Conference on Robotics and Automation (ICRA)*, London, United Kingdom, 2023, pp. 7378–7384, doi: 10.1109/ICRA48891.2023.10160353.
3. **M. Dragusanu**, D. Troisi, A. Villani, D. Prattichizzo and M. Malvezzi. HAPP: a Haptic Portable Pad for Hand Disease Manual Treatment. *In 2022 31st IEEE International Conference on Robot and Human Interactive Communication (RO-MAN)*, pp. 345–350, 2022, doi: 10.1109/RO-MAN53752.2022.9900810.

4. **M. Dragusanu**, Z. Iqbal, A. Villani, N. D'Aurizio, D. Prattichizzo and M. Malvezzi. HANS: a Haptic System for Human-to-Human Remote Handshake. *In 2022 9th IEEE RAS/EMBS International Conference for Biomedical Robotics and Biomechatronics (BioRob)*, pp. 1–8, 2022, doi: 10.1109/BioRob52689.2022.9925284.
5. **M. Dragusanu**, G. M. Achilli, M. C. Valigi, D. Prattichizzo, M. Malvezzi and G. Salvietti. The Wavejoints: A Novel Methodology to Design Soft-Rigid Grippers Made by Monolithic 3D Printed Fingers with Adjustable Joint Stiffness. *In 2022 International Conference on Robotics and Automation (ICRA)*, 2022, pp. 6173–6179, doi: 10.1109/ICRA46639.2022.9811548.
6. **M. Dragusanu**, Z. Iqbal, D. Prattichizzo and M. Malvezzi. Design of a Modular Hand Exoskeleton for Rehabilitation and Training. *Proceedings of the ASME 2021 International Mechanical Engineering Congress and Exposition*, Volume 5: Biomedical and Biotechnology. November 1–5, 2021, p. V005T05A067, doi: 10.1115/IMECE2021-70343.
7. **M. Dragusanu**, T. L. Baldi, Z. Iqbal, D. Prattichizzo and M. Malvezzi. Design, Development, and Control of a Tendon-actuated Exoskeleton for Wrist Rehabilitation and Training. *I2020 IEEE International Conference on Robotics and Automation (ICRA)*, Paris, France, 2020, pp. 1749–1754, doi: 10.1109/ICRA40945.2020.9197013.

Book Chapters

1. **M. Dragusanu,** D. Troisi, D. Prattichizzo and M. Malvezzi. Joint Stiffness Analysis and Regulation for Underactuated Soft Grippers Based on Monolithic Structure. *In: Petuya, V., Quaglia, G., Parikyan, T., Carbone, G. (eds) Proceedings of I4SDG Workshop 2023*. I4SDG 2023. Mechanisms and Machine Science, vol 134. Springer, Cham, doi: 10.1007/978-3-031-32439-0_56.
2. D. Troisi, **M. Dragusanu**, A. Villani, D. Prattichizzo, M. Malvezzi. HapticPalm: A Wearable Robotic Device for Haptics and Rehabilitative Hand Treatments. *In: Cavallo, F., et al. Social Robotics. ICSR 2022. Lecture Notes in Computer Science*, vol 13818. Springer, Cham, doi: 10.1007/978-3-031-24670-8_36.
3. **M. Dragusanu,** Z. Iqbal, D. Prattichizzo, and M. Malvezzi, Exploiting a wearable extra-finger for haptic applications. *In: Seifi, H., et al. Haptics: Science, Technology, Applications*. EuroHaptics 2022. Lecture Notes in Computer Science, vol 13235. Springer, Cham, doi: 10.1007/978-3-031-06249-0.

4. G.M. Achilli, S. Logozzo, M.C. Valigi, **M. Dragusanu**, M. Malvezzi. Theoretical and Experimental Characterization of a New Robotic gripper's Joint. *In: Niola, V., Gasparetto, A., Quaglia, G., Carbone, G. (eds) Advances in Italian Mechanism Science.* IFToMM Italy 2022. Mechanisms and Machine Science, vol 122. Springer, Cham, doi: 10.1007/978-3-031-10776-4_85.

Extended Abstract—Conference

1. **M. Dragusanu**, S. Marullo, M. Malvezzi, G. M. Achilli, M. C. Valigi, D. Prattichizzo, and G. Salvietti. Soft collaborative gripper for dress- ing assistance. *In I-RIM - Conferenza Italiana di Robotica e Macchine Intelligenti*, 7–9 ottobre, 2022, doi: 10.5281/zenodo.7531218.
2. **M. Dragusanu**, D. Troisi, A. Villani, D. Prattichizzo, and M. Malvezzi. Haptic portable pad for hand disease manual treatment. *In I-RIM - Conferenza Italiana di Robotica e Macchine Intelligenti*, 7–9 ottobre, 2022, doi: 10.5281/zenodo.753 1232.
3. **M. Dragusanu**, D. Troisi, M. Z. Iqbal, T. L. Baldi, D. Prattichizzo, and M. Malvezzi. Finger actuation of a modular wearable exoskeleton for hand/wrist rehabilitation and training. *In I-RIM - Conferenza Italiana di Robotica e Macchine Intelligenti*, 7–9 ottobre, 2022, doi: 10.5281/zenodo.7531288.
4. **M. Dragusanu**, A. Villani, D. Prattichizzo, and M. Malvezzi. Design of a wearable haptic device for hand palm cutaneous feedback. *In I-RIM - Conferenza Italiana di Robotica e Macchine Intelligenti*, 8–10 October, 2021, doi: 10.5281/zenodo.5900555.
5. **M. Dragusanu**, T. L. Baldi, Z. Iqbal, D. Prattichizzo, and M. Malvezzi. Development of a wearable exoskeleton for hand/wrist rehabilitation and training. *in I-RIM 3D - Conferenza Italiana di Robotica e Macchine Intelligenti*, 10–12 Dicembre, 2020, doi: 10.5281/zenodo.4781036.

Acknowledgements It is a pleasure to thank all the people who contributed in some way to the work described in this thesis. First and foremost my gratitude goes to my advisor, Prof. Monica Malvezzi for continuous guidance and support over these Ph.D. years. She has been an excellent mentor and fantastic professor that transmitted me the passion for the research. I really thank her for all the time that she has been close to me encouraging my research and allowing me to grow as a research scientist. A special thanks to my co-advisor Prof. Domenico Prattichizzo, a man able to make you love robotics, always full of great ideas. He believed in me from my bachelor's degree and together with Prof. Malvezzi they managed to bring out the best of me.

I would like to thank also all my lab mates for helping me every day in the lab, for the stimulating discussions, the sleepless nights spent together because of the deadlines, and for all the fun times we had together. Furthermore, I wish to acknowledge the help provided by the people of the Disability and DSA office of the University of Siena during my Ph.D.

Before the end, I wish to thank two people very close to me: Rita and Lorenzo, my acquired grandparents. Two special and magnificent people who have always been able to give me the right advice.

Reminding us that life is not made of work, I would like to thank all my friends with whom I have shared adventures and misadventures outside the university walls.

Finally, a very special thank goes to my family, for the love, support, and constant encouragement throughout my Ph.D. In particular, I am very grateful to my parents and my brother. Without them, I wouldn't have gotten this far and I wouldn't be the person I am today. This is why I dedicate the entire work to them.

Competing Interests The author has no competing interests to declare that are relevant to the content of this manuscript.

Contents

Acronyms

Roman Symbols

ABS	Acrylonitrile Butadiene Styrene
ADLs	Activities of Daily Living
AM	Additive Manufacturing
BLDC	Brushless DC Motors
CAD	Computer Aided Design
CAE	Computer Aided Engineering
CRPS-I	Complex Regional Pain Syndrome Type-I
CRSs	Comfort Rating Scales
DIP	Distal InterPhalangeal
DoFs	Degrees of Freedom
EE	Electromagnet-Embodiment
EEE	Electromagnet-Electromagnet-Embodiment
EMG	ElectroMyoGraphy
EPE	Electromagnet-Plate-Embodiment
FDM	Fused Deposition Modelling
FEM	Finite Element Method
FSR	Force Sensitive Resistors
GOS	General Opinion Score
GPU	Graphics Processing Unit
GUI	Graphical User Interface
HRI	Human-Robot Interaction
IMU	Inertial Measurement Units
IP	InterPhalangeal
IPCs	Interpenetrating Phase Composites
LA	Linear Actuator
MARG	Magnetic, Angular Rate, and Gravity
MCP	MetaCarpalPhalangeal
MEMS	Micro-Electro-Mechanical Systems
MOS	Mean Opinion Score

MT	Manual Therapy
NEP	No Electromagnet (nor) Plate
PCA	Principal Component Analysis
PE	Plate-Embodiment
PIP	Proximal Interphalangeal
RCM	Remote Center of Motion
RMS	Root Mean Square
RMSE	Root Mean Square Error
ROM	Range of Motion
ROS	Robotics Operating System
RPS	Revolute-Prismatic-Spherical
RPY	Roll-Pitch-Yaw
SCD	Single Case Design
SLA	Stereo-Lithography
SPI	Serial Peripheral Interface
TM	TrapezioMetacarpal
TPU	Thermoplastic Polyurethane
TSA	Twisted String Actuation
UCD	User-Centered Design
VR	Virtual Reality
WHO	World Health Organization

Chapter 1
Introduction

The technological advancements of recent years have lead to the revolution across various sectors, with robotic devices being increasingly adopted. These devices are now found in industries, agriculture, restaurants, public transport, homes, and many other aspects of human life. In this context, the medical and healthcare system has changed as well: the use of robotic devices has consolidated, becoming part of the so called assistive and rehabilitative technologies. Currently, two main factors are driving innovation in these technologies.

Firstly, as a result of improved quality of life, people are living longer, which has led to an increased number of individuals requiring support and rehabilitation. According to the World Health Organization (WHO) reports, global life expectancy at birth increased by approximately six years in 2019, reaching 73.3 years, meanwhile, healthy life expectancy increased by about five years, from 58.3 to 63.7 years, meaning that people live an average of nine years with health conditions [1].

WHO also highlights that over one billion people need an assistive device, such as a wheelchair, prosthesis, or hearing aid, but only 10% of those in need have access to those devices [2, 3]. Furthermore, the World Federation of Occupational Therapists estimates that a minimum of 750 occupational therapists per 1 million people is required to meet global rehabilitation needs [4]. Additionally, there is a need for at least five prosthetists and orthotists per 1 million people [5]. According to WHO, rehabilitation is clearly considered an essential solution for improving quality of life. Globally, more than 2 billion people are estimated to require rehabilitation at least once during the course of their illness or condition [6].

Secondly, technology is an essential tool for maintaining and enhancing the quality of life even for people with permanent or temporary disabilities. According to WHO, disability is not just a disadvantage affecting an individual but a complex phenomenon that relates a person's body and the environment in which he/she lives [7]. Nowadays, studies on disability follow a socio-relational approach, meaning that a person with a disability, depending on their clinical condition, may find themselves in an environment whose characteristics affect their physical and social abilities [8].

M. Dragusanu, *Design of Soft–Rigid Devices for Rehabilitative and Assistive Robotics*, Springer Theses, https://doi.org/10.1007/978-3-031-84823-0_1

Technological advancements in the assistive and rehabilitative medical field play a crucial role for people with disabilities, aiding in mobility, performing manual tasks, communication, learning, and increasing autonomy in Activities of Daily Living (ADLs). These technologies offer the opportunity to radically change their way of life and enhance integration into society.

Nevertheless, due to high costs and absent or insufficient financial channels, the ability to deliver assistive and rehabilitative technology is still constrained or nonexistent in many regions of the world. Many national healthcare systems urgently need improvement, particularly through increased investments in human and technical resources and enhanced collaboration [9]. Additionally to this, communication gaps between technology producers and end-users remain a significant challenge.

The work lead in the framework of the presented research activity, aims to address these issues by developing solutions that make assistive and rehabilitative technologies more accessible and affordable. Specifically, the focus of the presented research in case of assistive and/or rehabilitative robotics technologies fild is shifted to the upper limbs by proposing new hand/wrist exoskeletons and haptics devices systems. Upper limbs play a crucial role in ADLs and, especially the hand, represent one of the greatest engineering challenges both, from mechanical design and control strategy point of view, due to its complex anatomical structure and wide range of movements that can perform. Furthermore, these robotic devices must coexist with the human user, often for long periods, therefore they must respect fundamental requirements in terms of wearability, comfort, ease of use and safety.

Focusing on the assistive robotics technologies area only, the thesis shifts attention to robotic manipulators, particularly the end-effector, i.e. the so called robotic gripper, to assist users in performing ADLs. This research presents innovative solutions in this field, capable of adapting to human needs by exploiting the use of novel mechanical structures and actuation transmission systems.

Overall, this thesis represents an attempt to merge robotics with themes of personal assistance and rehabilitation, a central challenge in the Human-Robot Interaction (HRI) field. In this complex scenario, methods such as topological optimization, new mechanical designs combining rigid and soft structures, advanced materials, and rapid prototyping technologies together with the new emerging field of artificial intelligence, have been exploited to propose innovative and accessible solutions for assistive and rehabilitative technologies.

1.1 Robotic Devices for Rehabilitation and Assistance

The purpose of rehabilitation, guided by physiotherapists and physiatrists, is to maintain or restore physical abilities in individuals with temporary or permanent disabilities. The rehabilitation process aims to promote, at least in part, the recovery of user's functionality by exploiting all functional system that have remained intact, reducing the discomfort caused by limitations imposed by the disease, and helping the individual gain better control of themselves and their surrounding environment.

Currently, there is no clear information on the minimum amount of treatment required for rehabilitation to be effective, as it varies depending on the patient and the specific issue being addressed. According to guidelines from the Royal College, the amount of rehabilitation therapy for stroke patients should be as much as the patient can tolerate [10]. This approach is widely supported by the scientific community for all conditions requiring rehabilitation.

However, traditional physical rehabilitation is often associated with high costs, must be sustained over time, and is mostly done manually, requiring a significant workforce. In cases of temporary disability, rehabilitation is often interrupted when the user has already regained about 60–70% of functionality in the affected area, such as with upper limb injuries. In most cases, the patient requires further rehabilitation which is carried out by the patient himself or with the family help, posing significant economic and physical burdens.

Technological innovation is gradually transforming the rehabilitation environment, with robot-mediated therapy emerging as an effective approach to improve the current medical health environment [11]. This approach requires less workforce and allows for the possibility of rehabilitation tools to be available at home, making the technology more accessible and enabling users to be responsible for their own rehabilitation process.

Robot-mediated therapy combines robotics with neuroscience and rehabilitation to define novel systems that support individuals with neurological diseases [12–14]. The therapy performed by using robotic devices is a clinically proven method to improve rehabilitation outcomes in various neuromuscular disorders, such as spinal injuries [15].

The COVID-19 pandemic situation, broke out at the beginning of 2020, dramatically modified our habits. Medical and rehabilitation practices have adapted significantly, with services now being delivered remotely through audiovisual technologies. Rehabilitation and orthopedics have shifted from face-to-face visits to guided audiovisual sessions.

Telerehabilitation, initially considered difficult or nearly impossible to implement, has now been forced to be used and now it could further spread and become more common, even necessary [16]. Although there are still some limitations, the advantages of remote rehabilitation are evident, whether in synchronous sessions, where the user and physiotherapist collaborate in real-time, or asynchronous sessions, which involve a combination of therapist-guided phase and self-manage user rehabilitation phase (store-and-forward). These tools allow users to perform physiotherapy exercises autonomously, increasing the intensity and efficiency of rehabilitation, providing progress feedback, reducing the physiotherapist's workload, and decreasing the need for physical presence, thus encouraging autonomy and independence in people with disabilities. Although research in this area is ongoing, various benefits can be observed in the use of rehabilitation and assistive technologies [17].

Furthermore, the technological process we are witnessing is fundamental for enhancing the quality of life for individuals with disabilities. These technologies not only improve physical capabilities but also boost self-esteem by promoting inclusion and participation in society [18, 19]. As the population ages, functional limitations become more common, requiring higher levels of assistance from caregivers. Assistive technologies can reduce caregiver burden by improving the older adults independence. Positive outcomes are also evident from studies involving children with physical impairments and their caregivers [20, 21]. This impact is particularly evident in education: assistive technologies promote educational, psychological, and social benefits by providing tools for learning and communication [22].

Based on the physical iteration of the human-robot [23, 24], three primary approaches can be distinguished for the robotic devices presented in this thesis: robotic exoskeleton systems, rehabilitation robot systems, and assistive robotic manipulator systems.

1.1.1 Robotic Exoskeletons Systems

The exoskeleton is a wearable device[1] developed to assist, support, and replicate natural human movements. Typically, the mechanical joints of the robotic system align and couple with the human joints. Once the joint axes are defined within a range of motion, both joint position and orientation can be controlled, allowing the device to operate in either active or passive modes.

Robotic exoskeletons can be used either as a strength, endurance and speed augmentation device for healthy users in various military and industrial applications, as well as a device to be deployable for ADLs supporting patients with mobility and manipulation related permanent/temporary disabilities [25–28]. However, the focus of this research is limited to the second category, aimed at patient rehabilitation and support.

Robotic exoskeletal systems provide effective strategies to enhance and promote patient movement. They are increasingly used to accelerate recovery from disease and support in various manipulation tasks, such as power grasping and dexterous manipulation. These systems are designed for high-intensity rehabilitation, following specific protocols in a controllable and repeatable manner [29–31]. Exoskeletons are typically categorized into devices for lower limbs and upper limbs. While research on lower limb rehabilitation exoskeletons dates back to the 1960s, it was only after the work of Bernhardt et al. [32] that the field gained significant attention. To date, several good results have been achieved in this research area [33, 34].

As the focus of this work is on the upper limbs, the presented research on exoskeleton systems are for these human body parts, in particular for wrist and hand. These exoskeletons are particularly complex due to the challenges posed by HRI, hand size, and the high number of Degrees of Freedom (DoFs) that allow a variety of movements. Usually their realization exploits the use of electric motors and pneumatic chambers to induce the movement of the finger.

[1] Wearable devices are systems designed to be worn by humans, characterized by appropriate shape, kinematics, and weight, with the aim of assisting, augmenting, or restoring human functions. They can be viewed as advanced symbiotic systems between humans and robots.

Hand and wrist exoskeletons are one of the most promising solutions for improving rehabilitation procedures. After traditional rehabilitation, many patients, especially those recovering from strokes, may not fully regain hand function due to permanent disabilities [35]. In such cases, exoskeletons can assist in improving hand performance for ADLs. Although significant progress has been made in this field [36, 37], challenges remain. To date, the current generation of portable hand exoskeletons is limited by factors such as size, weight, type of actuation, and manipulation capabilities. As a result, most are still prototypes, available only in laboratory settings or specialized rehabilitation centers, making them inaccessible for home use at a moderate and accessible cost.

Given these challenges, designing hand supports, which exploit exoscheleton technologies, is a hot-topic for the scientific community and more in general is one of the most challenges in robotics.

1.1.2 Rehabilitation Robots Systems

Rehabilitation robots are now capable of compensating for, and in some cases replacing, traditional rehabilitation practices in individuals with neurological, coordination, and motion impairments such as stroke, spinal cord injuries, orthopedic surgeries, etc.

Among these robotic devices, exoskeletal technologies, as previously discussed, play an important role. However, there are additional robotic technologies that also enhance the medical rehabilitation system. These technologies are often categorized based on the nature of human–robot interaction: therapist–robot interaction, robot–patient interaction, and robot learning. The latter uses machine learning techniques, such as support vector machines, and more generally, the design of intelligent algorithms, to monitor patient progress during rehabilitation. This can lead to faster and more complete restoration of the lost individual's capabilities. For example, machine learning methods have been employed to suggest interventions based on patients' motor functions and health conditions [38], or for real-time monitoring of compensatory movements in post-stroke patients [39].

In robot–patient interaction, the system collects data on the patient's therapeutic performance, provides feedback on the rehabilitation process, and tracks the frequency and intensity of therapy. It also monitors the robot's response to the patient's movements. Therapist–robot interaction involves creating, monitoring, and adjusting the patient's customized rehabilitation plan.

User's progress information can be tracked in various ways, including muscle activity signals, body position tracking, and force sensors. For instance, in [40], a robotic hand rehabilitation system driven by surface electromyography (EMG) measurements is presented. Feedback to the patient can be delivered through multiple channels, such as monitors, virtual reality, neurostimulation, or haptics, as demonstrated in [41, 42].

This thesis focuses also on the use of haptic technologies to develop hand-centered assistive and rehabilitative solutions. Studies on these therapeutic assistive technologies for hands are presented in [43], while biofeedback systems are used in arm rehabilitation [44, 45]. However, it appears that none include telerehabilitation as a rehabilitation model.

Home-based rehabilitation is an emerging trend, but haptic technologies for hand home-delivered therapy appears to be uncovered. Addressing this gap is one of the significant challenges in the field of haptics.

1.1.3 Assistive Robotic Manipulators Systems

The field of human-robot interaction, specifically regarding assistive robotic manipulators, is always of great interest for the scientific community. This area deals with the development of different configurations, such as fixed desktops, wheelchair-mounted systems, and home automation solutions. The primary goal is to enhance individuals' independence and assist them in interacting safely with their environment. These robots are designed to adapt to and coexist with humans in unstructured and dynamically changing environments, while performing tasks such as opening doors, grasping and manipulating objects, dressing, eating, and cooking.

In most cases, the human maintains full control over the manipulator through customized interfaces. Current research focuses on developing improved interfaces to optimize manipulator control, such as those incorporating haptic feedback or advanced control algorithms. To date, the most commonly used interfaces are based on sensitive joysticks or intelligent medical aids, including smart wheelchairs equipped with portable robotic arms [46], smart walkers [47], or devices like the anklets described in [48] to guide blind individuals while walking.

Moreover, advances in technology and artificial intelligence have enabled the integration of powerful computing capabilities into manipulators, transforming them into intelligent machines that significantly improve users' quality of life. Voice control, speech recognition systems, vision-based gesture recognition algorithms, and bio-signal-based devices are increasingly being employed to allow users to control robots for performing specific tasks [49–51]. Unlike industrial manipulators, which are designed to carry out precise tasks in short time and are often placed in delimited, circumcised, and forbidden area to humans, assistive robots used in daily life must be designed to safely interact with people. In this context, predicting, detecting, and avoiding collisions is a critical requirement for these manipulators. As a result, they are limited in terms of speed, acceleration, and joint/end-effector strength to ensure safe human-robot collaboration. The end-effector, in particular, plays a key role in HRI and has garnered increased attention in recent years. This research activity framework focuses also on developing end-effectors that can enhance users' independence in daily activities. Even developing new end-effectors to perform precise tasks by reaching certain trajectories and adapting to different objects shapes represents one of the main challenges in this research field.

1.1.4 User Centered Design

User-Centered Design (UCD) refers to design processes in which the end-user's perspective is the key point in the development of new technologies. This methodology is usually divided into two types [52]. The first UCD type, which is more widespread, consults users on their needs and involve them only in specific moments, such as requirement gathering and usability testing. The second type, however, gives to the users a deeper impact on the design as they are involved during all the main design and prototyping phases.

In this research, the latter UCD approach was revised and adapted to allow users to participate in every phase of development. This began from the initial concept and continued through to the final prototyping stage, transforming the traditional process of developing medical and assistive devices thanks to the constant user feedback.

In addition to the technological and economic barriers mentioned above, it is worth noting that technologies designed without consistent input from the end-user, or a clear understanding of how they will be used, often face challenges in adoption. This disconnect can lead to the risk of developing technology that fail to meet the relevant needs of the user and the use case. For successful design, the technology must address the actual requirements of the user, considering utility, usability, occupational, and social factors [53]. Rehabilitation and assistive robotics, in particular, ought to be accepted and adopted into everyday practice by the users. To achive this goal, it is necessary to discern user's specific needs, as the quality of life, the feeling of being in control, dignity, and independence as well as deal with her/his perspective fears and expectations.

It has been argued that involving users in a participatory design process might help overcome conflicting values and expectations of developers and end-users [54, 55]. This collaborative approach can fill the gap between device developers and users, leading to better adoption and satisfaction with the technology.

1.2 Organization and Main Contribution of Thesis

The organization and the main results of the presented research activity are visible on the scheme of Fig. 1.1. The primary contribution of this work is to offer user-friendly devices that can be comfortably used at home by individuals with temporary or permanent disabilities, helping them improve autonomy in daily life activities. As illustrated, two main research paths have been followed, i.e. rehabilitation (denoted in blue) and assistance (denoted in orange). These paths explore three significant areas in robotics that are are currently receiving great interest from the healthcare system: exoskeletons, haptics focused on upper-limb rehabilitation and assistive home solutions, and robotic grippers, aimed at developing innovative end-effectors for personal assistance.

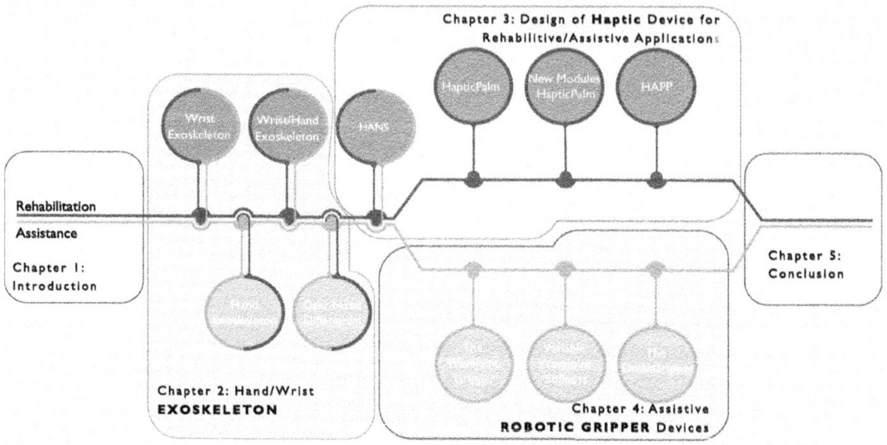

Fig. 1.1 Structure of the thesis

The research conducted during the Ph.D. period, as highlighted in Fig. 1.1, initially focused on the exoskeletons field. Starting from the existing literature, advanced wrist and hand exoskeleton systems were developed, providing improvements and new design strategies. These devices were designed with the user's needs in mind, paying close attention to human-robot interaction.

Exoskeleton systems capable of recording possible movements carried out by experts, which can later be replicated at home via easy-to-use graphical interfaces, were developed. An exoskeleton for the wrist was created to help and assist in home rehabilitation process. Simultaneously, solutions for the hand were explored based on user feedback. These started from a complex, novel solution with one DoF using a parallel mechanism to replicate finger trajectories, to a lighter, modular, and more user-friendly design where the kinematic chain is closed by the user's finger. A novel modular hand/wrist exoskeleton was also developed, equipped with an automatic closure mechanism for easy self-user wearing. To reduce overall weight and bulk, a differential transmission system was implemented, allowing a single actuator to control two fingers. Finally, studies on the modular exoskeleton's kinematics, adaptability, and performance were conducted, taking into account varying hand sizes.

By following the assistance and rehabilitation paths outlined in Fig. 1.1, it becomes evident how these paths converge to explore the field of haptics with the introduction of the first device able of providing both assistance and rehabilitation. After this point, the two paths diverge: one continues to focus on haptics for hand rehabilitation devices, while the other explores the development of assistive devices through the design of robotic grippers. During this PhD research, the field of grippers was preliminarily explored to identify rigid/soft structures, such as compliant mechanical structures, that can be used to create novel exoskeletons.

In this phase, a methodology was developed for designing a new type of robotic gripper composed of 3D-printed tendon-actuated fingers. Each finger was designed as a monolithic element with stiff segments (phalanges) connected by flexible, wave-shaped sections. This methodology allows for customizing the flexible parts by adjusting parameters such as thickness, length, wave amplitude, and phase. As a result, tendon-driven actuation can be used not only to generate finger flexion but also to create more complex finger movements. Additionally, in line with the research on assistive devices, a soft-rigid gripper was designed specifically for robot-assisted dressing, exploiting a novel synergistic inter-play between tendon-driven and magnetic actuations. Moreover, a new type of actuation system, Twisted String Actuation (TSA), was introduced and studied for varying joint stiffness. This was the first time TSA was applied in a compliant mechanism.

Throughout the research, the applicability of topology optimization techniques was thoroughly investigated. Topological optimization is relatively new in the field of HRI, especially for the wearable robotics. This approach enabled the possibility to create complex geometric shapes that would have been difficult to achieve with traditional methods. Leveraging the innovations of Additive Manufacturing (AM) process, advanced materials, and artificial intelligence allowed for significant achievements, which are presented in this thesis.

The following subsections briefly summarize the work grouped by the robotic fields in Fig. 1.1, which contributed to the manuscript. The structure of the thesis is as follows: Chap. 2 addresses rehabilitation and assistive exoskeletons for the hand and wrist. Chapter 3 focuses on haptics robotic field, presenting devices for hand assistance and rehabilitation, with a distinction between grounded and wearable systems. Chapter 4 covers robotic grippers designed to improve quality of life, including new actuation systems and compliant structures. Finally, Chap. 5 presents future work and the conclusion of the thesis.

1.2.1 Exoskeletons

1.2.1.1 Wrist

Robot rehabilitation is an emerging and promising topic that incorporates robotics with neuroscience and rehabilitation to define new methods for supporting patients with neurological diseases. As a consequence, the rehabilitation process could increase the efficacy exploiting the potentialities of robot-mediated therapies. Nevertheless, clinical effectiveness alone is no longer sufficient to widely integrate robotic technologies into social and healthcare contexts. This work takes a step further by presenting an innovative exoskeleton designed for wrist flexion/extension and adduction/abduction motion training [56]. It is designed to be wearable and easy to control and manage. It can be used by the patient in collaboration with the therapist or autonomously where a key aspect of the proposed exoskeleton is represented by the tracking of wrist movements. This section of the thesis introduces the key steps in the design and development of the wrist exoskeleton system and presents preliminary tests conducted with a user who has limited wrist mobility.

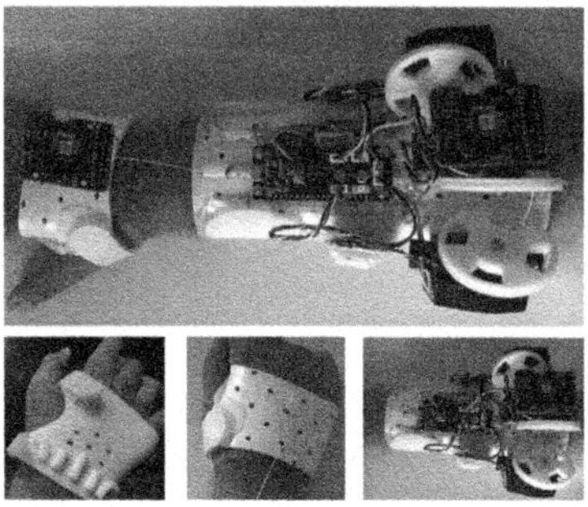

1.2.1.2 Hand

In this second chapter section it is presented the design of an innovative exoskeleton for hand finger flexion/extension motion rehabilitation and training [57, 58]. It is designed to be modular, wearable, and easy to control and manage. A user-centered design perspective has been employed in all the design and development phases. It can be used by the patient in collaboration with the therapist or autonomously. The kinematic structure of the finger actuation system has the peculiarity to present 3-DoFs when the exoskeleton is not worn and 1-DoF when it is worn, allowing better adaptability and higher wearability. The exoskeleton is able to actuate flexion/extension motion of the fingers and to apply bi-directional forces, i.e. it is able to both open and close the fingers. This part of the thesis introduces the main steps of device design and development and presents and compare three different solutions for hand exoskeleton system.

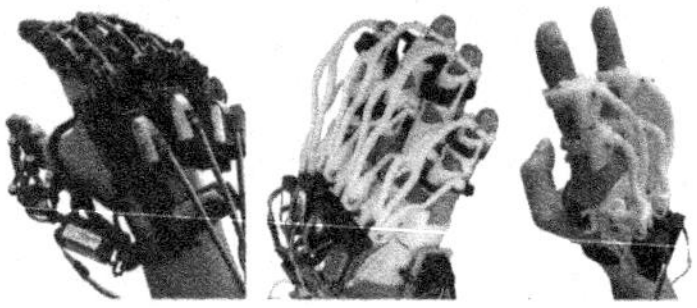

1.2.1.3 Hand/Wrist

Robotic devices for rehabilitation and training is a promising and challenging research topic with a potentially huge social impact. The availability of tools for autonomously performing physiotherapy exercises increases their efficiency, provides supplementary information about results and progress, reduces physiotherapist's efforts and the need of their physical presence during exercise sessions, and encourages autonomy and independence in people with disabilities. Nevertheless, supportive technologies developed without the inputs and feedback of the end-user throughout the design process, are less likely to be adopted for their intended purpose and use case. In this part of the thesis, a modular hand/wrist exoskeleton is presented, that actuates the wrist's flexion/extension and adduction/abduction motions and hand fingers' flexion/extension motions [59]. It is designed to be wearable and easy to control and manage and can be used by the patient in collaboration with the therapist or autonomously. The main features of the device and tests conducted with a user having limited hand and wrist mobility are presented. To our knowledge, the suggested technology is the first attempt to create a wearable hand/wrist exoskeleton that can record and replay motions while also storing data for future investigations.

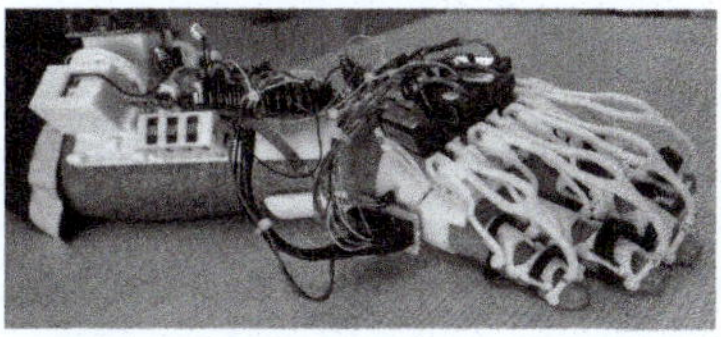

1.2.1.4 Underactuated Hand Exoskeleton

One of the main bottlenecks that constrain the complexity, weight, and costs of exoskeletons is represented by the actuators. This problem is particularly evident in devices designed for the upper limb, and in particular for the hand, in which dimension limits and kinematics complexity are particularly challenging. This thisis part presents the design and prototyping of a hand finger exoskeleton [60]. In particular, the focus is on the design of a gear-based differential mechanism aimed at coupling the motion of two adjacent fingers and limiting the complexity and costs of the system. The design of the gear-based differential is inspired by the mechanism widely employed in the automotive field, it allows to actuate two fingers with one actuator only, keeping their motions independent. The exoskeleton is able to actuate flexion/extension motion of the hand fingers and its design is based on the exoskeleton hand previously introduced with some improvements on the links for easy assembly and dissasembly.

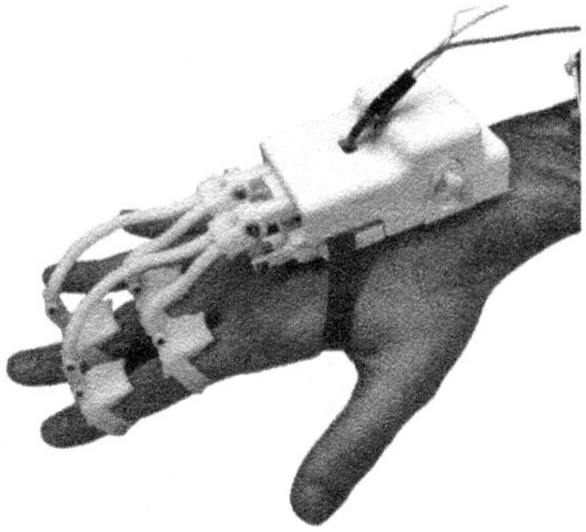

1.2.2 *Haptic Devices*

1.2.2.1 HANS: A Haptic System for Human-to-Human Remote Handshake

Handshake is a gesture used worldwide for greeting and communication purposes that is impossible in remote and forced distance contexts. In this thesis part the recent results in wearable haptics was exploited for designing HANS, a novel haptic system developed for reproducing a remote handshake and/or a hand hold between two users that can be used both for assistance and rehabilitation [61]. It consists of two modules: the sensing part composed of three rings developed for recording the handshake force and the actuation part a bracelet worn on user's palm, able to apply a pressure distribution that simulates the handshake action.

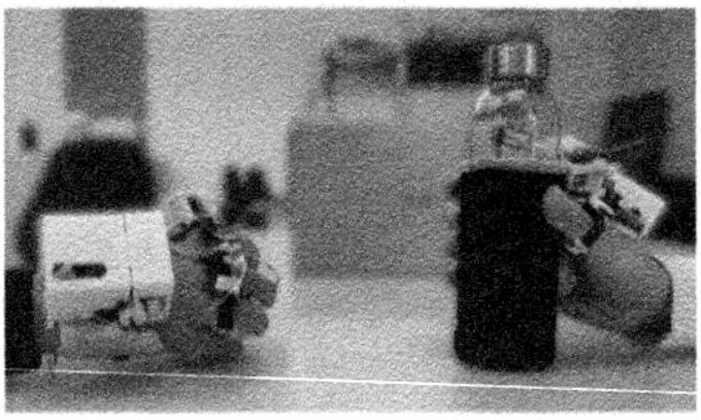

1.2.2.2 HapticPalm: Design and Evaluation of a Wearable Haptic Device for Hand Palm Cutaneous Feedback

The palm plays a fundamental role in many grasping, manipulation, and tactile exploration tasks. However, compared to areas like the fingertips, it remains less exploited in haptic applications. The HapticPalm is a novel haptic device designed to provide cutaneous stimulation to the palm [62, 63]. This wearable, palm-oriented device improve user interaction in virtual environments powered by various visual engines and is also suitable for rehabilitation purposes. The device uses a parallel tendon-based mechanical structure actuated by three motors positioned on the back of the hand. The HapticPalm is able of applying both normal and tangential forces, rendering the sensation of contact with surfaces of varying slopes. The end-effector can be easily swapped to simulate contact with surfaces of different curvatures. Since tendons can only apply tensile forces, a spring-based support was developed to keep the end-effector separated from the palm when not actuated or when no force is being applied.

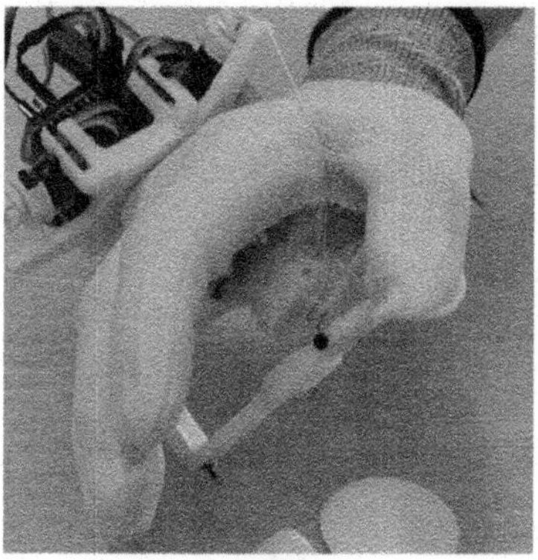

1.2.2.3 HapticPalm Modules for Rehabilitative Manual Treatments

In this part of the thesis, the HapticPalm, a wearable device based on a 3-DoFs parallel robotic structure, is improved to be used for rehabilitation of specific hand pathologies [64]. The thesis focuses in particular on the design of the contact interfaces between the device end effector and the palm, that have to simulate the interaction with different surfaces.

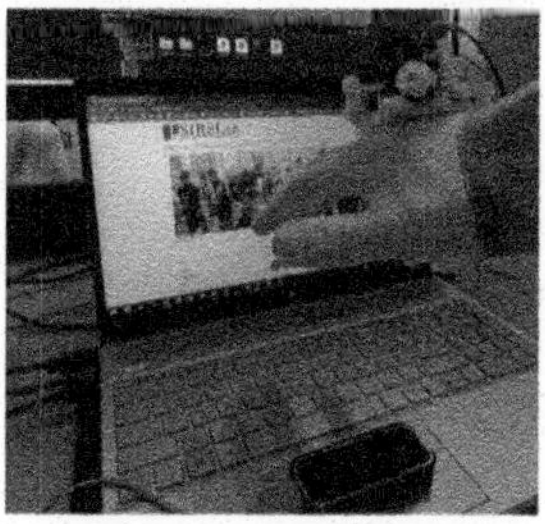

1.2.2.4 HAPP: A Haptic Portable Pad for Hand Disease Manual Treatment

Nowadays, researchers are focusing their efforts on the remote distribution of devices for rehabilitation, allowing users to perform the exercises without the presence of a doctor. Physiotherapists, usually, employ manual therapy to treat patients with musculoskeletal discomfort and/or impairments. In this case the purpose of the thesis is to introduce HAPP, a novel portable haptic device aimed to assist people suffering from various hand diseases, and more generally, to replicate the traditional mechanical and rhythmic stimulus features of manual treatments in order to study the effects of manual therapy in case of carpus and metacarpus problems [65]. Its structure is composed of a mobile plate, actuated by a 3-DoFs parallel robot, with a rack-and-pinion mechanism that activates the end-effector to stimulate the user's hand palm.

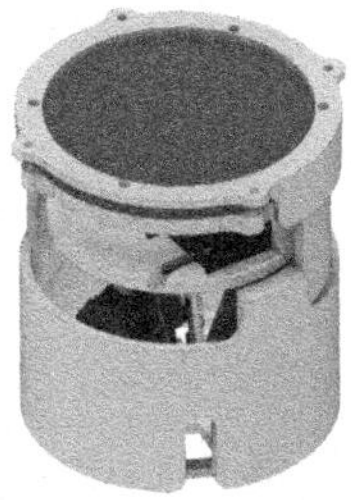

1.2.3 Robotic Grippers

1.2.3.1 The WaveJoints:A Methodology to Design Soft-Rigid Grippers Made by Monolithic 3D Printed Fingers with Adjustable Joint Stiffness

This work presents a novel methodology for designing soft-rigid grippers capable of performing various manipulation and assistance tasks [66]. The key innovation lies in the introduction of wave-shaped hinges, which can be tailored to achieve different three-dimensional stiffness behaviors. This design allows for the same tendon-driven actuation to be used across different tasks, including grasping objects of various shapes and performing in-hand manipulation of small items.

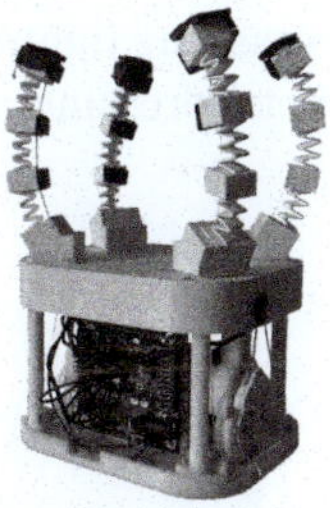

1.2.3.2 Compliant Finger Joint with Controlled Variable Stiffness Based on Twisted Strings Actuation

Underactuated tendon-driven fingers are a simple, yet effective solution, for realizing robotic grippers and hands. The lack of controllable degrees of actuation and precise sensing is compensated by the finger's deformable structure, which can adapt to objects during grasping and manipulation, and also implement grasping strategies by exploiting environmental constraints. However, a key drawback of these robotic fingers is that, due to the limited number of actuators, they can only perform a restricted range of movements. The finger's closure, driven by tendon activation, depends on its mechanical properties, particularly the stiffness of its elastic joints. Building on the concept of WaveJoints, this section introduces a passive elastic joint to be implemented in monolithic fingers in which, where the stiffness can be actively adjusted [67, 68]. This is achieved through a novel method that regulates joint rigidity by applying pre-compression to the structure, controlled by a twisted-string actuator (TSA).

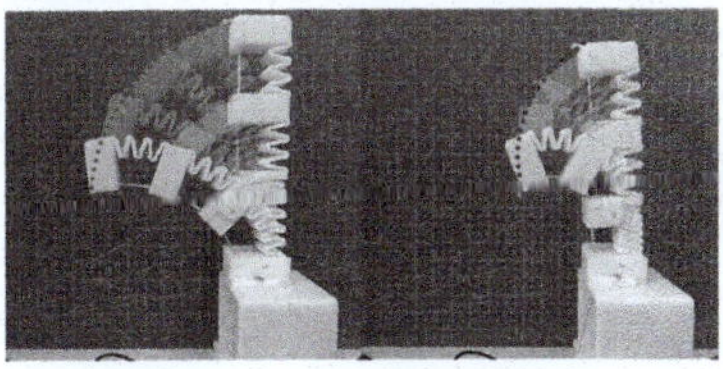

1.2.3.3 The DressGripper: A Collaborative Gripper with Electromagnetic Fingertips for Dressing Assistance

Finlly by following the assistance path in Fig. 1.1, this thesis presents the DressGripper [69], a collaborative gripper designed for safe interactions in wearing operations. The DressGripper accounts for the two main goals that have to be achieved by a robotic system designed for helping people to get dressed: (i) to be intrinsically safe and (ii) to keep firmly the cloth during the dressing operations. The DressGripper addresses these issues by combining a compliant and safe structure with an additional magnetic actuation at the fingertips. This solution allows a soft interaction with the robot and guarantees the grasping tightness. Preliminary experiments show the DressGripper suitability in robotic dressing assistance scenarios.

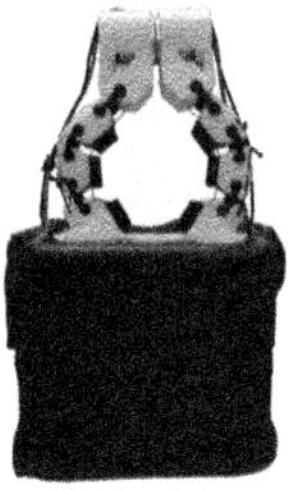

References

1. World Health Organization (2022) World health statistics 2022: monitoring health for the SDGD, sustainable development goals. World Health Statistics 2022
2. World Health Organization (2015) WHO global disability action plan 2014–2021: better health for all people with disability. World Health Organization
3. World Health Organization (2016) World health statistics 2016: monitoring health for the SDGs sustainable development goals. World Health Organization
4. Gimigliano F, Negrini S (2017) The World Health Organization "rehabilitation 2030: a call for action". Eur J Phys Rehab Med, 155–168
5. World Health Organization (2017) WHO standards for prosthetics and orthotics. World Health Organization
6. Cieza A, Causey K, Kamenov K, Hanson SW, Chatterji S, Vos T (2020) Global estimates of the need for rehabilitation based on the global burden of disease study 2019: a systematic analysis for the global burden of disease study 2019. The Lancet 396(10267):2006–2017
7. World Health Organization (2006) The world health report 2006: working together for health. World Health Organization
8. Leonardi M, Bickenbach J, Ustun TB, Kostanjsek N, Chatterji S (2006) The definition of disability: what is in a name? The Lancet 368(9543):1219–1221
9. World Health Organization (2020) World health statistics 2020. World Health Statistics 2020
10. Intercollegiate Stroke Working Party (2012) National clinical guideline for stroke, vol 25
11. Martinez-Martin E, Cazorla M (2019) Rehabilitation technology: assistance from hospital to home. Comput Intell Neurosci 2019
12. Peretti A, Amenta F, Tayebati SK, Nittari G, Mahdi SS et al (2017) Telerehabilitation: review of the state-of-the-art and areas of application. JMIR Rehab Assistive Technol 4(2):e7511
13. Díaz I, Catalan JM, Badesa FJ, Justo X, Lledo LD, Ugartemendia A, Gil JJ, Díez J, García-Aracil N (2018) Development of a robotic device for post-stroke home tele-rehabilitation. Adv Mech Eng 10(1):1687814017752302
14. Seron P, Oliveros M-J, Gutierrez-Arias R, Fuentes-Aspe R, Torres-Castro RC, Merino-Osorio C, Nahuelhual P, Inostroza J, Jalil Y, Solano R et al (2021) Effectiveness of telerehabilitation in physical therapy: a rapid overview. Phys Therapy 101(6):pzab053
15. Lum PS, Godfrey SB, Brokaw EB, Holley RJ, Nichols D (2012) Robotic approaches for rehabilitation of hand function after stroke. Am J Phys Med Rehab 91(11):S242–S254
16. Lim MA, Pranata R (2020) Letter to the editor regarding 'the challenging battle of mankind against covid-19 outbreak: is this global international biological catastrophe the beginning of a new era?'—is telehealth the future of orthopaedic and rehabilitation in post-covid-19 era?
17. Gorgey AS, Sumrell R, Goetz LL (2019) Exoskeletal assisted rehabilitation after spinal cord injury. Atlas Orthoses Assistive Dev, 440–447

18. Salvietti G, Hussain I, Cioncoloni D, Taddei S, Rossi S, Prattichizzo D (2016) Compensating hand function in chronic stroke patients through the robotic sixth finger. Trans Neur Syst Rehab Eng
19. Baldi TL, Spagnoletti G, Dragusanu M, Prattichizzo D (2017) Design of a wearable interface for lightweight robotic arm for people with mobility impairments. In: 2017 international conference on rehabilitation robotics (ICORR). IEEE, pp 1567–1573
20. Nicolson A, Moir L, Millsteed J (2012) Impact of assistive technology on family caregivers of children with physical disabilities: a systematic review. Disability Rehab Assistive Technol 7(5):345–349
21. Marasinghe KM (2016) Assistive technologies in reducing caregiver burden among informal caregivers of older adults: a systematic review. Disability Rehab Assistive Technol 11(5):353–360
22. McNicholl A, Casey H, Desmond D, Gallagher P (2021) The impact of assistive technology use for students with disabilities in higher education: a systematic review. Disability Rehab Assistive Technol 16(2):130–143
23. De Santis A, Siciliano B, De Luca A, Bicchi A (2008) An atlas of physical human-robot interaction. Mech Machine Theory 43(3):253–270
24. Mohebbi A (2020) Human-robot interaction in rehabilitation and assistance: a review. Curr Robot Rep 1(3):131–144
25. Van der Loos HFM, Reinkensmeyer DJ, Guglielmelli E (2016) Rehabilitation and health care robotics. In: Springer handbook of robotics. Springer, pp 1685–1728
26. Parietti F, Asada H (2016) Supernumerary robotic limbs for human body support. IEEE Trans Robot 32(2):301–311
27. Proud JK, Lai DTH, Mudie KL, Carstairs GL, Billing DC, Garofolini A, Begg RK (2022) Exoskeleton application to military manual handling tasks. Human Factors 64(3):527–554
28. Bai S, Virk GS, Sugar TG (2018) Wearable exoskeleton systems: design, control and applications. Institution of Engineering and Technology
29. Harwin WS, Patton JL, Reggie Edgerton V (2006) Challenges and opportunities for robot-mediated neurorehabilitation. Proc IEEE 94(9):1717–1726
30. Rosenstein L, Ridgel AL, Thota A, Samame B, Alberts JL (2008) Effects of combined robotic therapy and repetitive-task practice on upper-extremity function in a patient with chronic stroke. Am J Occup Ther 62(1):28–35
31. Banala SK, Kim SH, Agrawal SK, Scholz JP (2008) Robot assisted gait training with active leg exoskeleton (alex). IEEE Trans Neur Syst Rehab Eng 17(1):2–8
32. Bernhardt M, Frey M, Colombo G, Riener R (2005) Hybrid force-position control yields cooperative behaviour of the rehabilitation robot lokomat. In: 9th international conference on rehabilitation robotics, 2005. ICORR 2005. IEEE, pp 536–539
33. Shi D, Zhang W, Zhang W, Ding X (2019) A review on lower limb rehabilitation exoskeleton robots. Chin J Mech Eng 32(1):1–11
34. Pinto-Fernandez D, Torricelli D, del Carmen Sanchez-Villamanan M, Aller F, Mombaur K, Conti R, Vitiello N, Moreno JC, Pons JL (2020) Performance evaluation of lower limb exoskeletons: a systematic review. IEEE Trans Neur Syst Rehab Eng 28(7):1573–1583
35. Nakayama H, Jorgensen HS, Raaschou HO, Olsen TS (1994) Recovery of upper extremity function in stroke patients: the Copenhagen stroke study. Arch Phys Med Rehab 75(4):394–398
36. Sarac M, Solazzi M, Frisoli A (2019) Design requirements of generic hand exoskeletons and survey of hand exoskeletons for rehabilitation, assistive, or haptic use. IEEE Trans Haptics 12(4):400–413
37. Rehmat N, Zuo J, Meng W, Liu Q, Xie SQ, Liang H (2018) Upper limb rehabilitation using robotic exoskeleton systems: a systematic review. Int J Intell Robot Appl 2(3):283–295
38. Dolatabadi E, Taati B, Mihailidis A (2017) An automated classification of pathological gait using unobtrusive sensing technology. IEEE Trans Neur Syst Rehab Eng 25(12):2336–2346
39. Cai S, Li G, Enze S, Wei X, Huang S, Ma K, Zheng H, Xie L (2020) Real-time detection of compensatory patterns in patients with stroke to reduce compensation during robotic rehabilitation therapy. IEEE J Biomed Health Inf 24(9):2630–2638

40. Serpelloni M, Tiboni M, Lancini M, Pasinetti S, Vertuan A, Gobbo M (2016) Preliminary study of a robotic rehabilitation system driven by EMG for hand mirroring. In: 2016 IEEE international symposium on medical measurements and applications (MeMeA). IEEE, pp 1–6
41. Dawson-Elli AR, Adamczyk PG (2020) Design and validation of a lower-limb haptic rehabilitation robot. IEEE Trans Neur Syst Rehab Eng 28(7):1584–1594
42. Baldi TL, Paolocci G, Barcelli D, Prattichizzo D (2020) Wearable haptics for remote social walking. IEEE Trans Haptics 13(4):761–776
43. Choukou M-A, Mbabaali S, Hani JB, Cooke C (2021) Haptic-enabled hand rehabilitation in stroke patients: a scoping review. Appl Sci 11(8):3712
44. Shah VA, Risi N, Ballardini G, Mrotek LA, Casadio M, Scheidt RA (2018) Effect of dual tasking on vibrotactile feedback guided reaching—a pilot study. In: International conference on human haptic sensing and touch enabled computer applications. Springer, pp 3–14
45. Risi N, Shah V, Mrotek LA, Casadio M, Scheidt RA (2019) Supplemental vibrotactile feedback of real-time limb position enhances precision of goal-directed reaching. J Neurophysiol 122(1):22–38
46. Pana CF, Patrascu-Pana DM, Vladu IC, Manta LF, Petcu F-LB, Cismaru SI, Trasculescu AC (2021) Fuzzy control of the robotic arm for a smart electric wheelchair to assist people with movement disabilities. In: 2021 22nd international Carpathian control conference (ICCC), pp 1–6
47. Rizzon L, Moro F, Passerone R, Macii D, Fontanelli D, Nazemzadeh P, Corrà M, Palopoli L, Prattichizzo D (2016) c-walker: a cyber-physical system for ambient assisted living. In: Applications in electronics pervading industry, environment and society. Springer, pp 75–82
48. Rossi S, Baldi TL, Aggravi M, Ulivelli M, Cioncoloni D, Niccolini V, Donati L, Prattichizzo D (2020) Wearable haptic anklets for gait and freezing improvement in Parkinson's disease: a proof-of-concept study. Neurol Sci 41(12):3643–3651
49. Poirier S, Routhier F, Campeau-Lecours A (2019) Voice control interface prototype for assistive robots for people living with upper limb disabilities. In: 2019 IEEE 16th international conference on rehabilitation robotics (ICORR). IEEE, pp 46–52
50. Haseeb MA, Kyrarini M, Jiang S, Ristic-Durrant D, Gräser A (2018) Head gesture-based control for assistive robots. In: Proceedings of the 11th pervasive technologies related to assistive environments conference, pp 379–383
51. Schabron B, Reust A, Desai J, Yihun Y (2019) Integration of forearm SEMG signals with IMU sensors for trajectory planning and control of assistive robotic arm. In: 2019 41st annual international conference of the IEEE engineering in medicine and biology society (EMBC). IEEE, pp 5274–5277
52. Abras C, Maloney-Krichmar D, Preece J et al (2004) User-centered design. In: Bainbridge W (ed) Encyclopedia of human-computer interaction, vol 37, no 4. Sage, Thousand Oaks, pp 445–456
53. De Vito Dabbs A, Myers BA, McCurry KR, Dunbar-Jacob J, Hawkins RP, Begey A, Dew MA (2009) User-centered design and interactive health technologies for patients. Comput Inf Nursing: CIN 27(3):175
54. Lehoux P, Grimard D (2018) When robots care: public deliberations on how technology and humans may support independent living for older adults. Soc Sci Med 211:330–337
55. Achilli GM, Amici C, Dragusanu M, Gobbo M, Logozzo S, Malvezzi M, Tiboni M, Valigi MC (2023) Soft, rigid, and hybrid robotic exoskeletons for hand rehabilitation: roadmap with impairment-oriented rationale for devices design and selection. Appl Sci 13(20)
56. Dragusanu M, Baldi TL, Iqbal Z, Prattichizzo D, Malvezzi M (2020) Design, development, and control of a tendon-actuated exoskeleton for wrist rehabilitation and training. In: 2020 IEEE international conference on robotics and automation (ICRA). IEEE, pp 1749–1754
57. Dragusanu M, Iqbal Z, Prattichizzo D, Malvezzi M (2021) Design of a modular hand exoskeleton for rehabilitation and training. In: Proceedings of the ASME 2021 international mechanical engineering congress and exposition. Volume 5: Biomedical and biotechnology
58. Dragusanu M, Troisi D, Prattichizzo D, Malvezzi M (2024) Evaluating adaptability properties of a compact wearable hand exoskeleton. In: 2024 10th IEEE RAS/EMBS international conference for biomedical robotics and biomechatronics (BioRob), pp 1561–1566

59. Dragusanu M, Iqbal MZ, Baldi TL, Prattichizzo D, Malvezzi M (2022) Design, development, and control of a hand/wrist exoskeleton for rehabilitation and training. IEEE Trans Robot 38(3):1472–1488
60. Dragusanu M, Troisi D, Villani A, Prattichizzo D, Malvezzi M (2022) Design and prototyping of an underactuated hand exoskeleton with fingers coupled by a gear-based differential. Front Robot AI 9
61. Dragusanu M, Iqbal Z, Villani A, D'Aurizio N, Prattichizzo D, Malvezzi M (2022) Hans: a haptic system for human-to-human remote handshake. In: 2022 9th IEEE RAS/EMBS international conference for biomedical robotics and biomechatronics (BioRob), pp 1–8
62. Dragusanu M, Villani A, Prattichizzo D, Malvezzi M (2021) Design of a wearable haptic device for hand palm cutaneous feedback. Front Robot AI 8:254
63. Villani A, Dragusanu M, Prattichizzo D, Malvezzi M (2024) Validation and usability assessment of the hapticpalm, a wearable device for hand palm force feedback. In: 2024 IEEE haptics symposium (HAPTICS), pp 372–378
64. Troisi D, Dragusanu M, Villani A, Prattichizzo D, Malvezzi M (2022) Hapticpalm: A wearable robotic device for haptics and rehabilitative hand treatments. In: Cavallo F, Cabibihan J-J, Fiorini L, Sorrentino A, He H, Liu X, Matsumoto Y, Ge SS (eds) Social robotics. Springer Nature, Cham, Switzerland, pp 402–411
65. Dragusanu M, Troisi D, Villani A, Prattichizzo D, Malvezzi M (2022) Happ: a haptic portable pad for hand disease manual treatment. In: 2022 31st IEEE international conference on robot and human interactive communication (RO-MAN), pp 345–350
66. Dragusanu M, Achilli GM, Valigi MC, Prattichizzo D, Malvezzi M, Salvietti G (2022) The wavejoints: a novel methodology to design soft-rigid grippers made by monolithic 3D printed fingers with adjustable joint stiffness. In: 2022 international conference on robotics and automation (ICRA), pp 6173–6179
67. Dragusanu M, Troisi D, Prattichizzo D, Malvezzi M (2023) Compliant finger joint with controlled variable stiffness based on twisted strings actuation. In: 2023 IEEE international conference on robotics and automation (ICRA), pp 7378–7384
68. Dragusanu M, Troisi D, Prattichizzo D, Malvezzi M (2023) Joint stiffness analysis and regulation for underactuated soft grippers based on monolithic structure. In: Petuya V, Quaglia G, Parikyan T, Carbone G (eds) Proceedings of I4SDG workshop 2023. Springer Nature Switzerland, Cham, pp 492–499
69. Dragusanu M, Marullo S, Malvezzi M, Achilli GM, Valigi MC, Prattichizzo D, Salvietti G (2022) The dressgripper: a collaborative gripper with electromagnetic fingertips for dressing assistance. IEEE Robot Autom Lett 7(3):7479–7486

Chapter 2
Hand/Wrist Exoskeleton

For individuals with disabilities, technology plays a crucial role, since it offers the opportunity to have a life that in many cases is almost completely autonomous. Tools and assistive devices support ADLs, communication, education, and social integration. Today, numerous technologies in the medical and assistive fields enable people with disabilities to have a life that is almost completely "normal". In this context, robotic rehabilitation aids have demonstrated great potential by combining the high-intensity, long-duration interventions necessary for regaining motor function with quantitative metrics to assess therapeutic outcomes [1].

Technology in general and more specifically assistive robots will be effective if devices are accepted and regularly used by the people with physical disabilities in their everyday life, outside hospitals, laboratories and rehabilitation centers. Supportive technologies that are developed without incorporating user input and feedback throughout the design process are less likely to be adopted for their intended purpose. In this regard, the Cybathlon initiative, an international competition where individuals with physical disabilities compete in completing everyday tasks using latest robotic technology [2].

Robotic devices for rehabilitation and training is a promising and challenging research topic with a potentially huge social impact. The capacity of performing precise and repeatable therapeutic exercises, reducing the physiotherapists' physical burden, embedding virtual reality systems, collecting quantitative data that can be used to optimize therapy sessions, assess patient outcomes and the possibility of realizing the rehabilitation process in patient's home are the main advantages offered by rehabilitation robotics.

M. Dragusanu, *Design of Soft–Rigid Devices for Rehabilitative and Assistive Robotics*, Springer Theses, https://doi.org/10.1007/978-3-031-84823-0_2

2.1 State of the Art

Many researchers have focused on developing devices aimed at retraining impaired upper limbs [3, 4]. Regaining "pick and place" and "grasping" abilities enables patients to perform the majority of ADLs, leading to both functional improvement and greater independence. Therefore, successful upper arm therapy must address not only the arm but also the wrist and hand. In recent decades, hand therapy through exoskeletons and, more broadly, rehabilitation robotics has acquired increasing attention. Numerous robotic systems have been developed to provide upper-limb motor therapy, all with similar goals: to develop a training platform that helps patients regain hand range of motion and grasping ability, ultimately restoring the hand's participation in ADLs.

These devices widely differ in terms of cost, flexibility, size, weight, design philosophy, actuated DoFs, modularity, and range of motion. The following sections of the thesis highlight some of the most paradigmatic examples of hand exoskeletons relevant to this field.

Dovat et al. [5] introduced HandCARE, a hand exoskeleton that uses cable loops attached to the ends of each digit. A motor and pulley system applies forces to the fingers, while a clutch mechanism allows individual actuation of each finger and thumb. Similarly, the Rutgers Hand Master II, proposed in [6], is a force-feedback glove powered by pneumatic pistons positioned in the palm.

Lambercy et al. [7] adopted a different design philosophy, presenting a device with a parallelogram structure that involves two movable surfaces squeezed by the user. In contrast, many hand exoskeletons are based on rigid mechanical structures, using motors directly connected to the exoskeleton, that transmit motion to specific joints. The most popular designs in this category include systems based on remote centers of rotation [8], four-bar linkage mechanisms [9], base-to-distal devices with mechanical links in series [10], and matched-axis mechanical structures [11].

The hand module developed by Masia et al. [12] employs a double crank and slider mechanism driven by an electric motor, controlling the radius of a cylinder to guide grasping motions. A common disadvantage of these devices is their limited control over the proximal finger joints, which can result in physiologically inaccurate joint movements. To address this issue, Conti et al. [13] presented the kinematic synthesis of a hand exoskeleton based on a parallel mechanism, serving as the base stem for a robotic-assistive device designed for hand-opening disabilities. Control strategies for this exoskeleton, utilizing sEMG systems, are further explored in [14, 15].

Cable-driven devices have been developed to allow for individual control of the fingers and thumb using pulley systems that rest on the dorsal side of the hand [16, 17]. Bowden cables enable motors to be remotely located, reducing the overall weight, which allows these devices to be used in conjunction with arm movements. This cable mechanism is similarly employed by Randazzo et al. [18] and Marconi et al. [19]. In [20], the authors present a glove-type exoskeleton that actuates three fingers (excluding the little finger) and the thumb using tendon cables routed through a glove while in [21–23] a modular soft glove based on twisted string actuators and flexible structures are presented. Alternatively, [24] replaces tendons with air chambers and channels running along the palmar side of the hand digits, with an electropneumatic servovalve regulating air pressure to assist in digit extension.

The hand-wrist assistive rehabilitation device is presented in [25], where the exoskeleton directly controls finger rotation at the metacarpophalangeal (MCP) joint, thumb abduction/adduction, and wrist extension/flexion. The Hand Mentor (Kinetic Muscles, Inc., Tempe, AZ, USA) is a commercially available exoskeleton that uses artificial muscles to simultaneously extend and flex the fingers and wrist, with the thumb not actuated [26]. A 3D-printed system designed to assist stroke patients with rehabilitation exercises was also developed in [20]. Recently, a wearable soft exoskeleton for hand rehabilitation has been presented in [27], while [28] introduces a Bowden-cable-based bidirectional remote actuation system, noted for its high power-to-mass and power-to-volume ratios, as well as its compact and accessible design. An interested reader is referred to [29–31] for a more comprehensive review on hand exoskeletons.

In terms of wrist rehabilitation, Krebs et al. [32] introduced a robot designed to provide three rotational DoF for wrist rehabilitation. Similarly, Gupta et al. [33] presented the RiceWrist, a high-fidelity, 4-DoF wrist exoskeleton for training and rehabilitation, based on a parallel structure driven by linear actuators specifically designed for safety requirements. The RiceWrist is intended to provide kinesthetic feedback during motor skills training or rehabilitation of reaching movements. Cappello et al. [34] introduced a serial kinematics-based solution driven by gear motors to meet back-drivability requirement, while [35] presents a novel tendon-driven, 3-DoF wrist exoskeleton. A soft wrist orthosis exoskeleton, capable of assisting users across all DoFs, is detailed in [36]. Furthermore, wrist actuation systems are frequently integrated into upper-limb exoskeletons, which also include elbow and shoulder actuation, as seen in [37–40].

A key feature of the exoskeleton systems developed during this PhD is the tracking of hand and wrist movements. Several techniques for human body tracking are available, with optical trackers, camera-based systems, and fabric integrated sensors being the most common.

Optical tracking systems like Optitrack (NaturalPoint Inc., USA) and Vicon (Vicon Motion Systems, UK) exploit markers to estimate human posture in real time with high precision and accuracy. However, they require a structured environment, making them neither wearable nor portable, and unsuitable for outdoor scenarios. To address portability, camera-based tracking algorithms have become a popular solution, driven by advances in computer vision and GPU computational capabilities.

In [41], a commercial RGB camera was used to reconstruct the human kinematic chain. For upper body tracking, commercial devices like Leap Motion (Leap Motion Inc., USA) can estimate full hand and wrist configurations simultaneously. However, camera-based systems face limitations in outdoor environments due to lighting interference, and body occlusions can lead to inaccurate estimations.

Another method for estimating human pose uses Micro Electro-Mechanical Systems (MEMS) technology. MARG (Magnetic, Angular Rate, and Gravity) sensors, which include gyroscopes, accelerometers, and magnetometers, can be integrated into wearable devices to reconstruct body pose. The main drawback of MARG sensors is that the majority of the algorithms rely on the magnetometer to estimate the orientation, thus they are sensitive to local variations in the magnetic field. Despite this, tracking systems based on this technology are commercially available and allow to accurately track the whole body, both outdoor and indoor, in unstructured environments, under different lighting conditions, and free from grounded/bulky hardware [42]. For hand and arm tracking, inertial sensor-based systems were proposed in [43, 44], with whole-hand tracking achieved by placing sensors on the phalanges. A similar system using triaxial accelerometers was developed by Kim et al. [45], while [46] introduced a sensing glove with inertial and magnetic sensors for each finger.

Considering these tracking methodologies, the thesis focus on inertial MEMS technology to estimate hand pose. This approach meets the requirements for a wearable, robust, low-cost sensing system capable of functioning indoors and outdoors without lighting limitations. Additionally, by not relying on magnetometers for orientation, the system offers reliable estimates even in the presence of magnetic disturbances, such as those generated by motors.

2.2 Wrist

This section presents an exoskeleton for wrist actuation that can be used both for daily activities as well as for long term rehabilitation process (Fig. 2.1). The patient, even with limitation in upper limb motion capabilities, can wear the device and use it also without the need of external support. The exoskeleton is made of thermoplastic material, which can be customized to meet the user's specific needs. Wrist actuation is achieved through a tendon-driven mechanism, with a focus on minimizing the number of components. All actuators, electronic components, and batteries are housed in the forearm section of the exoskeleton, with data transmission to and from a PC managed wirelessly. A graphical user interface allows users to select exercises, set parameters, and monitor progress during execution.

A key feature of the exoskeleton is the tracking of wrist movements, as the hand and arm parts are not mechanically constrained. For this purpose, a balance was struck between achieving accurate motion estimation and ensuring ease of use. The tracking system utilizes two Inertial Measurement Units (IMUs), which are low-cost devices that integrate an accelerometer and gyroscope on a single board. This work developed the data acquisition and processing system for the IMUs, translating sensor information into biomechanical data and enabling real-time monitoring. The resulting tracking system records user movements (e.g., an exercise suggested and guided by the physiotherapist) monitors exercises controlled by the exoskeleton, and tracks the patient's range of motion and improvements over time. To the best of our knowledge, this is the first attempt to combine all of these features in a single wearable device.

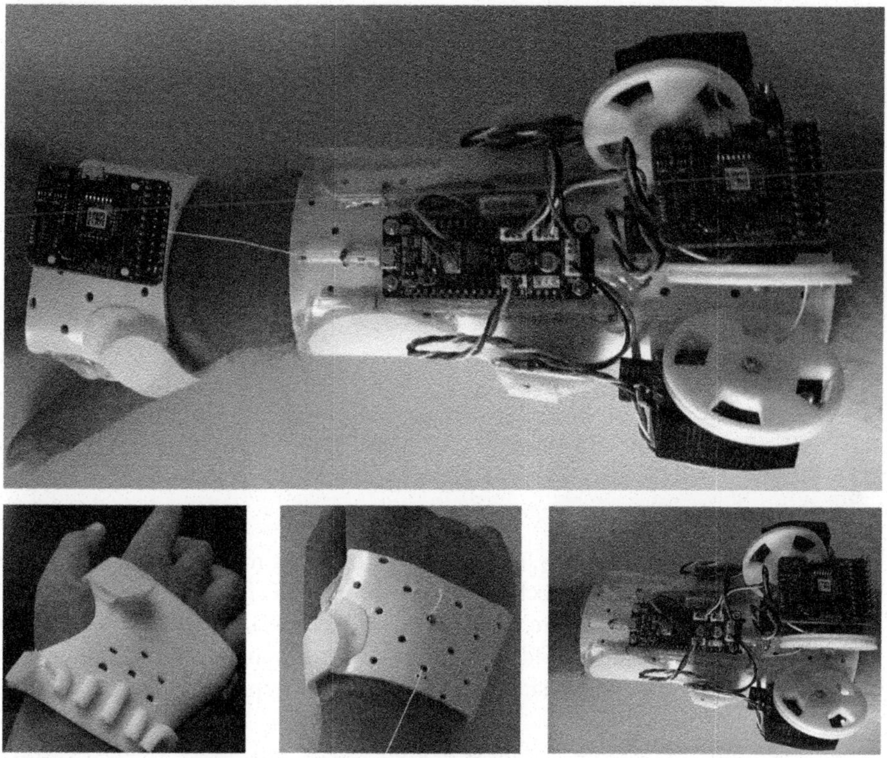

Fig. 2.1 Exoskeleton prototype. Top figure: the exoskeleton worn by the user. Bottom figures: two versions of the hand support and forearm support

2.2.1 Design Requirements

The exoskeleton consists of two independent rigid parts: one worn on the hand and the other attached to the forearm. These parts are connected by three tendons, which are anchored to the hand on one end, and wrapped around pulleys connected to the shafts of three motors on the other. The motors themselves are mounted on the forearm support. Given that the wrist can be modeled as a 2-DoF joint, three tendons are the minimum required to actuate both degrees of freedom, as demonstrated in previous research [47].

Let us indicate with θ_a and θ_e the adduction/abduction and flexion/extension rotations, respectively. Based on the desired motion capabilities, the following variation ranges are considered:

$$-45° < \theta_a < 20°, \quad -65° < \theta_e < 65°$$

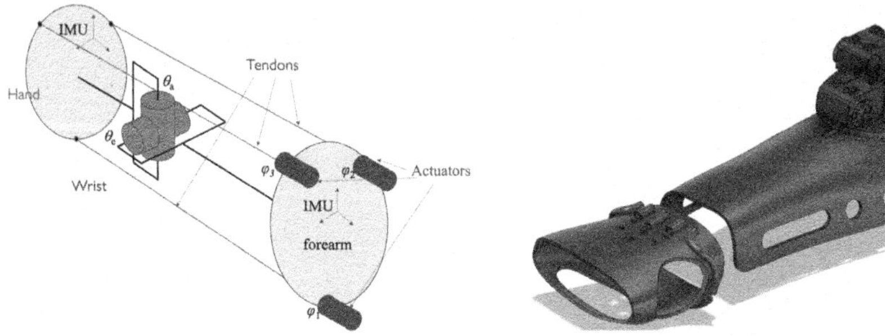

(a) (b)

Fig. 2.2 **a** Wrist and exoskeleton scheme. The wrist is modelled as a 2-DoFs universal joint, enabling the flexion/extension θ_e and adduction/abduction θ_a of the hand w.r.t. the forearm. Three tendons connect the exoskeleton hand and forearm supports and are actuated with three motors. Their angular rotation is indicated with ϕ_i. **b** CAD model of exoskeleton supports on the hand and on the forearm

We indicate with $\phi = [\phi_1, \phi_2, \phi_3]^T$ a vector collecting motor rotation angles and with $\theta = [\theta_a, \theta_e]^T$ a vector collecting wrist rotation angles.

The wrist/exoskeleton system can be modeled as a 2-DoF parallel mechanism with three actuators, as illustrated in Fig. 2.2a. By analyzing the system, an inverse kinematics relationship can be established. This relationship can be considered linear with good approximation

$$\boldsymbol{\phi} = J_i\theta \tag{2.1}$$

Inverse kinematics Jacobian matrix J_i is 3×2 and its terms depend on wrist and exoskeleton parameters. It is interesting to notice that ϕ values cannot be randomly selected, but need to belong to the 2-dimensional subspace $\mathcal{Q}$ whose basis is defined by J_i columns. If $\tilde{\phi} \in \mathcal{Q}$, we can solve the direct kinematic problem

$$\theta = J_i^{\#}\tilde{\boldsymbol{\phi}}, \tag{2.2}$$

where $^{\#}$ indicates the pseudo-inverse.

Indicating with $\tau_w = [\tau_a, \tau_e]^{\mathrm{T}}$ the adduction/abduction and flexion/extension wrist torques applied by the exoskeleton and with $\tau_m = [\tau_1, \tau_2, \tau_3]^{\mathrm{T}}$ the torques applied the motors, the following static relationship can be set:

$$\tau_w = J_i^T \tau_m \tag{2.3}$$

2.2.2 *Mechanical Design*

Supports: In the initial phase of the mechanical design, it was compared and evaluated different solutions and manufacturing processes. Producing the entire exoskeleton (both the hand and forearm components) using additive manufacturing was not ideal, particularly for the forearm component. This approach required a relatively complex process to tailor the structure to the user's forearm, including tasks such as 3D scanning the upper limb, adjusting the 3D-CAD files to match the specific user arm anatomy, and then proceeding with the manufacturing process. For the forearm support, a more practical solution was to adapt an existing approach used for orthoses. This involved shaping a thermoplastic plate directly onto the user's forearm [49]. Regarding the hand support, this part required a more compact design, a more complex geometry, and had to withstand higher mechanical stresses compared to the forearm support. Therefore, the advantages of using thermoplastic material were not evident. For these reasons, different designs were created, with some components produced using Acrylonitrile Butadiene Styrene (ABS) material via 3D printing, starting from a 3D-CAD model of the hand. Various shapes and assemblies were tested to identify the optimal solution in terms of wearability. A 3D-CAD model of the supports is reported in Fig. 2.2b.

Actuators, sensors, electronic components: Three Dynamixel XL-320 motors were used, each capable of generating a stall torque of up to 0.39 Nm at 7.4 V, which is suitable for the exoskeleton application. The motors' placement and the routing of the tendons on the forearm were carefully designed to ensure both user comfort and efficient transmission. The exoskeleton range of motion depends on the rotation q_i ($0 \leq q_i \leq 360°$) of each motor, resulting in a more effective control strategy. A 32 bit Arm Cortex-M3 microcontroller controls the motors by means of a library provided by the suppliers of the OpenCM9.04 board. While a RN42 Bluetooth module embedded in the board, communicates data with a PC application that allows the user to select and monitor the exercise.

Overall, the forearm support includes the following components: a board OpenCM9.04 C-Type; a Bluetooth module RN42; three Dynamixel XL-320 Motors; two batteries of 3.7 V, 500 mA; one IMU sensor (Xsens MTi-3). The hand support includes only one IMU sensor. The hand support contains a single IMU sensor, which is powered by the batteries located in the forearm. Raw data from the IMUs is transmitted to a remote PC using Xbee modules.

Overall features: An image of the exoskeleton prototype, worn by the user, is reported in Fig. 2.1, whereas its main features are summarized in Table 2.1. It can be noticed that the overall weight is quite low, about 300 g, and also the overall encumbrance is quite small, compared to other devices for the same purpose [33, 34].

2.2.3 *Device Control*

As mentioned in the introduction, a practical way to estimate hand orientation is through IMU sensors. The wrist angles, or the orientation of the hand relative to the forearm, are calculated using two IMUs: one placed on the back of the hand and the other attached to the exoskeleton. To compute the orientation of each board, the

Table 2.1 Main features of the wrist exoskeleton

Parameter	Value	Unit
Range, flexion/extension	± 65	°
Range, adduction	45	°
Range, abduction	20	°
Weight	300	g
Actuator stall torque	0.39	Nm
Actuator dimensions	$24 \times 36 \times 27$	mm
Actuator weight	16.7	g
Actuator no load speed	114	rpm
Max yield stress, forearm support	26	MPa
Max yield stress, hand support	34	MPa
Max tendon force	15	N

Reproduced from [48] with permission from IEEE. © IEEE 2020

algorithm from [50] was adapted. This algorithm determines the current orientation of each IMU relative to its initial pose. Raw sensor data is wirelessly transmitted to an external PC, where the necessary computations are performed. The system operates with an update rate of 1 kHz.

The following sections describe the calibration procedure for the sensing glove and briefly outline the IMU-based hand tracking algorithm.

Calibration: Each IMU board requires an initial calibration, which consists of two steps. In the first step, the user is asked to displace the hand in a known a-priori position, e.g., the user places the hand in a flat surface. In this phase, each IMU board collects 200 samples to estimate the gyroscope bias. The second step computes the offset quaternion between the hand and the forearm.

Hand tracking algorithm: In what follows, it is summarized the joint angles estimation, for more details, the interested reader is referred to [50]. This work employs quaternions to estimate the orientation of a single IMU sensor relative to a reference frame. Using quaternions helps overcome issues associated with Euler angles, such as gimbal lock and complications from trigonometric functions. Throughout this algorithm and the entire work, the following convention is used to represent a quaternion: $q = [w \; x \; y \; z]$, where w is the real number.

Let ${}^{S}q_H(t)$ and ${}^{S}q_F(t)$ be the quaternions that express the orientation, with respect to the Sensor reference frame Σ_S, of the frames associated to the hand, and to the forearm, respectively. Let ${}^{F}\hat{q}_H$ be the offset quaternions between the hand and the forearm, estimated during the aforementioned calibration phase. At a certain time instant t, the orientation of the hand referred to the forearm can be computed as

$$ {}^{F}q_H(t) = {}^{F}q_S(t) \otimes {}^{S}q_H(t), $$

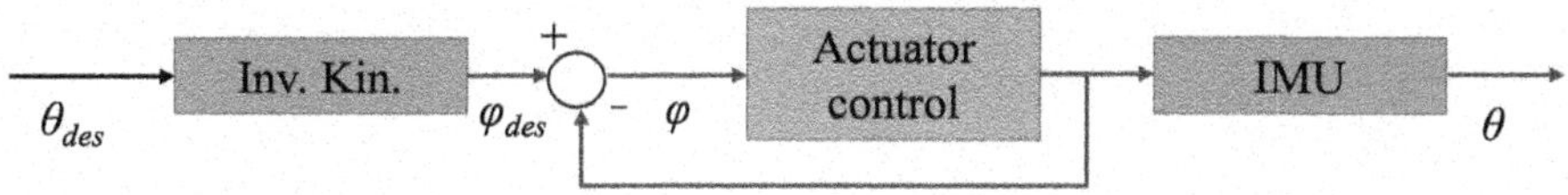

Fig. 2.3 Exoskeleton control scheme

where ${}^{F}q_{S}(t)$ is the conjugate quaternion of ${}^{S}q_{F}(t)$. Then, the quaternion that describes the orientation of the hand with respect to the initial configuration results

$$q_H(t) = {}^{F}q_H(t) \otimes {}^{H}\hat{q}_F$$

As a final step, the result is converted into *Euler Angles*.

2.2.3.1 Control

Exoskeleton control scheme is reported in Fig. 2.3. The input for the control scheme is the desired trajectory $\theta_{des} = [\theta_{a,des}, \theta_{e,des}]$, that can be assigned by the user through the graphical user interface or previously recorded by IMU sensors. θ_{des} values can be recorded for example during the execution of an exercise in which the exoskeleton is not actuated and wrist motion is manually guided by the physiotherapist. Through inverse kinematic analysis, wrist desired rotation angles are θ_{des} transformed in references for the actuators' control systems ϕ_{des} (Eq. (2.2)). Actual wrist movement θ is monitored by the tracking system based on IMU sensors during the exercise execution.

2.2.3.2 User Interface

A Matlab GUI interface (Fig. 2.4) has been developed to set exercise parameters and monitor them. When opening the application, the device has to be connected to the PC through the Bluetooth module. Once the exoskeleton is connected, the user can set a home position or start the exercise. The user can also choose between automatic or manual control of the device.

Several predefined wrist exercises, such as flexion/extension and abduction/adduction, are available through the interface. For each exercise, the user can select one of three speeds (low, medium, or high) and set a duration, using the respective drop-down menus. Alternatively, they can manually input a specific speed and time for the exercise.

When the *start* button is activated, the software takes all the user-defined parameters and sends them to the exoskeleton via Bluetooth communication. As the exercise begins, the software reads the motors' rotation angles and torque values, displaying them in a diagram on the interface.

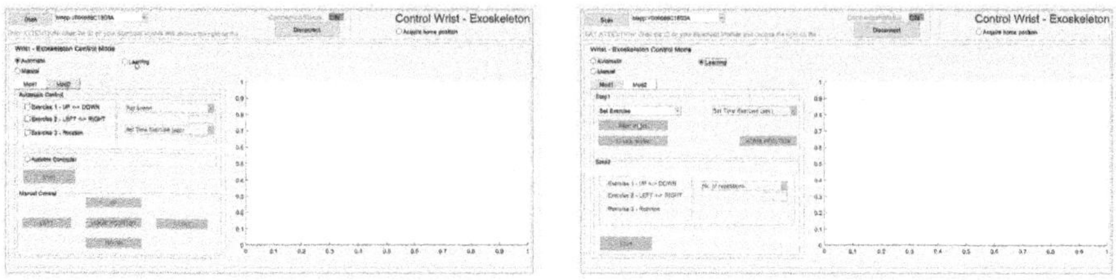

(a) (b)

Fig. 2.4 Graphical user interface realised for device control. **a** Automatic mode. **b** Learning mode

Manual control of the device is available through four interface buttons: flexion (*DOWN*), extension (*UP*), ulnar adduction (*LEFT*) and radial abduction (*RIGHT*). While a button is pressed, the corresponding motion is executed until preset maximum thresholds are reached.

Finally, the *disconnect* button terminates the Bluetooth connection and closes the program.

2.2.4 *Tests*

Test 1: The system was evaluated on a subject with severe limitations in extension motion (movement in flexion are with reduced problems) and some restrictions in radial adduction and ulnar abduction. Two types of exercises, recommended by the physiotherapist, were used as validation methods.

The first set of tests aimed to assess how well the motors followed a specific desired motion. Flexion/extension movements were achieved by assigning the same motion profile to actuators 2 and 3, while applying the opposite profile to actuator 1. To simulate the flexion/extension movement, the following reference values were set for the actuators:

$$\phi_{2,des} = \phi_{3,des} = \alpha \sin(\omega t), \ \phi_{1,des} = -\alpha \sin(\omega t)$$

with $\alpha = 1$ rad, $\omega = 1.1624$ rad/s and $0 < t < 10$ s. Each trial lasted 10 s. References and measured values of rotation angles of a representative trial are reported in Fig. 2.5. The figure shows how the actuators are able to follow the profile for the entire duration of the exercise. Ten repetitions of the trial were performed and for each reference actual value of the motors were recorded. It is observed that the average error in following the reference is 9.06°. Then I simulated the ulnar adduction and radial abduction. To reproduce this motion, motor 1 is maintained steady, whereas motors 2 and 3 pull their tendons with opposite movements. To recreate this behavior the following reference profiles were used to control the motors:

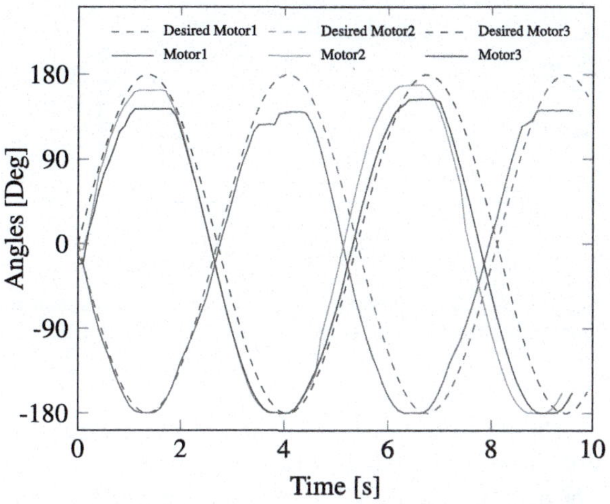

Fig. 2.5 Test 1, flexion/extension representative trial. Dashed curves show the desired angular position of the motors, solid ones represent the actual values. Desired motion of motors 2 and 3 are overlapped. Reproduced from [48] with permission from IEEE. © IEEE 2020

$$\phi_{1,des} = 0, \ \phi_{2,des} = \alpha \sin(\omega t), \ \phi_{3,des} = -\alpha \sin(\omega t)$$

with $\alpha = 1$ rad, $\omega = 1.1624$ rad/s and $0 < t < 10$ s. Ten consecutive trials were performed. For each repetition desired rotation angle and real value of the motors were recorded. It can be observed that the average error in tracking the angular profile was 9.94°.

Test 2: Another set of tests aimed to verify the system's ability to record an exercise performed by a physiotherapist and reproduce it using the exoskeleton. As shown graphically in Fig. 2.4, the system can record hand motion relative to the forearm through the tracking system. The recorded movement is then transformed into reference values for the actuators, allowing the exoskeleton to replicate the motion.

A physiotherapist and a patient with limited mobility participated in this test. The physiotherapist was asked to gently move the patient's hand for twelve seconds while the system recorded the hand's orientation relative to the forearm. Ten adduction/abduction and ten flexion/extension exercises were conducted. A representative trial from these tests is shown in Fig. 2.6.

2.3 Hand

This section presents the design of an exoskeleton for hand flexion/extension motion assessment and training. The device has been designed starting from the user's point of view, aiming to be easily and independently wearable, simple to control, modular, and versatile. It can be used by the patient either in collaboration with a therapist or autonomously.

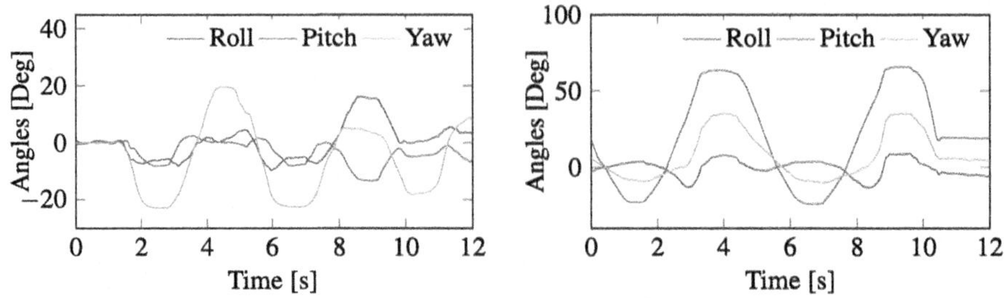

Fig. 2.6 Test 2 representative trials. (left) Adduction/abduction motion, (right) flexion/extension motion. Reproduced from [48] with permission from IEEE. © IEEE 2020

This thesis section presents and compares three different solutions for finger actuation. All the solutions are modular and designed to control each finger independently. The modules for the index, middle, ring, and little fingers share the same mechanical structure but vary in dimensions. The thumb module, not detailed in this part of the thesis, uses a different mechanism due to the unique kinematic structure of the thumb. Actuators, which typically have the greatest impact on the overall device weight and bulk, are positioned on the back of the hand to reduce weight and minimize inertial loads that could fatigue the user. Motion is transmitted to the finger joints through an efficient transmission system. Each finger is actuated by a single linear actuator that controls both the proximal and intermediate phalanges. This design allows for bi-directional force application, enabling both flexion and extension of the finger. The mechanical transmission is based on the concept of postural synergies, as introduced by the neuroscientific studies in [52]. Specifically, the position and dimensions of the exoskeleton linkages have been optimized to replicate the first postural synergy.

2.3.1 Design Requirements

The device is designed to assist the user in performing flexion and extension motions of all fingers, with adjustable amplitude throughout the full physiological range. The fingers can be controlled both independently and in a coordinated manner. The exoskeleton does not control, nor constrain, the adduction and abduction movements of the fingers.

The human hand (see Fig. 2.7) can be represented as a mechanism composed of five serial kinematic chains, the fingers, with a common base on the wrist.

Each finger can be represented as a 4-DoFs serial kinematic chain: the MCP joint of the index, middle, ring and pinky fingers is the joint connecting the finger to the hand and can be approximately modeled as a 2-DoFs joint, composed of two revolute joints with perpendicular and incident axis: one of them is needed to model adduction/abduction and the other one models flexion/extension. The remaining joints, the proximal interphalangeal (PIP) and distal interphalangeal (DIP) joints can be

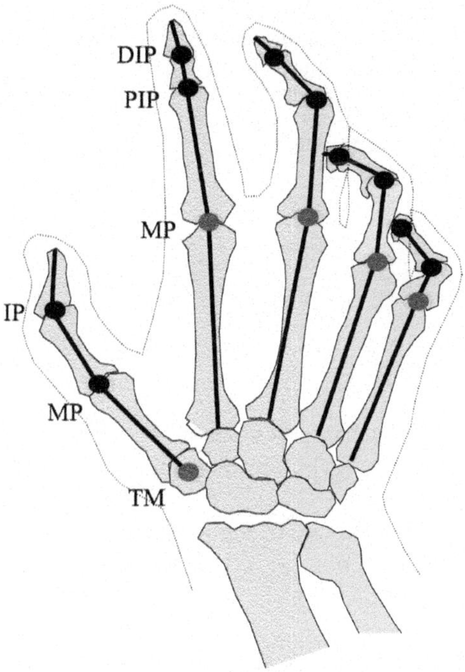

Fig. 2.7 Structure of the hand, fingers, bones and joints. Copyright © 2021 American Society of Mechanical Engineers (ASME) [51]

approximately represented as a single DoF revolute joint. If the hand is not affected by particular pathologies, it can be assumed that the rotation axes of PIP, DIP and the flexion/extension one of the MCP can be considered approximately parallel.

In this presented thesis work it is consider only the four fingers (index, middle, ring and little), and it is neglect the thumb, due to the complexity of its motion. Human object manipulation skills are highly dependent on thumb kinematics and its ability to oppose the other fingers, due to its unique structure. The thumb has at least five degrees of freedom DoFs: two in the trapeziometacarpal (TM) joint, two in the metacarpophalangeal (MCP) joint, and one in the interphalangeal (IP) joint. A more detailed analysis of the thumb is omitted here for the sake of brevity.

Finger structure and kinematics: The kinematic chains for the index, middle, ring, and little fingers consist of three links, representing the phalanges, connected by three parallel revolute joints, corresponding to the MCP, PIP, and DIP joints. The exoskeleton presented in this work actuates the flexion/extension motion of the fingers, while the adduction/abduction motion is neither actuated nor constrained. Therefore, the finger model considered in this study is planar.

The scheme of the index finger is represented in Fig. 2.8. Points K, N and L represent the axes of MCP, PIP, and DIP joints, respectively, point Q represents the fingertip. θ_1, θ_2 and θ_3 indicates their relative rotation angles. We furthermore indicate with l_{KN}, l_{LN} and l_{LQ} the lengths of the links representing the proximal, intermediate and distal phalanges, respectively.

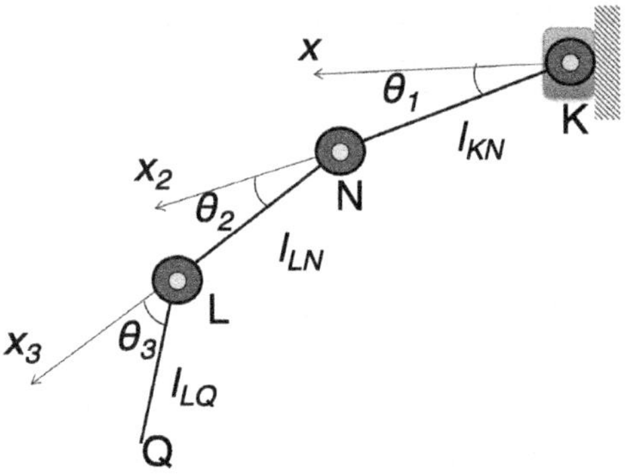

Fig. 2.8 Kinematic model of the index/middle/ring/little fingers considering only the flexion/extension motion. Copyright © 2021 American Society of Mechanical Engineers (ASME) [51]

For a given set of angles $\boldsymbol{\theta} = [\theta_1, \theta_2, \theta_3]^{\mathrm{T}}$ the evaluation of fingertip coordinates $\mathbf{r_b} = \left[x_p, y_p\right]^{\mathrm{T}}$, i.e., the solution of the forward kinematics problem, is straightforward.

The velocity of the fingertip $\mathbf{v}_P$ can be expressed as a function of joint angular velocities $\dot{\boldsymbol{\theta}} = \left[\dot{\theta}_1, \dot{\theta}_2, \dot{\theta}_3\right]^{\mathrm{T}}$ by introducing the finger Jacobian matrix $\mathbf{J}_f$:

$$\mathbf{v}_P = \mathbf{J}_f \dot{\boldsymbol{\theta}} \tag{2.4}$$

where $\mathbf{J}_f$ is a 2×3 matrix representing the finger Jacobian matrix. In a static equilibrium condition, the transpose of $\mathbf{J}_f$ matrix relates the force applied to the fingertip $\mathbf{f}_P$ to the torques $\boldsymbol{\tau} = [\tau_1, \tau_2, \tau_3]^{\mathrm{T}}$ applied to joints, i.e. :

$$\boldsymbol{\tau} + \mathbf{J}_i^{\mathrm{T}} \mathbf{f}_P = 0 \tag{2.5}$$

Hand synergies Neuroscience studies [52] have shown that, despite the human hand's complex mechanical structure with many degrees of freedom, a limited set of variables can represent a wide range of hand poses used in everyday tasks. More recently, these concepts have been applied to robotics [53, 54], inspiring the development of a new generation of underactuated robotic hands.

In robotic hands, postural synergies represent a method for controlling the whole hand, having n_q DoFs, through a lower dimension set of input variables $n_z \leq n_q$: indicating with $\dot{\mathbf{q}}$ hand joint velocities, the following relationship can be defined

$$\dot{\mathbf{q}} = \mathbf{S}\dot{\mathbf{z}} \tag{2.6}$$

where $\mathbf{S}$ is the so-called *synergy matrix* and $\dot{\mathbf{z}}$ represents synergy velocities. Columns of the matrix of synergies $\mathbf{S} \in \Re^{n_q \times n_z}$ represent the so-called *postural synergies*, also referred as *eigengrasps* in the literature, in other terms the joint velocities that are obtained acting on each single synergy $\dot{z}_i$.

In human hands, synergies can be evaluated by analyzing hand posture measurements, for example through Principal Component Analysis (PCA) of hand postures during grasping operations, as described in [52]. In robotic hands, where mechanical coupling between joints creates postural synergies, these synergies can be derived from the kinematic analysis of joint couplings and constraints [55]. In artificial systems, hand synergies can also be introduced at the control level, where the coupling between joints is managed by the hand's control system. For instance, in [56], a procedure is proposed and discussed to map human hand synergies onto robotic hands, even when the robotic hand's kinematic structure differs significantly from that of an anthropomorphic hand.

The first version of the exoskeleton, described in [57] and further developed in the initial solution of this work, applied the results of our previous studies on synergies [54, 58] to set the reduction ratio between θ_2 and θ_1. Specifically, the value of this ratio was based on the first postural synergy. The data used for developing this exoskeleton were sourced from the HandCorpus database [59]. In [57], a kinematic synthesis procedure for designing an exoskeleton structure that constrains finger movement according to the first postural synergy is detailed. This design aims to ensure that, even though the joint rotations are coupled, the constraint feels intuitive and natural to the user.

Exoskeleton requirements: This section summarizes the main requirements that guided the design of the exoskeleton for hand finger actuation.

- *Modularity*: modular exoskeleton, each finger can be independently actuated and controlled, the user can choose to actuate the whole hand or only one or some fingers.
- *Wearability*: the exoskeleton should be easily worn by the user, possibly without the need of external assistance.
- *Encumbrance*: the encumbrance of the exoskeleton should be as contained as possible, the bottom surface of the fingers should not be constrained, to allow the user to grasp and manipulate objects.
- *Number of actuated DoFs*: for each finger module, only one actuator is employed, the motion of MCP, PIP and DIP should therefore be coupled by the mechanical structure of the exoskeleton.
- *Type of motion*: the exoskeleton will actuate the flexion/extension motion of each finger only. The flexion/extension range for the MCP joint is [0°–90°].
- *Maximum force*: the developed exoskeleton will be able to apply a maximum equivalent force at the fingertip of 20 N both in flexion and extension.

These requirements guided the design process from the earliest stages, including the selection of the actuation type and the definition of the main structure. For example, the need to actuate both flexion and extension motions, while minimizing the weight and bulk of the device, led to the choice of a linear electromechanical actuator and a rigid link-based mechanism for motion transmission.

2.3.2 Exoskeleton Mechanical Structure: Proposed Solutions

Hand exoskeletons are complex devices composed of multiple intricate parts that require precise and intuitive control architecture. Achieving perfect alignment between the exoskeleton joints and the wearer's joints is crucial but challenging. Various design strategies are employed to ensure proper alignment of all components, as human hands have many joints in a small space.

Devoting a separate actuator to each degree of freedom would result in a complex and heavy device. Therefore, most hand exoskeletons use joint coupling systems or underactuation to simplify the design. When fewer actuators are used, a transmission system is required to convert actuator motion into the desired finger or hand movement. In this work, three different mechanisms were developed, investigated, and compared.

First solution A prototype of the first solution, introduced in [57], is shown in Fig. 2.9, which presents the complete CAD design, and Fig. 2.9b, which details the CAD model for the index finger. As seen in Fig. 2.9a, the design consists of five assemblies: four for each finger and one for the thumb. The mechanism for all fingers is the same, with minor variations in link dimensions to accommodate different finger sizes. The thumb assembly, however, consists of a 2-DoFs mechanism for both flexion/extension and abduction/adduction.

In Fig. 2.9b, the mechanism used for index finger flexion and extension is depicted, showing that one linear actuator controls these movements for each finger. For the thumb, two linear actuators are used, one for flexion/extension and another for abduction/adduction. The flexion and extension mechanism consists of 10 links and, as described in [57], is designed to replicate the closure motion generated by the first postural synergy.

Referring to Fig. 2.9b, the pair of links labeled MB connects Link A to the middle phalanx, while the PB links connect Link A to the proximal phalanx. Link A is the first link attached directly to the actuator. All flexion/extension mechanisms-whether for fingers or the thumb-share the same structure, with only minor changes in link dimensions. The thumb's abduction/adduction mechanism includes an additional linear actuator to provide an extra DoF.

The mechanism has 1-DoF, so the position of the linear actuator can be used to estimate the posture of the finger, by means of a standard forward kinematics procedure and no external measurement systems are needed.

Second solution The second solution is illustrated in Fig. 2.10. Similar to the first solution, it consists of five assemblies: four for each finger and one for the thumb, as shown in Fig. 2.10a. All modules appear very similar, with the only difference being the geometric dimensions adjusted for the varying lengths of human fingers. Each finger is actuated by one actuator for flexion and extension. To maintain a simpler design, abduction and adduction motions are not implemented, restricting the thumb to flexion and extension only. The assembly for the index finger is shown in Fig. 2.10b. Compared to the first solution, this design undergoes a complete redesign, removing

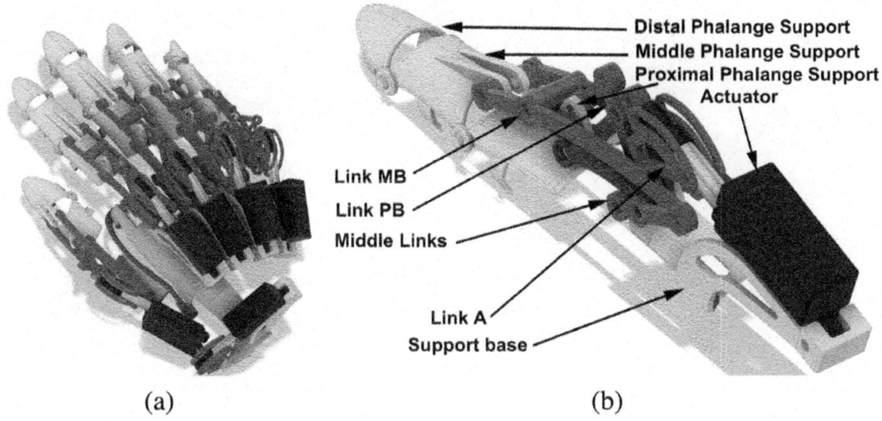

Fig. 2.9 **a** CAD model of the first exoskeleton, worn on the back of the hand, **b** CAD model of the index finger module. Copyright © 2021 American Society of Mechanical Engineers (ASME) [51]

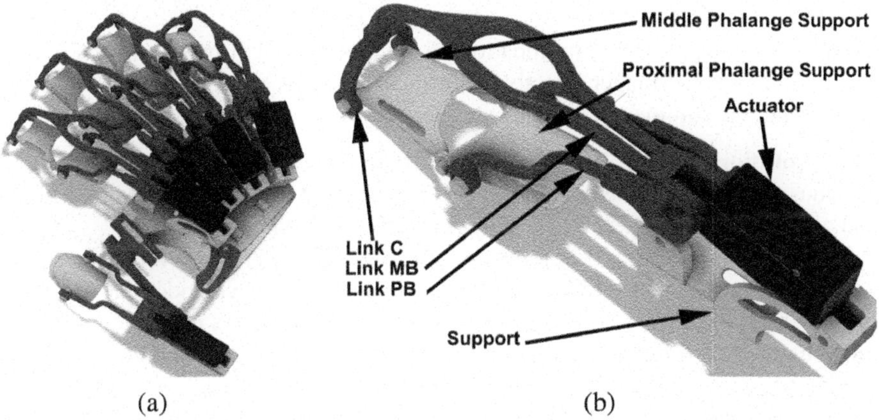

Fig. 2.10 **a** CAD model of the second exoskeleton, worn on the hand; **b** CAD model of the index finger mechanism. Copyright © 2021 American Society of Mechanical Engineers (ASME) [51]

many complexities from the previous version. Link MB connects the middle phalanx to the actuator, while Link PB connects the proximal phalanx to the actuator. Link C serves as a secondary link, connecting Link MB to the middle phalanx support.

From a mechanical perspective, a key difference in this solution is that it is under-actuated when not worn. The kinematic structure is *closed* by the finger, enhancing wearability and adaptability to the user's specific finger dimensions. While the previous solution was suitable for only a specific finger and could not be adjusted for different users, each module of this second development accommodates a range of finger dimensions and tolerates misalignments and small variabilities.

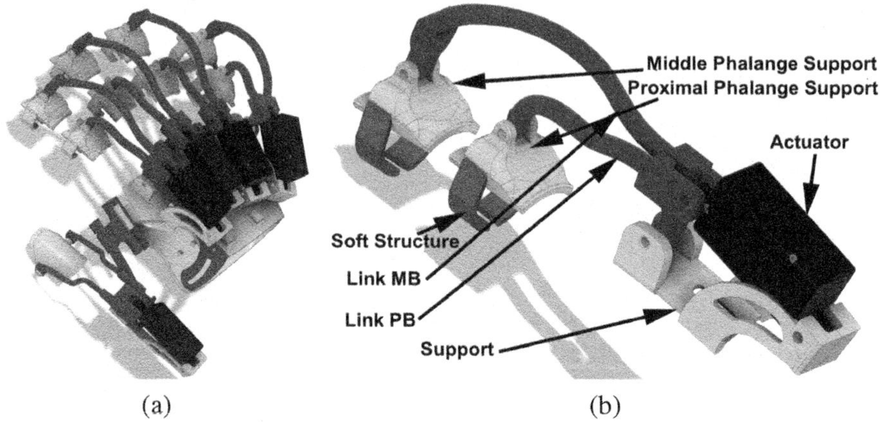

Fig. 2.11 **a** CAD model of the third exoskeleton, worn on the hand; **b** CAD model of the index finger mechanism. Copyright © 2021 American Society of Mechanical Engineers (ASME) [51]

The drawback of this simplification of the mechanical structure means that the finger's posture is no longer directly related to the actuator's displacement. Therefore, an external measurement system or an initial calibration procedure is necessary.

Third solution Finally, Fig. 2.11 illustrates the third exoskeleton design. Like the previous designs, this one consists of five independent modules: four for the fingers and one for the thumb. Each assembly is actuated by a single actuator.

This third solution was developed to address issues with the second design, which was not easy for users to wear independently and required a considerable amount of time for assembly. This complexity could reduce the device's effectiveness during rehabilitation or training. Additionally, for users with smaller hand sizes, it was challenging to assemble all the fingers onto the back support.

To address hese complexities, a redesign of the finger assemblies was carried out, as shown in Fig. 2.11b. In this design, only two links are used to actuate the proximal and distal phalanges, resulting in a simpler mechanism. Link MB connects the middle phalanx to the actuator, while Link PB connects the proximal phalanx to the actuator. To ensure a secure fit on the fingers, a soft structure is included with each phalanx support, taking the form of a half ring that allows for easy attachment to each phalanx.

As with the previous designs, the finger's posture is not directly related to the actuator's displacement due to the underactuated structure of the mechanism. Therefore, an external measurement system or an initial calibration procedure is necessary for accurate finger posture estimation.

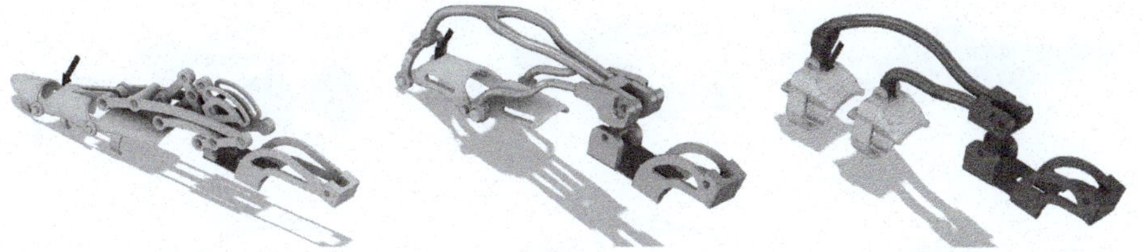

Fig. 2.12 Three CAD models of the index modules used for FEM analyses. Blue arrows represent the applied forces while the area highlighted in blue indicates the constraints. **a** CAD model of the first solution, where the mechanism and the finger's support are defined with the ABS material. **b** CAD model of the index module of the second solution, where the mechanism is made with aluminum and the finger supports in ABS; **c** CAD model of the third solution, where the mechanism is made of steel and the rings are realised in ABS and soft plastic. Copyright © 2021 American Society of Mechanical Engineers (ASME) [51]

2.3.3 Design Development and Evaluation

In the previous section, a qualitative assessment of the solutions in terms of ease of use, wearability, and mechanical simplicity was presented. In this section, I will further analyze the solutions from a mechanical perspective. Structural analyses have been conducted to compare the proposed designs in terms of mechanical robustness and to select the most suitable materials for the manufacturing phase. The materials considered for the mechanical structure and actuator support were ABS, steel, and aluminum. In the first two models, ABS was used for the finger phalanges' support. In the third model, a combination of ABS and soft plastic was used for the rings that connect the device to the phalanges. For this study, I used Autodesk® Fusion 360, a 3D-CAD/CAE simulation software. While the mechanical structures of the three exoskeleton designs differ, they all use the same linear actuator. Therefore, the analysis focused on the mechanical structure, excluding the actuator itself.

Figure 2.12 shows the three different CAD models of the index finger modules, each using different material combinations. For this work it is selected the index finger for all three models to perform a consistent comparison under similar conditions. The figure also indicates the points where the force is applied, shown with blue arrows, and highlights the constrained areas, specifically the base of the linear actuator's support, marked in blue.

We conducted these analyses using different materials, i.e. ABS, steel, and aluminum, and different magnitudes of the applied forces (20, 10 and 5 N). All forces were applied to the extremity of the structure, as it represents the most critical point during hand rehabilitation and is likely to experience the highest stress.

The results were reported both in terms of stress and displacement. Figures 2.13 and 2.15 show some of the analysed cases, while Table 2.3 collects the main results from all the considered configurations. Finally Table 2.2 reports the weight of each of the index module finger.

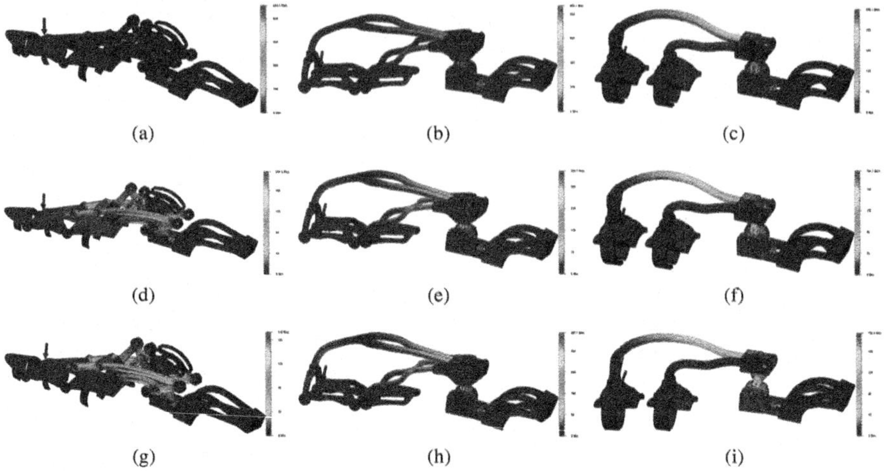

Fig. 2.13 Results of the FEM analyses, stress distributions. The applied force has magnitude of 20 N. **a–c** show the results of the FEM analysis when the material used for the mechanism is ABS. **d–f** report the stress results when the material used for the mechanism is aluminum while for the results in **g–i** the material for the mechanism is steel. Copyright © 2021 American Society of Mechanical Engineers (ASME) [51]

Table 2.2 Mass of the three models

Material	Weight	Weight	Weight
	Model 1 (g)	Model 2 (g)	Model 3 (g)
ABS	27.979	28.456	31.242
Steel	81.394	84.512	86.350
Aluminum	40.88	44.411	44.552

Copyright © 2021 American Society of Mechanical Engineers (ASME) [51]

It is worth noting that the maximum stress that ABS can withstand is upto 60 MPa. Among the models analyzed, only the third model, with an applied force of 5 N, produces results close to this limit, yielding a maximum Von Mises stress of 74.78 MPa. These results indicate that none of the three models can be manufactured using ABS unless the applied forces are significantly reduced. The maximum stress of that can be resisted by steel is much higher, upto 500 MPa. Using steel for the mechanical structure all the models have an acceptable Von Mises stress, the models that have the better results are the first and the third. Aluminum has a maximum resistance coefficient that is slightly lower than the steel, i.e. upto 500 MPa. Different Young's modules, i.e. 210 GPa for the steel and 75 GPa for aluminum lead to different maximum displacements that is approximately three time larger for the aluminum with respect to steel.

The weight of each module, depending on the material, is reported in Table 2.2. It's evident that ABS is the lightest material while steel the heaviest. From the Finite

Table 2.3 Synthesis of the FEM analysis results

Model	Force (N)	ABS		Steel		Aluminum	
		Von Mises (MPa)	Displ. (mm)	Von Mises (MPa)	Displ. (mm)	Von Mises (MPa)	Displ. (mm)
1	5	171.1	4.907	43.25	0.729	51.4	1.119
2		217.3	15.09	96.93	0.812	88.66	2.193
3		74.78	15.12	48.79	0.192	48.66	0.597
1	10	342.2	9.814	86.5	1.459	102.8	2.239
2		434.6	30.17	193.9	0.406	177.3	1.096
3		149.6	30.24	97.58	0.386	97.33	1.194
1	20	684.3	19.63	173.0	2.918	205.6	4.478
2		869.1	60.35	387.7	0.812	354.7	2.193
3		299.1	60.48	195.2	0.771	194.7	2.388

Element Method (FEM) analyses, it results that the ideal material for the exoskeleton structure is aluminum.

Considering the quantitative factors highlighted in this section and the qualitative ones introduced earlier, the third model provides the best overall results. A graphical comparison is shown in Fig. 2.14, where the three solutions are evaluated based on six criteria: (i) wearability, (ii) lightness, (iii) mechanical strength, (iv) deformation, (v) finger posture estimation, i.e. if it's possible to estimate finger posture from actuator position (vi) adaptability to different finger dimensions. Each criterion is ranked from 1 to 5 based on the considerations discussed previously.

The overall evaluation demonstrates that the third solution meets most of our design requirements, i.e. wearability, strength, weight, and simplicity, scoring the highest in 4 out of 6 criteria. The first prototype excels in mechanical strength and provides precise finger posture estimation due to its fully-actuated structure. The second prototype performs similarly to the third but with slightly lower scores.

2.3.4 *Prototypes*

This section present three exoskeleton prototypes developed on the basis of the solutions previously presented. All the exoskeletons are developed to be worn on the back of the hand, facilitating the user in flexion and extension motions.

Prototype 1 The first prototype corresponds to the initial solution, shown in Figs. 2.9 and 2.16a. The exoskeleton consists of five separate mechanisms: four for the fingers and one for the thumb. Each finger mechanism features a single linear actuator connected to a 1-DoF articulated system, specifically designed to reproduce the first postural synergy.

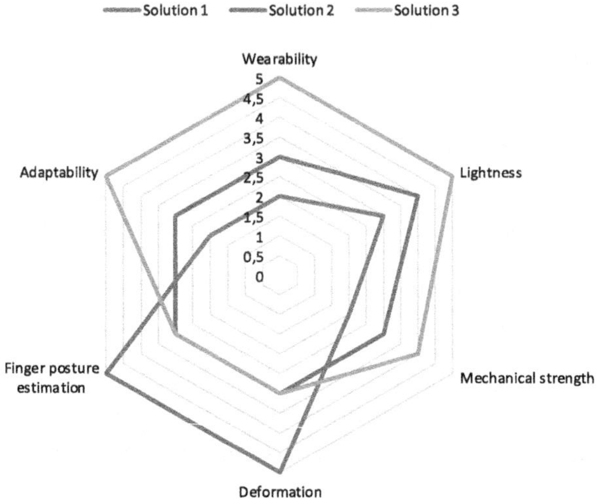

Fig. 2.14 Overall comparison of the proposed solutions. Copyright © 2021 American Society of Mechanical Engineers (ASME) [51]

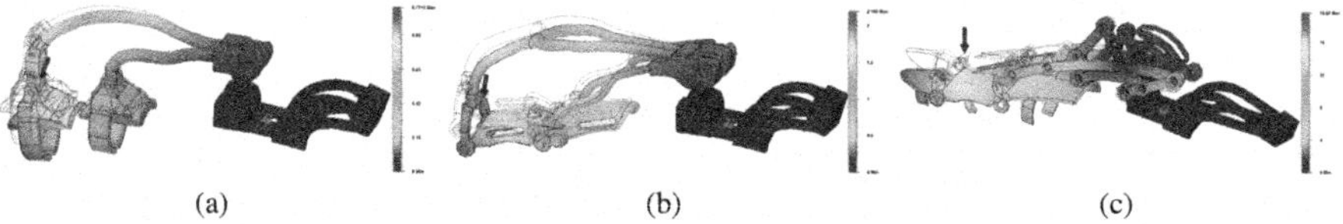

Fig. 2.15 Results of the FEM analyses for the three index models in terms of displacements. The applied force has a magnitude of 20 N in all the cases, while the materials for the mechanism used is steel in (**a**), aluminum in (**b**) and ABS in (**c**). Copyright © 2021 American Society of Mechanical Engineers (ASME) [51]

For actuation, the device uses an Actuonix PQ12-63-6-R linear actuator from Actuonix Motion Devices Inc. for each finger. This actuator incorporates a DC motor coupled with a worm gear to generate linear motion, with a gear reduction ratio of 63. Rated at 6VDC, it can be used similarly to a simple servo.

This actuator offers several features that are particularly useful for our application, such as low voltage operation, simple control, symmetric push and pull forces, precise feedback, and a compact miniature size. Other key characteristics are summarized in Table 2.4. A simple position control with adjustable proportional gain is implemented, with the Arduino Uno serving as the controller. A dual-cell LiPo battery is used as the power source. The circuitry is integrated into an arm band that can be easily worn, with a total weight of 90 g. For this demonstrative prototype, the entire exoskeleton structure was manufactured using ABS via additive manufacturing. The total weight of the exoskeleton is 250 g.

Prototype 2 The second prototype consists of four finger assemblies and one thumb assembly, as shown in Fig. 2.16b. Each finger assembly is treated as an independent

Table 2.4 Linear actuator main characteristics

Technical features	
Max. force (lifted)	45 N
Mass	15 g
Stroke	20 mm
Stall current	550 mA @ 6V
Feedback potentiometer	5 kΩ
Max speed (no load)	15 mm/s
Feedback potentiometer resolution	0.5 mm

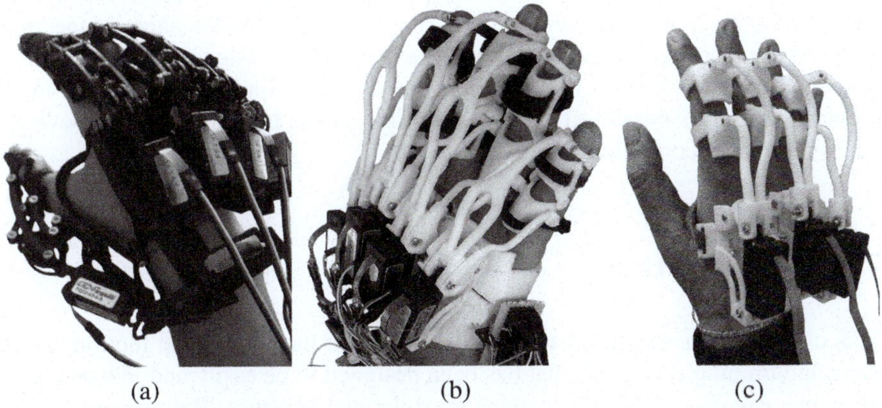

Fig. 2.16 First and secondo prototype. **a** Prototype 1: Hand exoskeleton, each finger uses on linear actuator that create flexion and extension by moving proximal and middle phalanges. It produces the first postural synergy. **b** Prototype 2: Hand exoskeleton, each finger uses one linear actuator that create flexion and extension by moving proximal and middle phalanges. **c** Prototype 3: Hand exoskeleton, showing only two fingers structure, each finger uses on linear actuator that create flexion and extension by moving proximal and middle phalanges

module that can be controlled separately. The modules for the index, middle, ring, and little fingers share the same structure but vary in size, as previously described. The corresponding 3D-CAD model is presented in Fig. 2.10.

The same actuator of Prototype 1 is used, and the same strategy of transmitting the motion using mechanical linkage systems is used. For each finger, the transmission mechanism is designed to replicate the coordinated movement between the proximal and middle interphalangeal joints, as observed in the first postural synergy. This allowed us to reduce the number of actuators to one per finger. Two LiPo batteries, each rated at 3.7 V, are connected in series to provide a 7.4 V power source. A Teensy 3.6 microcontroller manages different hand opening and closing exercises. Each finger module is equipped with two small Force Sensitive Resistor (FSR) sensors (Ohmite FSR04), placed under the hand's back support, which assist in physiotherapist-guided manual exercises. Since the linear actuators are not back-drivable, the FSR sensors detect signals when the physiotherapist pushes or pulls the fingertip, allowing the actuator to move accordingly. The exercise or movement is recorded by the microcontroller and transmitted to a PC, enabling the user to replay or save the recorded motion for future exercises, even without a physiotherapist's assistance.

Prototype 3 The third prototype also consists of five finger modules and features a simplified design with a minimal number of linkages. Like the previous versions, the exoskeleton can be worn on the entire hand or on individual fingers, depending on the user's needs. Two of the finger modules are shown in Fig. 2.16c, highlighting the simplicity of this structure, which reduces many complexities compared to the earlier designs. As with the other prototypes, the linkages are designed to closely replicate the first postural synergy. A soft ring structure provides stable connections to the finger phalanges, enabling smooth flexion and extension movements. Power is supplied by two 3.7 V LiPo batteries, and the same linear actuator used in the previous designs is employed here as well. The system is controlled by a powerful Teensy 3.6 microcontroller.

2.4 Wrist and Hand

This part of the thesis, proposes an exoskeleton for hand and wrist motion assessment and training (Fig. 2.17) that has been designed to be easily and independently wearable, easy to control and manage, modular and versatile. The proposed device can be used by the patient in collaboration with the physiotherapist or autonomously, and is composed of two independent and modular elements: the wrist actuation and the hand actuation systems. To the best of our knowledge, the proposed device represents the first attempt to realize a wearable hand/wrist exoskeleton able to record and play back motions and, at the same time, store data for further analyses.

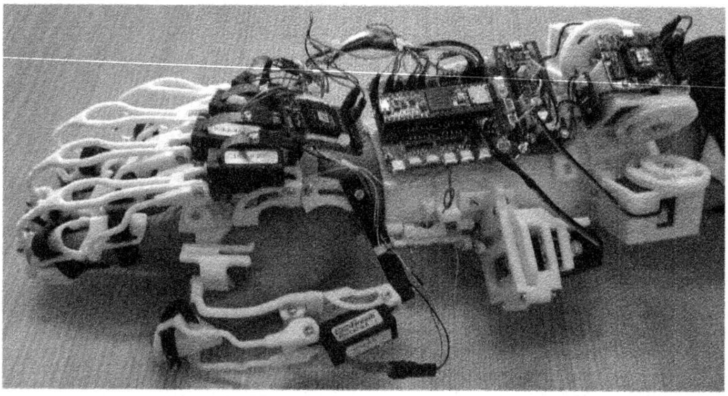

Fig. 2.17 Prototype of the hand/wrist exoskeleton for rehabilitation and training worn by a user

2.4.1 Design Requirements

The goal of this work is to develop an actuated hand/wrist exoskeleton for upper limb rehabilitation and training, suitable for both clinical use and home-based therapy for individuals with long-term impairments. As mentioned earlier, the design process was user-centered, involving a potential user from the early stages [60]. Based on their needs, an appropriate set of design requirements was established. The design aimed to meet these requirements as fully as possible. The user also contributed during the development phase, providing feedback and suggestions, which were used to refine the requirements. This thesis part outlines the main requirements that guided the device's design.

2.4.1.1 Identification of the Target Application

It is challenging to define a comprehensive set of design guidelines for assistive and rehabilitation hand and upper limb exoskeletons due to the wide variability in impairments and disabilities (e.g. , stroke, muscular dystrophy, brachial plexus injury, SCI). These conditions can cause significant differences in range of motion, muscle tone, joint stiffness, etc. Additionally, even within the same condition, factors such as severity, injury level, time since injury, and the subject's age contribute to this variability [61]. In [62], a study aimed at identifying design criteria for an assistive powered hand exoskeleton is presented. This study was based on structured interviews with clinicians and patients with hand impairments, along with assessments of patients' hand capabilities. The findings revealed a wide range of needs and expectations.

The device developed during the PhD is designed for a specific application: rehabilitation and training for subjects with low residual strength, limited active control of the hand and wrist, low spasticity, and reduced muscle tone. Although the device was developed to meet the needs of a representative user, as I will detail in the following sections, its modular structure makes it adaptable to a range of users and varying needs.

Mechanical requirements

Wrist module: Wrist articulation allows the following motions: (i) flexion/extension, (ii) radial deviation or adduction and ulna deviation or abduction: (iii) pronation/supination. Starting from an initial reference configuration, typical values for the amplitude of both flexion and extension motions are 85°, 40°–45° for the adduction, and less than 20° for the abduction. Pronation/supination motion has not been considered in this work, since it involves the whole forearm and would need the device to be extended at least upto the elbow.

The wrist module is requested to support the patient in the execution of the following exercises: (i) full or partial Flexion/Extension with pre-defined profiles or guided by the physiotherapist, with an amplitude that can be selected in the physiological range previously mentioned; (ii) full or partial Abduction/Adduction with pre-defined profiles or guided by the physiotherapist with an amplitude that can be selected in the physiological range previously mentioned; (iii) coupled Flexion/Extension and Abduction/Adduction guided or pre-recorded by the physiotherapist. In the guided exercises, both the amplitude and the speed can be varied.

Hand module: The human hand has a complex mechanical structure that can be modeled as a 30-DoF system [63]. Each finger can be represented as a kinematic chain, with a universal joint (composed of two intersecting, orthogonal revolute joints) at the MCP joint, and two hinges for the PIP and DIP joints. In cases where the hand is not affected by specific pathologies, the rotational axes of the PIP, DIP, and the flexion/extension axis of the MCP can be assumed to be parallel. The thumb, however, has a more intricate structure with at least 5-DoFs: 2-DoFs at the TM joint, 2-DoFs at the MCP joint, and 1-DoF at the IP joint. In this work, the focus is on reproducing the opening/closing motion of the hand, which primarily involves finger flexion and extension, with limited adduction and abduction. To minimize the complexity of the exoskeleton and reduce the number of actuators, only the flexion/extension motion is actuated, while the adduction/abduction movement is left unconstrained.

The hand exoskeleton features two coupled bending DoFs to exercise the MCP and PIP joints of the fingers. During tripod grasping, typical MCP, PIP, and DIP flexion angles are approximately 46°, 48°, and 12° for the index finger, and 46°, 54°, and 12° for the middle finger [64, 65]. Regarding speed, physiotherapists recommend, as noted in [66], that the time for a complete flexion/extension cycle of a finger joint should be less than 20 s, with hyperextension of these joints carefully avoided. As for the required forces, [65] highlights that in typical grasping tasks, forces below 20 N are sufficient. In summary, the hand module of the device is designed to assist users in performing flexion and extension motions of all fingers, with a range that covers the full physiological movement described. The fingers should be capable of being controlled both independently and in coordination. The adduction/abduction motion of the fingers is neither controlled nor constrained by the exoskeleton's mechanical structure.

2.4.1.2 Requirements for Wearability and Adaptability

Preliminary studies and initial prototypes of the device were introduced in [48] for the wrist and in [57] for the hand. Early user feedback revealed that one of the primary limitations of these prototypes was the inability for users to put them on independently. One key requirement to address, therefore, is ensuring that even users with limited upper limb mobility can wear and operate the device autonomously. Another important consideration is the device's adaptability to the user's specific characteristics, such as anthropometric measurements. To achieve this, the parts of the device that come into contact with the user's hand, fingers, and forearm were developed using a parametric approach. This allows for automatic adjustments to different users based on a limited number of easily obtainable measurements. Regarding the hand part, to limit as much as possible any interference during ADLs, the mechanical transmission system has to be constrained to be on the back of the fingers and the palm, the width of the finger modules should not exceed too much the finger width. Additionally, the exoskeleton should be as lightweight as possible, with its inertia distributed to avoid causing fatigue for the user.

The solution presented in this work includes two modules: one for the hand and one for the wrist. The hand module can be further divided into finger sub-modules, designed for a user needing to train both wrist and hand movements. However, the structure and control systems are developed so that each module can be used and controlled independently. For instance, if the user only wants to train the wrist, they do not need to wear the hand module.

2.4.1.3 Requirements for Control

The device allows users to perform pre-defined exercises, such as wrist flexion/extension, adduction/abduction, and hand opening/closing, following customizable profiles (e.g. , sinusoidal, trapezoidal). Users can adjust parameters like amplitude, time-frequency, and duration. Another requested feature was the ability to record an exercise guided by a physiotherapist, store it, and replay it autonomously, for example, at home. Given the modular structure of the device, the control system and GUI were developed to manage both the entire system and each individual module independently.

2.4.2 Device Description

As previously mentioned, the device consists of two modules: a wrist module and a hand module. The wrist module uses a tendon-actuated system with two main components worn on the hand and forearm. The hand module enables opening/closing motions through five finger modules, each powered by its own actuator. CAD models of both the hand and wrist modules are shown in Figs. 2.18 and 2.20. In what follows, before tackling the algorithmic development and experimental evaluation, it is described in detail all the mechanical part comprising the exoskeleton.

2.4.2.1 Wrist Actuation

The wrist module builds on a preliminary prototype introduced in [48]. While that system was simple and low-cost, it was unsuitable for users with limited motion capabilities, and the Velcro-based closure system led to unwanted or unfeasible relative motion between the device and the forearm.

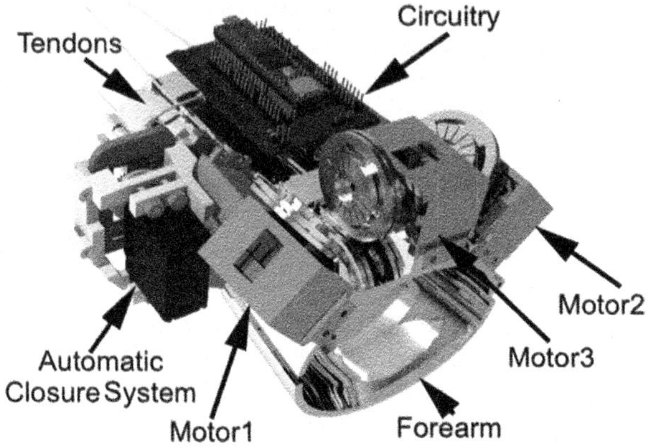

Fig. 2.18 Exoskeleton prototype wrist CAD renderings module. Reproduced from [67] with permission from IEEE. © IEEE 2022

In the version presented here, significant improvements have been made, particularly to the forearm section. The most notable upgrade is the addition of an automatic closure system, designed to enhance wearability. The complete forearm CAD model is shown in Fig. 2.18. The support was modeled using Autodesk® Fusion360, tailored to the user's anatomical features. The forearm support employs a parametric approach, allowing for easy customization based on three key measurements: (i) forearm circumference near the wrist, (ii) forearm circumference near the elbow, and (iii) the distance between the wrist and elbow. Similarly, the 3D-CAD model of the hand support can be adjusted for different users based on (i) palm width near the finger MCP joints and (ii) palm length (distance from the MCP joints to the wrist).

The section of the wrist actuation system connected to the hand, shown in Fig. 2.20, was also customized to the user's anatomical features and serves as the support for the hand actuation system. Further details on this component are provided in Sect. 2.4.2.2.

The structural components of the wrist module, both on the hand and forearm, were constructed from ABS material using Fused Deposition Modeling (FDM) technology.

The wrist joint actuation design has been completely completely redesigned to enhance wearability and fit. The user's wrist movement during exercises is guided and supported by a 3-DoF tendon system actuated by three servo motors (Dynamixel XL-320).

Two tendons are connected to the upper part of the hand to control extension motion, with the corresponding motors referred to as *Motor1* and *Motor2*. The third tendon, connected to the palm of the hand, actuates downward (flexion) motion and is labeled *Motor3*.

When *Motor1* and *Motor2* rotate in the same direction, and *Motor3* rotates in the opposite direction, they facilitate flexion/extension motion. Conversely, when *Motor1* and *Motor2* rotate in opposite directions, they achieve radial/ulnar deviations. As mentioned in Sect. 2.4.1, wrist pronation and supination motions are not activated.

The actuator placement on the forearm and tendon routing were chosen based on the understanding that flexion is typically easier than extension for users with

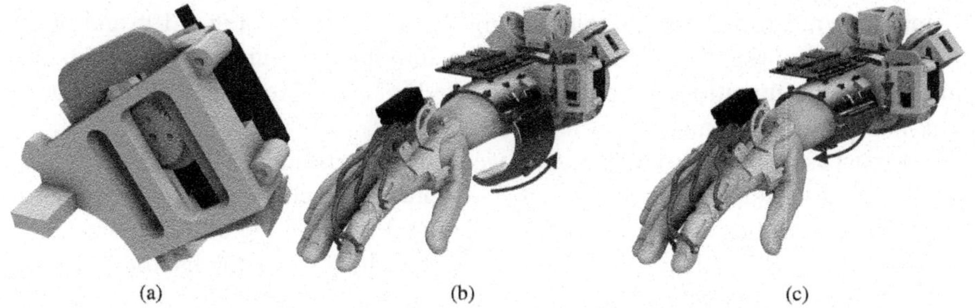

Fig. 2.19 Exoskeleton rendering highlighting the automatic closure mechanism: **a** detail of the rack and pinion mechanism used for ensuring a tight closure and allowing batteries to last longer; **b** open configuration; **c** close configuration. Reproduced from [67] with permission from IEEE. © IEEE 2022

low residual force and low muscle tone, the target application for this work (see Sect. 2.4.1). This is particularly relevant in exercises where the palm side of the hand faces down, as the weight of the hand aids in flexion. Therefore, tendon and actuator positioning on the forearm considers that more effort is required for extension than for flexion.

Additionally, the pulleys connected to the motor shafts have been redesigned compared to [68]. The pulley diameter has been reduced to save space while maintaining the desired range of motion. An external support with a thread-fixing system has been added to manage excess wire length, allowing for adjustment of tendon length based on each user's anatomical dimensions. Furthermore, the tendon routing has been designed to prevent the tendon from slipping off the pulley during exercises.

One of the key innovations introduced in this work is the automatic closure system of the forearm module, which allows users to wear the device easily and autonomously. The assembly shown in Fig. 2.19a is connected to the lower part of the forearm support. As the motor rotates the pinion, the rack translates, causing the lower part of the forearm support to rotate and wrap around the arm. This system securely holds the complete forearm assembly in place. Additionally, since the rack-and-pinion structure is not easily driven back without actuating the servo, keeping the motor active continuously is unnecessary.

In general, the automatic closure motors operate only during the opening and closing phases when the exoskeleton is being worn, which helps extend battery life compared to other solutions. Users can control the opening and closure of the forearm fastening mechanism via the software GUI developed for the exoskeleton, which will be detailed in subsequent sections. The system ensures a comfortable opening and closure process that can be autonomously managed by the user.

The rack-and-pinion mechanism is actuated by a servo motor (HS-422, Hitec RCD Inc., USA). The pinion gear, which drives the rack, is connected directly to the motor's output shaft. The pinion gear is designed to provide a rack stroke suitable for device closure and to withstand the torque applied by the motor. The motor's maximum rotation range is limited to $10° - 170°$, corresponding to a rack stroke of

20 mm. The mechanism is illustrated in Fig. 2.19; specifically, Fig. 2.19b and c show the complete exoskeleton rendering with the automatic closure mechanism in open and closed configurations, respectively, while Fig. 2.19a provides a close-up of the rack-and-pinion mechanism.

To assist users in easily and correctly wearing the wrist module, the tendon system provides flexible support for alignment. Two tendons are connected to the dorsal part of the hand module, while a third tendon, routed through the closure mechanism, connects to the palm. This helps users insert their hands into the hand-exoskeleton module, ensuring that the two lateral tendons on the wrist-exoskeleton remain above the hand, while the central tendon goes beneath it. The basic principle behind using the tendon-actuated wrist exoskeleton is to maintain tension in the tendons. Once users feel comfortable with the device in place, they or their physiotherapists can use the GUI to lock the exoskeleton in position and set it to the initial state, activating the automatic closure mechanism to pull the tendons tight. It's important to note that because the wrist actuation system is tendon-based and inherently underactuated, it can adapt to various user characteristics and compensate for misalignment or improper positioning.

2.4.2.2 Hand Actuation

The hand actuation system consists of five modules, one for each finger, allowing for both joint and independent control. The hand exoskeleton module is made up of two primary components: the support structure for the finger modules, which also connects to the wrist exoskeleton's tendons, and the individual finger modules. Users can wear the hand exoskeleton by inserting their hand into the support, designed specifically to accommodate the user's hand shape and dimensions. The interior of the support is lined with a spongy material for comfort, while the exterior is made of ABS plastic. Two design options have been developed for this support.

The first option features two separate pieces, i.e., one for the dorsal side of the hand and another for the palm, secured with Velcro straps. The second option is a single-piece design, which eliminates the need for Velcro and enhances resistance to the forces exerted by the wrist actuation system. Users have better rated the second version. At the top of the support, a horizontal slot allows for the attachment of individual finger modules, while the bottom section is designed to keep the palm uncovered. Both components feature a series of holes for connecting the tendons from the wrist module.

The position of the finger modules can be adjusted laterally within the horizontal slot on the hand support and can also be moved back and forth, thanks to a motor support that runs along the base. The modules for the index, middle, ring, and little fingers share the same mechanical structure but differ in dimensions. The thumb module employs a unique mechanism due to its specific kinematic structure [69]. Figure 2.21a and b illustrate the rendered CAD models of the fingers and thumb, respectively.

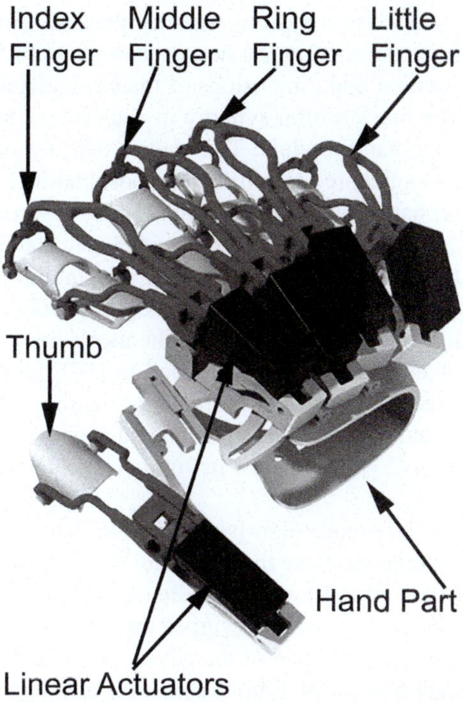

Fig. 2.20 Exoskeleton prototype, hand CAD module renderings. Reproduced from [67] with permission from IEEE. © IEEE 2022

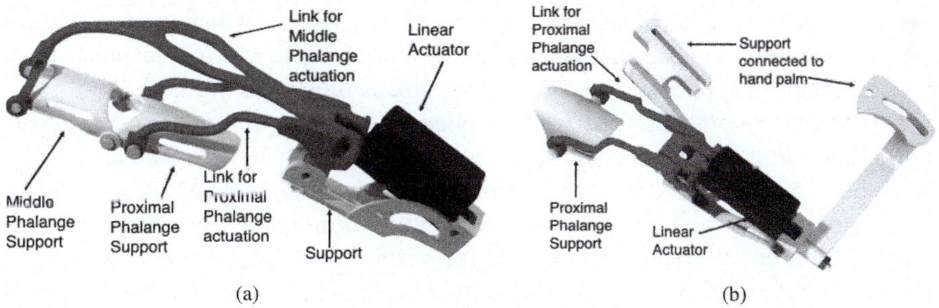

Fig. 2.21 Hand module. **a** CAD model of single finger part. **b** CAD model of thumb part. Reproduced from [67] with permission from IEEE. © IEEE 2022

In exoskeletons, actuators typically contribute the most to the overall weight and bulk of the device. To minimize the inertial loads that may lead to user fatigue, the actuators are positioned on the back of the hand, with motion transmitted to the joints through a mechanical linkage system, as shown in Fig. 2.21a and b.

One linear actuator PQ12-63-6-R from Actuonix has been used for each finger. It moves both the proximal and intermediate phalanges, and it is able to apply bi-directional forces. The main characteristics of this linear actuator are summarized in Table 2.4.

The mechanical transmission system was designed to implement the concept of postural synergies, as outlined in the neuroscientific studies referenced in [52]. Specifically, the positioning and dimensions of the exoskeleton linkages have been tailored to replicate the first postural synergy in each finger while preserving their independence within the hand module. This means that, for each finger, the transmission mechanism is engineered to mimic the coordination between the proximal and intermediate interphalangeal joints seen in the first postural synergy, yet allows for independent control of each finger. This design choice enables the use of a single actuator for each finger, offering flexibility and adaptability due to the independence of finger movements. Automatic synthesis procedures facilitate the accurate determination of linkage dimensions based on the user's hand anthropometric measurements, such as phalange lengths, as detailed in [57]. Moreover, the kinematic structure of the finger actuation system-particularly the mechanism that couples the metacarpophalangeal and proximal interphalangeal joints-has been modified from the version presented in [57] to enhance its lightweight design and adaptability to the user's fingers.

Linear actuators are inherently non-back-drivable, which means that a physiotherapist cannot freely open or close the hand, i.e., flexing or extending the fingers, while the patient is wearing the hand exoskeleton. To address this limitation, the exoskeleton is equipped with a system designed for active tracking and cancellation of the forces exerted on it by the hand or the physiotherapist. The approach involves estimating the force applied to the fingertip when a physiotherapist interacts with the hand, either by opening or closing it. This is achieved by measuring the reaction force on the support that connects the exoskeleton to the back of the hand. To facilitate this, two Force Sensitive Resistors (FSRs) are placed beneath the base of the linear actuator. The forces measured by these FSR sensors are then used to generate a reference position signal that guides the linear actuator to move in response to the physiotherapist's applied forces on the fingertip, as illustrated in Fig. 2.22.

It is worth noticing that the force applied to the fingertip can be estimated by measuring the reaction force and moment at the point where the actuator connects to the back of the hand. This can be validated through a quasistatic analysis of the system comprising the finger and the exoskeleton. Additionally, an estimation of the reaction force can be obtained using two force sensors, as demonstrated in Fig. 2.22. This estimation approach is further supported by the results of a stationary structural analysis conducted using FEM on the CAD model of one of the finger modules, as shown in Fig. 2.23a. In this analysis, external forces of 5 N are applied at the fingertip in opposite directions. Specifically, Fig. 2.23 presents the results in terms of displacement. The aim of this structural analysis was to verify the overall exoskeleton stress/deformation distribution when an external force is applied, but the outcomes of the analyses highlighted how the physiotherapist force is transmitted through the different elements of the exoskeleton and in details how it can be measured with force sensors on the back part of hand palm (Fig. 2.23). This result is exploited to control the linear actuator in both directions, allowing for motion guided by the physiotherapist. For each finger, two small Force Sensitive Resistor (FSR) sensors (Ohmite FSR04, with an active area diameter of 5.60 mm) are strategically positioned at the points

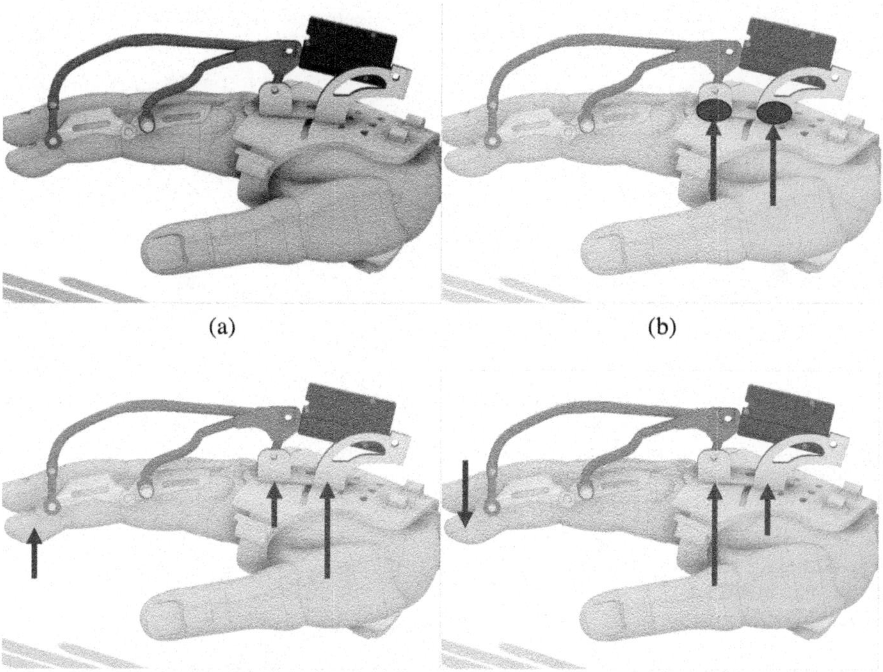

(a) (b) (c) (d)

Fig. 2.22 **a** CAD rendering representing the finger module worn by the user; **b** Red dots indicate where FSR sensors are positioned, when the no external forces are applied by the actuator or externally to the finger, can be assumed that the reaction force between the actuator support and the hand back support, measured by the FSR sensors, are constant and equal; **c** When a force is applied to the fingertip to open the finger (extension), the reaction forces on the support are different, and the one farther from the MPC joint increases; **d** When a force is applied to the fingertip to close the finger (flexion) the reaction force on the support closer to the MPC increases. Reproduced from [67] with permission from IEEE. © IEEE 2022

identified through the FEM analysis, situated between the motor support and the hand shell. These sensors exhibit a decrease in electrical resistance as the force applied to their surface increases. Specifically, the selected sensor is capable of measuring normal forces ranging from 0.2 to 50 N, has a long-term drift of less than 2%, and demonstrates a repeatability of 2% when a force of 10 N is applied. The measurable force range, reliability, and compact size of these sensors make them well-suited for controlling the linear actuator in the backward mode.

A detailed view of the prototype, showcasing the embedded sensors, is presented in Fig. 2.24. For a single finger, it is expected that when no forces are applied to the fingertip, the output from the sensors remains consistent. On the contrary, when pushing or pulling forces are exerted by the physiotherapist on the distal phalanx, the sensors experience varying degrees of compression, allowing for an estimation of the force based on the sensor output. Thus, a PD controller has been implemented

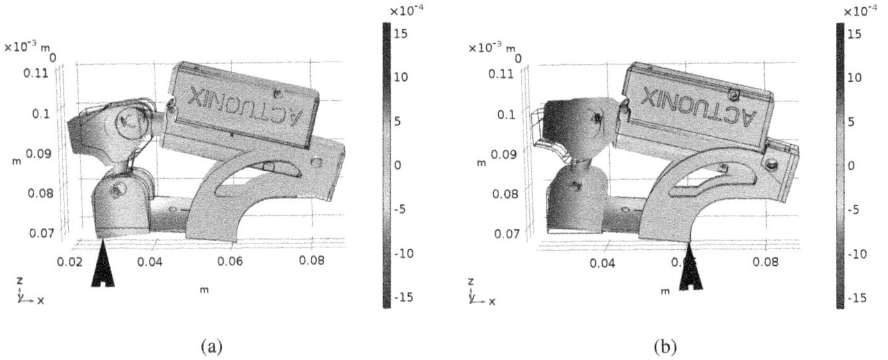

Fig. 2.23 Results of FEM analysis on finger module support to evaluate force distribution generated by physiotherapist pulling and pushing action on the fingertip. **a** Result generated by a pulling force applied on the fingertip of the index finger. **b** Result generated by a pushing force applied on the middle finger pulp. Black arrows represent the placement of pressure sensors. Reproduced from [67] with permission from IEEE. © IEEE 2022

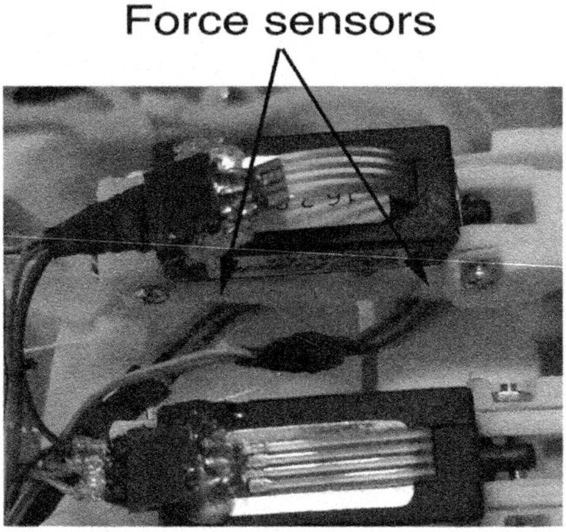

Fig. 2.24 FSR sensors positioning in the index finger module. Reproduced from [67] with permission from IEEE. © IEEE 2022

to maintain the forces detected by the sensors at zero. This allows the fingers to smoothly follow the desired motion in both directions. The position of each joint can be inferred from the actuator stroke, thanks to the kinematic structure of the mechanism. This control strategy, aimed at minimizing discrepancies between the forces measured by the FSR sensors, is designed to be robust against errors caused by device misalignment. Additionally, a calibration procedure is available to address any force offsets induced by unintended sources, ensuring accurate measurements.

As a preliminary experimental test devoted to device kinematic validation, it was evaluated the capability of the proposed fingertip actuation mechanism in following the first synergy trajectory. The kinematic structure of the exoskeleton worn by a user is shown in Fig. 2.25. The linear actuator LA is connected to the hand back support by means of a hinge joint indicated with O, and by means of the link BC.

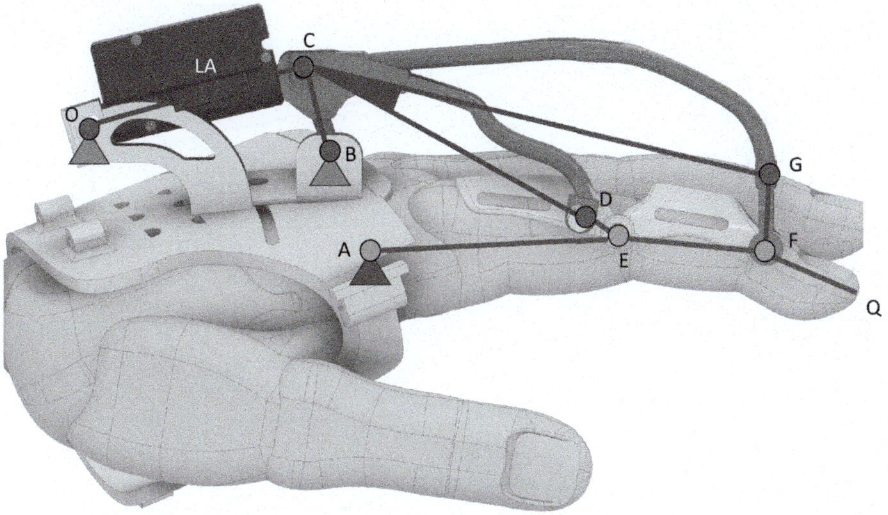

Fig. 2.25 Kinematics model of the finger exoskeleton worn by a user. Reproduced from [67] with permission from IEEE. © IEEE 2022

Through the hinge joint indicated with C, the actuator moves the main element of the exoskeleton (two links rigidly connected). The first one, indicated with CD, is connected to the link fixed on the proximal phalanx, while the second one, indicated with CG, is connected to the link GF and then to the link EF fixed on the middle phalanx. The main difference between this structure and most existing designs in the literature lies in its unique DoFs. When the exoskeleton is not worn on the finger, it exhibits three DoFs, therefore it is underactuated. However, once it is worn on the finger, the biomechanical structure closes the mechanism and reduces the number of DoFs to one. This design eliminates the need for a Remote Center of Motion (RCM) at the MCP joint, leading to a significant simplification of the mechanical structure.

In the synthesis of the finger exoskeleton, an approach similar to the one described in [57] and based on the reproduction of the first postural synergy of the human hand, has been adopted.

Initially, a kinematic simulation was conducted for each finger, as illustrated in Fig. 2.26, which depicts the index finger's response to varying MCP rotation angles ranging from 1° to 45°. Following the theoretical feasibility assessment, I validated the prototype's accuracy using an optical tracking system. Specifically, we utilized a Vicon tracking system comprising ten Bonita cameras and 6.4 mm retro-reflective markers to monitor the motion of the exoskeleton. For comparison, Fig. 2.27 presents a representative trajectory captured by the index finger.

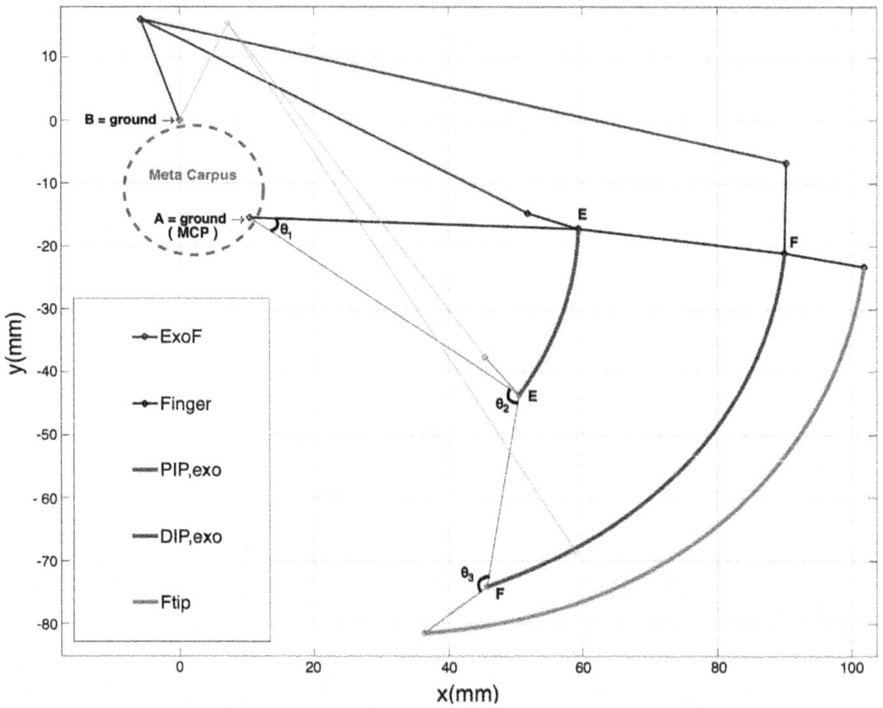

Fig. 2.26 Kinematic simulation of the index finger module for different values of the MCP rotation angles, varying from 1° to 45°. The PIP joint is represented by point E trajectory while the DIP joint is represented point F trajectory. Reproduced from [67] with permission from IEEE. © IEEE 2022

2.4.3 *Device Control*

2.4.3.1 Tracking

A key aspect of controlling the device is the tracking of hand and wrist motions. The chosen solution utilizes multiple IMUs, which are low-cost electronic devices that integrate an accelerometer and a gyroscope on a single board. This approach strikes an optimal balance between estimation accuracy, wearability, and lightweight design. Specifically, we developed data acquisition and processing software capable of translating real-time IMU measurements into biomechanical information, such as the orientation of the hand relative to the forearm. The resulting algorithm is able to: (i) record the user's motion (e.g., wrist exercises suggested and guided by the physiotherapist); (ii) monitor/control exercises played back by the exoskeleton; and (iii) analyze patient's wrist articulation range of motion and consequential improvements. To this end, it is exploited two Xsens Mi-3 (Xsens, NL) embedding an accelerometer, a gyroscope, and a magnetometer in a single chip. For the purpose of this work, it was

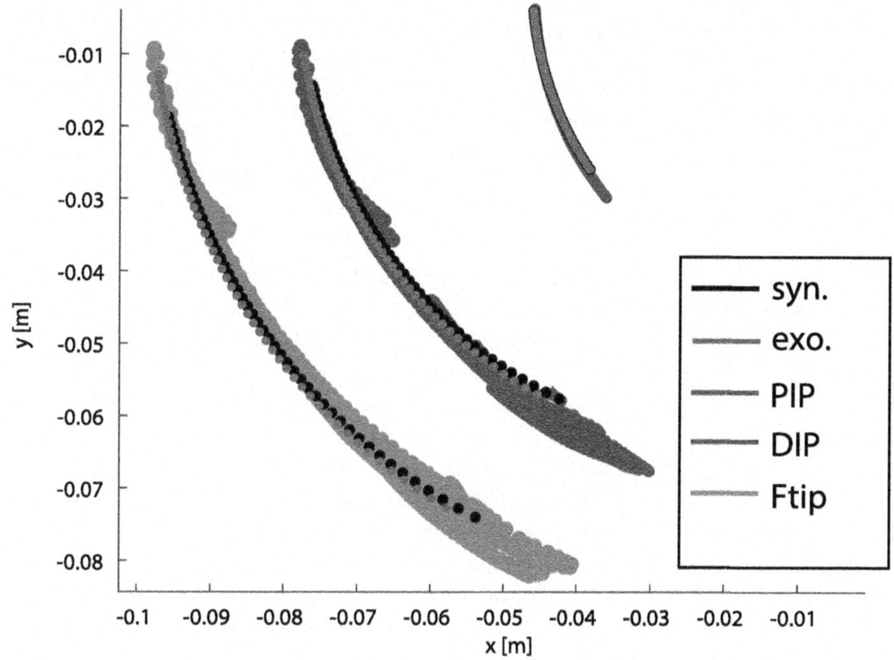

Fig. 2.27 Representative trajectories comparison: in red trajectories of points E (corresponding to the PIP joint position), in blue F (corresponding to the DIP joint position), and in green Q (corresponding to the fingertip position) for different values of MCP angle. Trajectory are acquired using the optical tracking system. Black dots represent the theoretical exoskeleton trajectory, while magenta dots correspond to the first postural synergy [52]. Reproduced from [67] with permission from IEEE. © IEEE 2022

decided not to use readings provided by the magnetometer since the magnetic flux in the surrounding of the exoskeleton is not reliable. The orientation of the hand with respect to the forearm (i.e., the wrist angles) is computed by means of two sensors board. An IMU is placed on the back of the hand exoskeleton structure, whereas a second one is firmly attached to the forearm exoskeleton support (as visible in Fig. 2.17).

To estimate the orientation of each board, it was adapted the algorithm presented in [50]. Raw data from the sensors are collected and processed by the worn micro-controller in charge of all the mathematical computations. The update rate for the system is 1 kHz.

The following sections provide a brief overview of the procedure for calibrating the sensors and outline the tracking algorithm. Each IMU board requires an initial calibration consisting of two steps. In the first step, the user is instructed to keep their hand stable for one second, such as resting it on a flat surface. During this phase, each IMU board collects 500 samples to estimate the gyroscope bias. The second step involves computing the offset quaternion between the hand and the forearm.

In this work, quaternions are employed to estimate the orientation of each IMU sensor, as described in Sect. 2.2.3. Utilizing quaternions helps to mitigate issues associated with Euler angles, such as the gimbal lock problem and complications related to trigonometric functions.

2.4.3.2 Actuators' Control

The complete control scheme for the wrist and hand module is illustrated in Fig. 2.28. Users can select various options through the software GUI, with the data transmitted to the device via Bluetooth. Two RN42 Bluetooth modules facilitate communication between the PC and the device. A Teensy microcontroller oversees the movement of the motors and the autonomous closure mechanism. It also receives data related to wrist exercises and generates a set of commands for the Open CM 9.04 control board to actuate the three XL-320 motors.

In terms of controlling the hand actuation system, finger motion is constrained by the mechanical structure of the exoskeleton. Consequently, the hand configuration is directly related to actuator displacements, following standard forward kinematics relationships. It is worth to observe that for this type of mechanism the forward kinematic procedure depends on the user's specific biometric dimensions (e.g. the lengths of phalanges) and on displacements of finger modules. A calibration procedure included in the GUI solves this issue. Both the hand and wrist actuators utilize position control. Users can select the proportional gain within a predefined range to adjust the device's stiffness. The input for the control scheme is the desired movement, denoted as $\boldsymbol{\theta}_{des}$ which can be assigned by the user via the graphical user interface or recorded by the tracking system. This desired movement is represented as a 7×1 vector, consisting of two rotation angles for the wrist and one rotation angle for each finger.

The values for $\boldsymbol{\theta}_{des}$ can be recorded during exercises when the exoskeleton is not actuated and the physiotherapist manually guides the hand and wrist motions, or they can be retrieved from an exercise database through the user interface. Using inverse kinematic analysis, the desired configurations are converted into reference signals for the actuator control systems, denoted as $\boldsymbol{q}_{des}$. This reference is represented as an 8×1 vector (three motor rotation angles for the wrist module and five linear actuator strokes for the hand).

During exercise execution, actual hand and wrist movements, represented as $\boldsymbol{\theta}$, are monitored by the tracking system and linear actuator encoders. This data is displayed on the GUI and logged for further analysis. In this initial version of the device, position-based control is implemented instead of the more commonly used impedance or admittance control strategies in robotic rehabilitation. Position control was chosen due to its simplicity, making it easier for users to manage through the GUI.

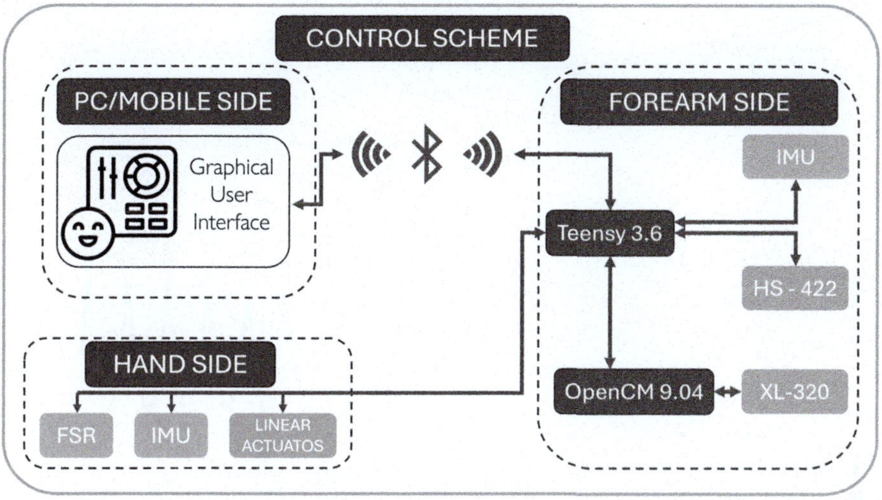

Fig. 2.28 Control scheme for wrist and hand exoskeleton modules

2.4.3.3 Graphical User Interface

Together with the hardware design and prototyping, GUI has been developed to manage the exoskeleton and fully exploiting its features. The main goal of the GUI is to provide users with a straightforward and intuitive method for controlling the device, which was achieved by incorporating feedback and requirements from the target users during its development.

The interface is organized into various sections (or pages): an initial overview page that presents the overall system, followed by several more specific pages dedicated to the individual functions of the exoskeleton. Each page includes navigation buttons, allowing users to switch between sections effortlessly. Additionally, every page is equipped with tools to control the different functions of the exoskeleton. A set of *default* parameters, chosen on the basis of user's feedback, has been defined for each function of the exoskeleton. If the parameters are not properly selected, the exoskeleton will not initiate any actions. For instance, when a user attempts to activate an exercise in automatic mode with the wrist exoskeleton, it will remain inactive until all parameters, such as speed, duration, and mode, are correctly set.

Additionally, the GUI facilitates the storage and replay of hand and wrist motions for training and rehabilitation purposes in real time. This stored data can be utilized to monitor the effectiveness of the rehabilitation process. A cross-platform Python-based application connects to the exoskeleton system via Bluetooth and presents users with options to record and replay wrist and finger movements. A screenshot of the GUI is shown in Fig. 2.29.

The user interface is organized into three main pages that assist users in selecting their desired features:

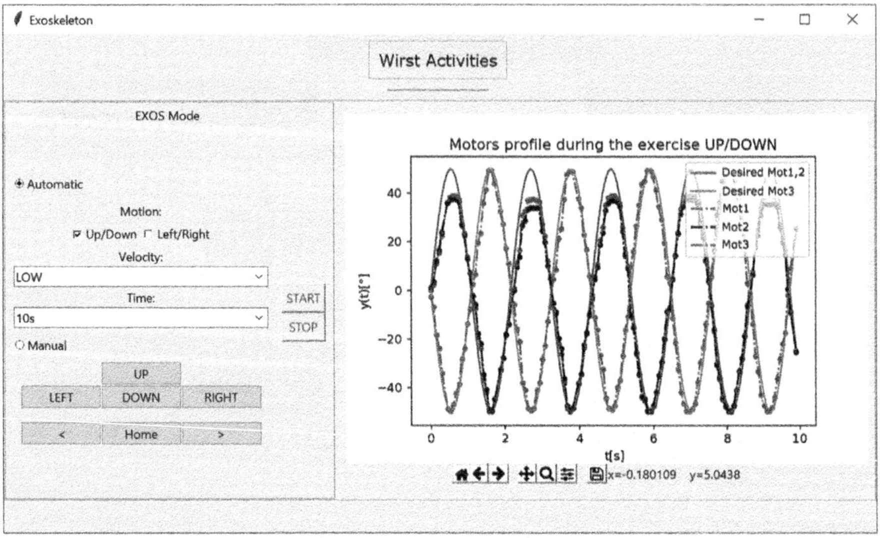

Fig. 2.29 Graphical user interface display during an automatic exercise layout for wrist flexion/extension

Activities for Hand: The aim of this page is to control the hand-exoskeleton. Two modes are available: *Learning Mode* and *Reproduce Mode*. *Learning Mode* is further divided into *Motion Mode* and *Grasp Mode*. The former allows to control and move one finger at a time (selectable via five checkboxes). The *Grasp* option lets the user to control all the fingers by moving only the index finger and exploiting the first postural synergy. Both modalities can be recorded and played back on demand in the *Reproduce Mode*.

Activities for Wrist: Here the user is allowed to select two modes of use: *automatic* or *manual*. The *manual* modality enables 4 buttons for controlling the motion of the wrist: DOWN for flexion, UP for extension, LEFT for ulnar adduction and RIGHT radial abduction. Conversely, the *automatic* mode allows the user to perform some typical exercises for the wrist, such as abduction/adduction and flexion/extension movements. Paradigmatic exercises are already available in the interface. For each exercise the user can select a running time and three different speeds (high, medium, and low). Moreover, the GUI allows also to set manually a specific time span and a certain speed value for the exercise.

Learning Mode for Wrist: The aim of this page is to let the exoskeleton learn exercises, performed for example by a physiotherapist, and then play back them. During the *Learning* phase, wrist exoskeleton motors are disabled. In this way, the physiotherapist can freely move the wrist while the exoskeleton tracking system records these movements. Regarding wrist exercises IMU data are acquired and elaborated with frequency 200 Hz and the saved in a file by GUI software. In *Reproduce* mode, a profile previously recorded and saved is loaded from the archive and played back.

The Learning/Reproduce modes are available also for hand module, and also in this case in *Learning* mode the system acquire samples at 200 Hz. In fingers Learning mode the linear actuators are moved using the FSR-based control detailed before.

It is important to note that the wrist and hand modules are managed differently. Specifically, the *Activities for Hand module* does not include an Automatic Mode. Given the complexity of the hand structure and the distinct actuation methods employed, the design team, in consultation with the user and their physiotherapist, determined that the ability to execute exercises with a pre-recorded profile was unnecessary.

The GUI homepage provides several general functions, including options to connect or disconnect from the exoskeleton's Bluetooth, navigate through all available pages, and control the closure mechanism. In particular, users can activate or deactivate the closure mechanism through the homepage using two dedicated buttons. Furthermore, through this page the user or the physiotherapist can reset the initial position of the exoskeleton, and set/deactivate the initial position of all actuators, including the motors used to control the closure mechanism. A flowchart reporting all the GUI components is reported in Fig. 2.30.

Both hardware and software development considered patient's safety in the event of exoskeleton malfunctions or any physical issues experienced by the user. The exoskeleton can be deactivated at any time by pressing a button on the Teensy board, which immediately disables all motors and removes torque from each one. This command can also be executed via software using the Stop button, which is available

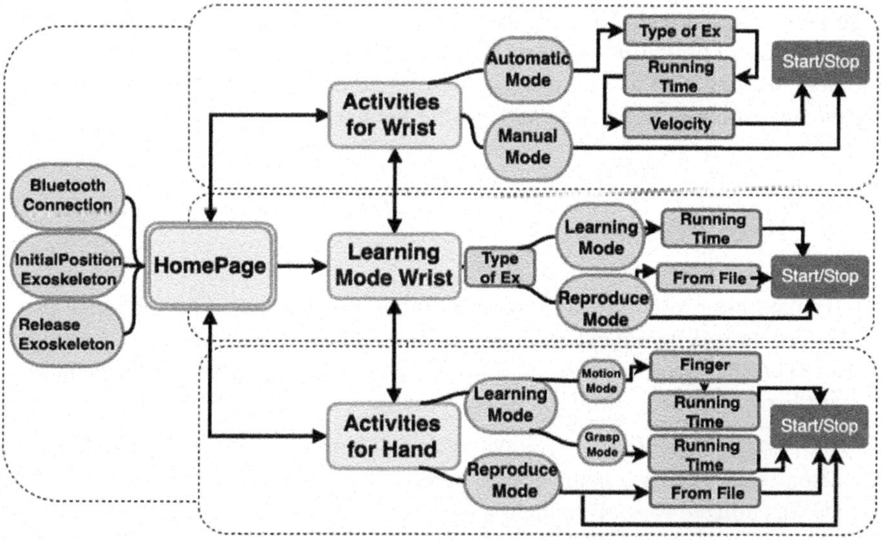

Fig. 2.30 Graphical user interface flow chart for Wrist and hand exercises. Light yellow blocks represent GUI pages, orange blocks are the operations inside the page and light blue blocks shows editable and selectable options

on all GUI pages. Additionally, the motor controlling the closing mechanism is disabled as soon as the mechanism is opened. In the case of motor failures, torque is instantly disengaged, allowing for manual opening of the mechanism.

2.4.4 Tests and Evaluation

The exoskeleton modules were tailored to the specific characteristics and needs of the user, thus during the testing and evaluation phase, a single patient was involved in accordance with the Single-Case-Design (SCD) methodology. This approach is commonly used in clinical settings, where an individual serves as the sole unit of data analysis, providing rigorous experimental evidence [70].

The tests aimed to assess the device's performance regarding accuracy in executing specific exercises. Various exercises, recommended by the physiotherapist and involving both the hand and wrist, were evaluated.

The subject gave his written informed consent to participate and was able to discontinue participation at any time during experiments. The experimental evaluation protocols followed the declaration of Helsinki, and there was no risk of harmful effects on subject' health. Data were recorded in conformity with the European General Data Protection Regulation 2016/679, stored locally, and used only for the post processing evaluation procedure. Please note that no sensible data were recorded.

A stepwise validation process was implemented. The initial phase focused on wrist tracking and actuation, followed by an assessment of finger functionality. Finally, both the wrist and hand were evaluated together. The system was tested on a subject with severe limitations in wrist extension motion (flexion movements were less problematic), as well as restrictions in radial adduction and ulnar abduction, and significant difficulty in opening and closing the hand.

2.4.5 Wrist Evaluation

To evaluate the proposed exoskeleton in wrist-based exercise performance it was conducted three different experiments. In all the experiments, precision in following a desired profile was considered as a metric and measured by means of the Root Mean Square Error (RMSE). Similarly to [71], for each trial it is defined this quantity as $RMSE_t = \sqrt{\frac{1}{N}\sum_{i=1}^{N}(y_{t,i} - y_i)^2}$, where N is the number of samples in a trial, y_i is the actual value, and $y_{t,i}$ is the corresponding target value. The mean of the RMSE values was utilized to analyze the tracking performance throughout the experiment. Notably, the tracking RMSE is an effective metric for assessing both the speed and accuracy of the robot's movements. This is because the RMSE increases not only when the exoskeleton is slow to update the control variables but also when it fails to reach the target values.

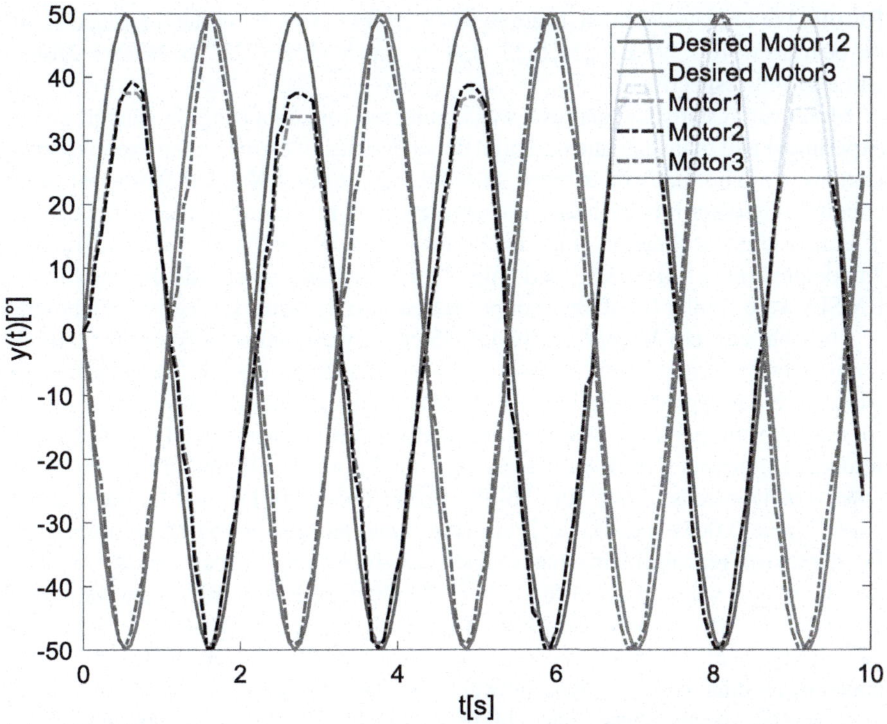

Fig. 2.31 Wrist test 1: automatic wrist flexion and extension. Reference and actual motor rotations during one of the trials. Reproduced from [67] with permission from IEEE. © IEEE 2022

Wrist test 1: flexion/extension A set of tests was conducted to assess the system's accuracy in following a specific desired motion. To cover the full range of motion of the patient's wrist, a predefined set of movements was generated. Three different motion speeds were evaluated. As described in Sect. 2.4.2, wrist flexion and extension are achieved by applying the same profile to actuators *Motor1* and *Motor2*, while the opposite profile is applied to actuator *Motor3*. To simulate a realistic flexion/extension exercise typically performed by a physiotherapist, the following reference values were established for the actuators:

$$\varphi_{1,des} = \varphi_{2,des} = \alpha \sin(\omega t), \ \ \varphi_{3,des} = -\alpha \sin(\omega t)$$

with $\alpha = 50°$, $\omega = 3.0, 4.0$ or $5.0\,\text{rad}\,\text{s}^{-1}$ and $0 < t < 10\text{s}$. The three values of ω represent "low", "moderate", and "high" speed of wrist flexion/extension, respectively. The internal encoder of the motors was used to record the actual angular value. Twenty trials for each speed were repeated, each one lasted 10 s. Desired and measured values of rotation angles of a representative trial are reported in Fig. 2.31, the figure shows how the actuators are able to follow the profile for the entire duration of the exercise.

Results We observed that the average RMS errors in following the reference among the 60 trials were $5.39° \pm 0.25°$, $5.25° \pm 0.24°$ and $5.55° \pm 0.25°$ for *Motor1*, *Motor2*, and *Motor3*, respectively.

Moreover, a statistical analysis was conducted for supporting the outcome of the experiment and to investigate potential dependencies of errors on the exercise speed. Data were not normally distributed, thus for each motor, a Kruskal-Wallis H test was conducted to determine if there were differences in root mean square errors between actuating the exoskeleton with different values of ω: "low" ($\omega = 3.0\,\mathrm{rad\,s^{-1}}$), "moderate" ($\omega = 4.0\,\mathrm{rad\,s^{-1}}$) and "high" ($\omega = 5.0\,\mathrm{rad\,s^{-1}}$) speeds. Distributions of RMSEs were similar for all the groups, as assessed by visual inspection of a boxplot.

For what concern *Motor1*, median RMS errors were statistically significantly different between groups, $\chi^2(2) = 47.79$, $p < 0.001$. Subsequently, pairwise comparisons were performed using Dunn's (1964) procedure with a Bonferroni correction for multiple comparisons. This post hoc analysis revealed statistically significant differences in median RMSE values between the "low" (3.69) and "moderate" (4.97) ($p = 0.004$) speeds, "low" and "high" (6.32) ($p < 0.001$), and "moderate" and "high" ($p = 0.001$) speeds. Such test was exploited also in the next comparisons. For the sake of readability in what follows it is referred only as 'pairwise comparison'. Similar results were obtained for *Motor2*. Medians of RMS errors were statistically significantly different between different values of ω, $\chi^2(2) = 46.81$, $p < 0.001$. The subsequent pairwise comparison analysis revealed statistically significant differences in median RMSE values between the "low" (3.67) and "moderate" (4.68) ($p = 0.005$) speeds, "low" and "high" (6.11) ($p < 0.001$), and "moderate" and "high" ($p = 0.001$) speeds. As expected, also *Motor3* follows the same behaviour of *Motor1* and *Motor2*. RMSE medians were statistically significantly different considering the three speeds, $\chi^2(2) = 48.04$, $p < 0.001$. Also in this case, pairwise comparisons were performed using. The post hoc test revealed statistically significant differences in median RMSE values between the "low" (3.86) and "moderate" (5.14) ($p = 0.004$) speeds, low and "high" (6.48) ($p < 0.001$), and "moderate" and "high" ($p = 0.001$) speeds.

2.4.5.1 Wrist Test 2: Adduction/Abduction

Then the simulation of ulnar adduction and radial abduction was conducted. To achieve this movement, *Motor3* was kept stationary while *Motor1* and *Motor2* pulled their tendons in opposing directions, as detailed in Sect. 2.4.2. The desired and measured rotation angles for a representative trial are illustrated in Fig. 2.32. As in the previous experiment, with the aim at evaluating the exoskeleton in the whole range of motion of the wrist, the following reference profiles were used as motors control input:

$$\varphi = \alpha \sin(\omega t), \; \alpha = \begin{cases} 30° \text{ if } \sin(\omega t) > 0 \\ 20° \text{ if } \sin(\omega t) < 0 \end{cases}$$

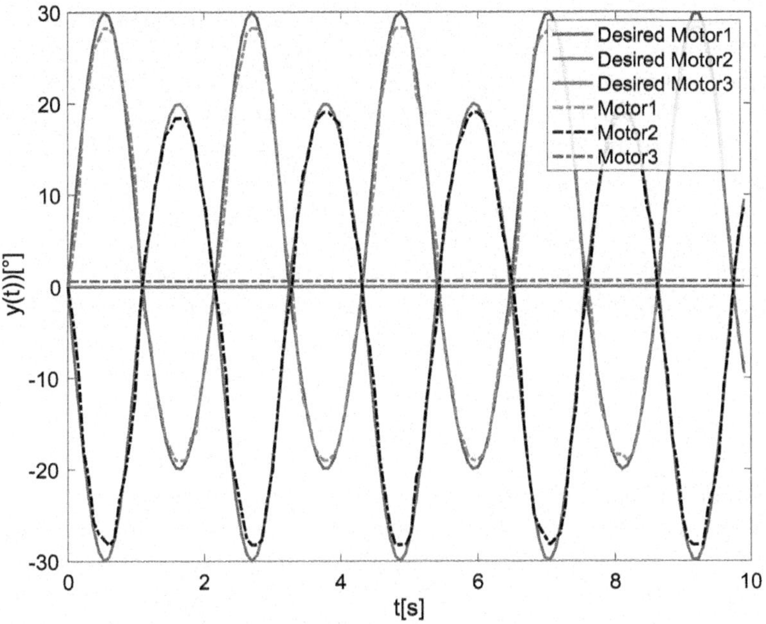

Fig. 2.32 Wrist test 2: ulnar adduction and radial abduction. Reference and actual motor rotations during one of the trials. Reproduced from [67] with permission from IEEE. © IEEE 2022

$$\varphi_{1,des} = \varphi, \ \varphi_{2,des} = -\varphi, \ \varphi_{3,des} = 0$$

$\omega = 3.0, 4.0$ or $5.0\,\text{rad}\,\text{s}^{-1}$ and $0 < t < 10\text{s}$. Twenty consecutive trials were repeated for each value of ω, for a total of 60 repetitions. Desired rotation angle and real motor value were recorded and analysed.

Results We observed that the average RMS errors among all the trials in tracking the requested profile were $4.06° \pm 0.14°$, $3.64° \pm 0.15°$ and $0.17° \pm 0.12°$ for *Motor1*, *Motor2*, and *Motor3*, respectively.

The same statistical analysis conducted in the previous experiment was repeated to analyse also results concerning adduction/abduction movements. Data of *Motor3* were excluded from the analysis since the motor was maintained stable and the recorded errors are due only to measurement noise. The mean among all the trials is $0.17°$ with a standard deviation less of $0.12°$, this means that the motor remained stable for all the trials, the recorded error is due to the mechanical resolution of the encoder. Data of *Motor1* and *Motor2* were not normally distributed, thus a Kruskal-Wallis H test was conducted to determine if there were differences in root mean square errors between moving the motor with different values of ω, i.e. , "low" ($\omega = 3.0\,\text{rad}\,\text{s}^{-1}$), "moderate" ($\omega = 4.0\,\text{rad}\,\text{s}^{-1}$) and "high" ($\omega = 5.0\,\text{rad}\,\text{s}^{-1}$) speeds. Distributions of RMSEs were similar for all the groups, as assessed by visual inspection of a boxplot.

Regarding *Motor1*, median RMS errors were statistically significantly different between groups, $\chi^2(2) = 49.72$, $p < 0.001$. Multiple pairwise comparisons were performed and revealed statistically significant differences in median RMSE values between the low (3.00) and moderate (4.03) ($p < 0.001$) speeds, low and high (5.04) ($p < 0.001$), and moderate and high ($p = 0.003$) speeds. Comparable results were obtained analysing results of *Motor2*. Medians of RMS errors were statistically significantly different between different the three values of ω, $\chi^2(2) = 50.37$, $p < 0.001$. Following pairwise comparisons revealed statistically significant differences in median RMSE values between the low (2.43) and moderate (3.63) ($p = 0.001$) speeds, low and high (4.73) ($p = 0.002$), and moderate and high ($p < 0.001$) speeds.

2.4.5.2 Wrist Test 3: Record/Playback

An additional test was conducted to verify the system ability to record an exercise performed by a physiotherapist and subsequently reproduce it with the exoskeleton. In this test, a physiotherapist worked with the previously mentioned patient, who had severe limitations in wrist mobility. The physiotherapist gently moved the patient's hand for ten seconds while the system recorded the hand's orientation relative to the forearm (i.e. , the wrist angles). This included ten adduction/abduction and ten flexion/extension exercises.

A representative trial from this test is depicted in Fig. 2.33, demonstrating the system's capability to record hand motion in relation to the forearm via the tracking system and to playback those motions using the exoskeleton. Ten consecutive trials were performed using the same profile recorded by the physiotherapist, and for each repetition, the actual values of the motor rotation angles were documented.

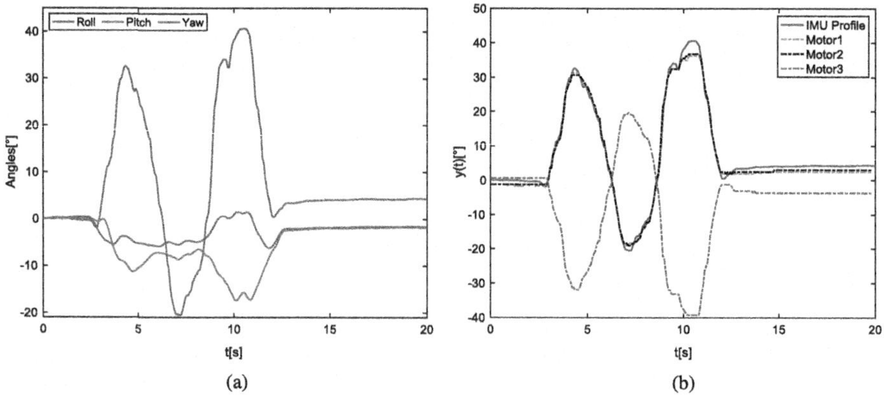

Fig. 2.33 Wrist test 3: record/playback. **a** Roll, pitch, yaw angles measured by the tracking system. **b** Learning Mode: Flexion and extension angles as recorded by the physiotherapist and corresponding motor rotations. Reproduced from [67] with permission from IEEE. © IEEE 2022

Results The average RMS errors in tracking the trajectory previously recorded by the physiotherapist were $3.15° \pm 0.54°$ for *Motor1*, $3.51° \pm 0.62°$ for *Motor2*, and $2.59° \pm 0.76°$ for *Motor3*.

2.4.6 Hand Evaluation

As second stage, performance of the hand part of the exoskeleton has been considered.

2.4.6.1 Hand Test 1: Single Finger

We started evaluating the hand module by assessing the exoskeleton's capability to follow therapeutic exercises using four fingers. The first experiment involved an individual finger exercise performed by the physiotherapist. During this exercise, the physiotherapist moved a finger (i.e., index, middle, ring, or little finger) by either pulling it downward or pushing it upward. The force-sensitive resistors (FSR) installed beneath the base of the finger (as shown in Figs. 2.23 and 2.24) detected these movements, prompting the linear actuator to respond accordingly.

To accurately recognize genuine finger movements and minimize issues related to misalignment or improper positioning of the finger module on the hand, two threshold values were established. These thresholds represented a balance between responsiveness and reliability in identifying finger motion. A threshold window that is too wide (i.e., the distance between the upper and lower thresholds) would require the physiotherapist applying relatively high forces to move the exoskeleton, potentially resulting in forced finger motion. Conversely, a threshold window that is too narrow could be overly sensitive to noise and sensor errors.

The optimal threshold values for the sensors depend on several factors, including sensor characteristics, assembly accuracy, and the user's specific attributes. To address this, a calibration procedure is incorporated into the graphical user interface (GUI), allowing users to assess and modify the threshold values at the beginning of each exercise or whenever necessary. In the experiments described in this study, conducted with a single user during the same exercise session, the lower threshold (measured in FSR output voltage) was set to 1 V, while the upper threshold was established at 1.9 V. Finger movements were recorded, and upon completion of the exercise, all data were saved for future analysis or for repeating the exercise. Figure Fig. 2.34a illustrates the data acquired during the recording phase, where the orange curve represents the FSR readings as the physiotherapist pushes and pulls the fingertip, while the blue curve indicates the position of the actuator. The trial began with the finger in a starting position, almost straight but relaxed, resulting in both FSRs recording a force within the designated threshold limits. When the physiotherapist pressed the fingertip upward, the FSR located beneath the back end of the finger base detected a force that triggered the linear actuator to move backward, causing the finger to lift, as shown by the initial downward slope of the blue line. Conversely,

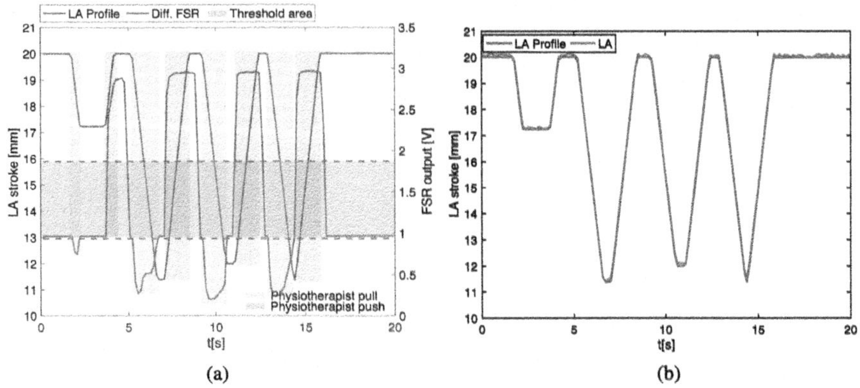

Fig. 2.34 Hand test 1: single finger exercise guided by a physiotherapist. **a** Recording phase: the differential FSR sensors measure (red line), threshold values for generating linear actuator reference (orange area), and corresponding linear actuator reference (blue line). **b** Reference (blue line) and real actuator displacement (red line). Reproduced from [67] with permission from IEEE. © IEEE 2022 (color figure online)

when the physiotherapist pressed the fingertip downward, the FSR under the front end of the finger base registered the force, prompting the linear actuator to move forward, which resulted in the finger moving downward, evident in the upward slope of the blue line. The physiotherapist could halt the upward or downward pressure at any point, allowing for varied motions. Figure 2.34b displays the profile recorded by the physiotherapist during the up-and-down movement of the finger by pushing or pulling the fingertip. The blue curve represents the recorded data, while the red plot illustrates the trajectory followed by the linear actuator, demonstrating that the actuator accurately followed the recorded trajectory.

Results To assess the accuracy and fidelity of the system in replicating the physiotherapist's movements, we compared the desired positions of the linear actuators (as recorded during the initial phase) with the positions achieved during the playback phase. For this quantitative evaluation, we focused on three of the five linear actuators used in the exoskeleton to maintain conciseness, as their behaviors were comparable. A total of forty trials of recording and playback were conducted for each of the selected motors. The resulting average RMS error was 0.34 ± 0.07 mm for LA1. Similarly for LA2 and LA3 the RMSE was 0.50 ± 0.04 mm and 0.38 ± 0.05 mm, respectively.

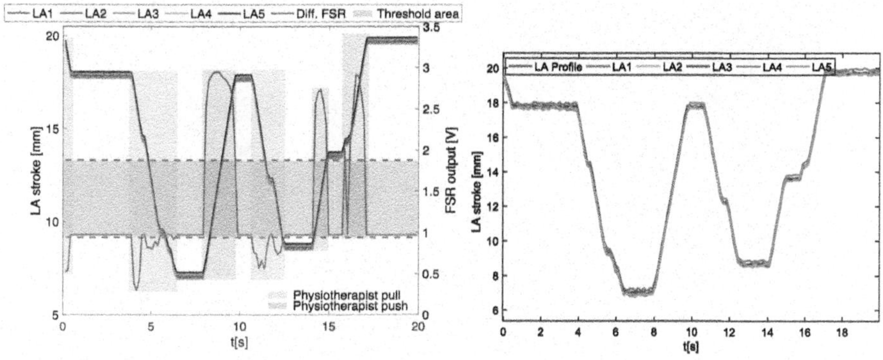

(a) (b)

Fig. 2.35 Hand test 2: synergy based actuation of all the fingers, guided by a physiotherapist. In **a** the differential FSR sensors measure (red line), threshold values for generating linear actuator reference (orange area), and corresponding linear actuator reference for all the fingers. **b** Reference (blue) and real actuator displacements for all the fingers. Reproduced from [67] with permission from IEEE. © IEEE 2022 (color figure online)

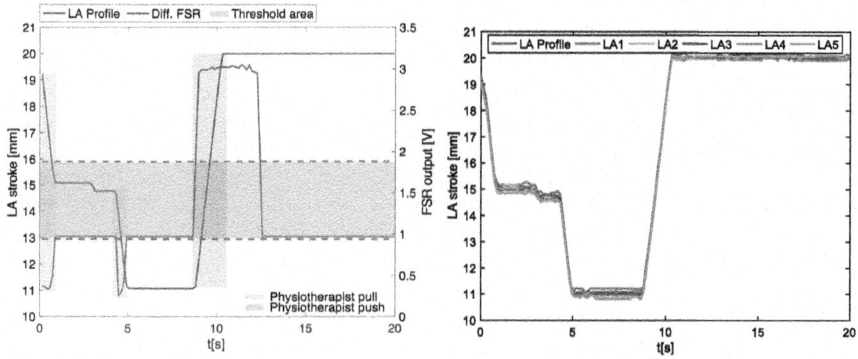

(a) (b)

Fig. 2.36 Hand test 3: grasp exercise perfomed by physiotherapist. **a** Recording phase: the differential FSR sensors measure (red line), threshold values for generating linear actuator reference (orange area), and corresponding linear actuator reference (blue line). **b** Grasp exercise reproduced without physiotherapist: reference (blue line) and real displacements of the linear actuators. Reproduced from [67] with permission from IEEE. © IEEE 2022 (color figure online)

2.4.6.2 Hand Test 2: Synergy Based Hand Motion

In this experiment, the physiotherapist guided the finger as in the previous single-finger motion exercise, but this time the actuation involved the entire hand, including all fingers and the thumb, moving in accordance with the first postural synergy. The data collected during this session were saved for later use in standalone exercises. As illustrated in Fig. 2.35a, the plot demonstrates that whenever the physiotherapist

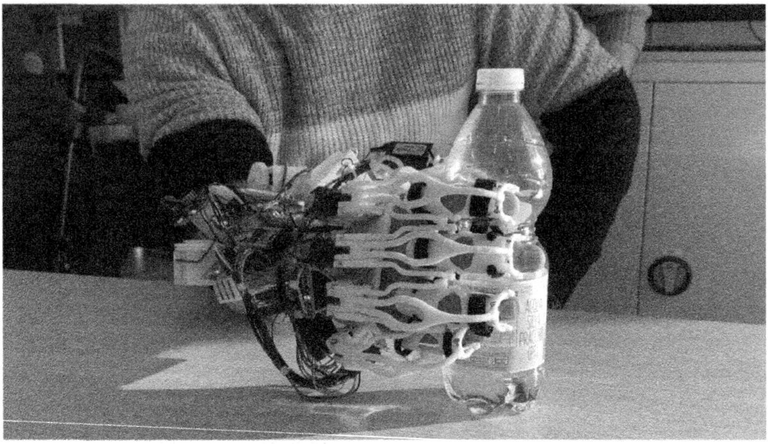

Fig. 2.37 Grasp exercise autonomously reproduced by the patient without physiotherapist

applied a downward or upward force on the finger, the FSR sensors detected this force and activated all the linear actuators accordingly, causing the fingers to move down or up, respectively. The orange line in the plot (Fig. 2.35a) represents the FSR readings, while the other five lines depict the movements of each finger. Additionally, Fig. 2.35b presents the stroke profile followed by the linear actuators, as recorded during the physiotherapist's guidance.

Results Following the approach of Hand test 1, 40 trials were recorded and analysed also in this experiment. Root Mean Square Error in following the desired position was 0.42 ± 0.12 mm, 0.54 ± 0.13 mm, and 0.53 ± 0.11 mm for LA1, LA2, and LA3, respectively.

2.4.6.3 Hand Test 3: Grasping Task

This experiment simulated a real-life scenario in which a physiotherapist assisted the patient in grasping an object, such as a bottle. The physiotherapist began by moving a single finger using the previously described method and then positioned it at the desired location. During this experiment, the physiotherapist had the option to either move each finger individually to facilitate grasping or utilize the first postural synergy, i.e., manipulating one finger to control the entire hand. As with previous exercises, all data from this session were recorded for reproduction in future therapy sessions. Figure 2.36a shows the FSR measures when physiotherapist formed a stable grasp and blue line shows the resulting linear actuator position. Similarly, Fig. 2.36b reports the comparison between the desired trajectory and the one followed by all the linear actuators to play back the physiotherapist movement. Finally, Fig. 2.37 shows the action of grasping a bottle with the exoskeleton using the physiotherapist recordings. It is worth noticing that the patient without the exoskeleton would not have been able to grasp the object due to the hand muscles limitations.

Results Analysis of the RMSE of the motors was conducted also at the end of '*Hand Test 3*' experiment. LA1 reported an RMS error of 0.31 ± 0.03 mm, LA2 0.36 ± 0.03 mm, whereas LA3 0.35 ± 0.02 mm.

In conclusion, for all the conducted hand tests the RMS error of the motors is comparable with the error given by the resolution of the feedback potentiometer and the mechanical properties of the hardware (see Table 2.4). These results support the hardware choice and the mechanical design of the exoskeleton that is able to reproduce the desired motion with high precision and accuracy.

It's worth to notice that while the errors measured in the linear actuators are minimal, these errors pertain solely to the actuators and do not consider the overall deformation of the transmission system. A comprehensive evaluation of the actual displacement errors in the hand module and their relationship with the structural properties of the mechanical transmission would necessitate extensive analysis and experimental work. Furthermore, the results would vary based on individual user characteristics, such as residual muscle capabilities or the presence of spasticity. This area will be a primary focus of future research.

2.4.7 Summary of User's Evaluation

The exoskeleton is designed for comfort, minimizing strain on the user thanks to its lightweight construction (approximately 500 g), optimal inertia distribution, and the use of soft materials in certain areas. For example, the rings connecting the finger module components to the phalanges are made from TPU. The system operates for about three hours on battery power, a duration deemed sufficient for training sessions. If extended rehabilitation time is necessary, the device can be connected to a power source via USB.

Compared to the preliminary version presented in [48], the new iteration of the exoskeleton features significantly improved wearability, largely due to the automatic closure system. To validate this improvement, I sought feedback from a potential user with reduced mobility regarding the time required to don the exoskeleton. In a preliminary qualitative assessment, it was found that the user spends less than half the time putting on the new model compared to the earlier version discussed in Sect. 2.2. This reduction in time is primarily attributed to the automatic closure system.

The device can now be worn autonomously by users with little to no mobility impairment. While those with limited arm mobility may still require some external assistance, the process has been significantly simplified and shortened.

The user provided positive feedback on the training process, noting increased freedom of movement in the hand and wrist following sessions, indicating that the device is an effective tool for rehabilitation. He appreciated the user-friendly GUI, which facilitates exercise control, and valued the wireless capability afforded by the batteries and Bluetooth connection. The availability of a range of pre-recorded exercises was also highlighted as a beneficial feature, enabling independent use of the device without external assistance. Additionally, he found it helpful to visualize exercises through diagrams on the GUI.

However, the user also identified areas for improvement. Despite the advantages of the automatic closure system, achieving complete autonomy in wearing the device remains challenging for individuals with reduced mobility. There is a need to further minimize the overall bulkiness by optimizing the size of the mechanical and electronic components. Lastly, he suggested streamlining the assembly and disassembly procedures for the modules, making it manageable with one hand.

2.5 Differential Mechanism

In this section it is presented the design and characterization of a modular hand finger exoskeleton, in which the number of actuators has been reduced by exploiting a gear-based miniaturized differential mechanism, in order to limit the weight, complexity and costs. One of the advantages of this kind of mechanism is that it is contained in a small box, while other solutions, such as tendon-based mechanisms, need a larger structure that could be uncomfortable for the user [64]. The developed hand exoskeleton is shown in Fig. 2.38. It is able to both flex and extend two adjacent fingers in an independent way, with an actuator only. If one of the coupled fingers finds an obstacle in its movement, the other one can still continue its motion. The second contribution presented in this part of the thesis is an improvement of the mechanical transmission between the actuators and the phalanges, with respect to the hand exoskeleton previously developed and summarized in Sect. 2.3, that is a part of a wider modular system that also includes the wrist. The device has been designed to be adopted in rehabilitation and tele-rehabilitation applications and to be used by the patient both in collaboration with the therapist or autonomously.

2.5.1 Design Requirements

The design of the exoskeleton started from analysis of the human hand structure and finger kinematics.

For simplicity, this discussion employs a streamlined kinematic model of the hand. In this model, the carpus is treated as a single rigid body, while each finger is represented as a planar kinematic chain consisting of two revolute joints located at the proximal interphalangeal (PIP) and distal interphalangeal (DIP) joints, with two degrees of freedom at the metacarpophalangeal (MCP) joint, as detailed in Sect. 2.3. The thumb exhibits a distinct kinematic structure: a comprehensive model would account for two degrees of freedom (DoFs) at the trapeziometacarpal (TM) joint, two at the MCP joint, and one at the interphalangeal (IP) joint. However, due to the limited range of motion for abduction-adduction movements of the thumb, this model can be simplified to a structure with four degrees of freedom. As a result, the

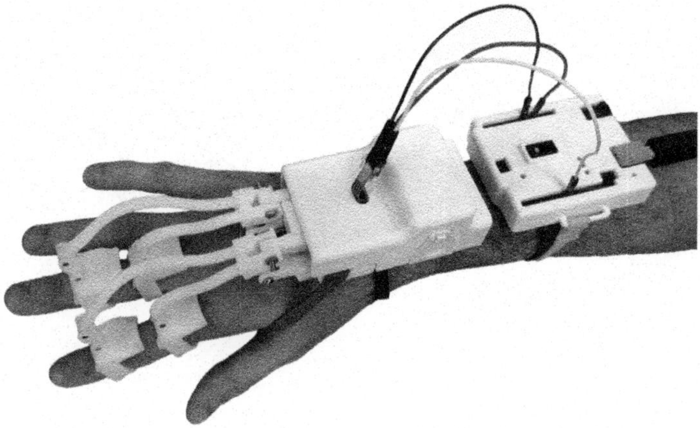

Fig. 2.38 Prototype of the exoskeleton worn by the user. Copyright © 2022 Dragusanu, Troisi, Villani, Prattichizzo and Malvezzi [72]. This is an distributed under the terms of the Creative Commons Attribution License (CC BY)

reference hand model comprises a total of 20-DoFs [54, 58]. Figure 2.39 illustrates the Syngrasp model in its simplified graphical representation, displaying the hand in its reference open configuration as well as activated in the first postural synergy for the flexion motions of the index and middle fingers.

However, various studies in the literature indicate that the intricate kinematics of the human hand can be simplified by considering joint coordination. For example, Cobos et al. in [73] demonstrated that the motion of the distal interphalangeal joint of each finger corresponds to a fixed fraction of the motion at the proximal interphalangeal joint. As detailed in Sect. 2.3, the research on exoskeleton hand design in this study is grounded in the concept of postural synergies, which allows for a reduction in the number of actuators. Specifically, each module of the exoskeleton corresponds to the third solution discussed in Sect. 2.3.2. Furthermore, the kinematic structure of the thumb is notably different from that of the other fingers and has not been incorporated into this solution. Additionally, the developed device is designed to assist users primarily in flexion and extension movements of the fingers, while adduction and abduction motions are not actively actuated.

2.5.1.1 Independent and Coupled Actuation of Fingers

A variety of actuating methods, both active and passive, have been developed and implemented for hand exoskeletons. Among the active actuation methods, electric motors, such as DC motors, brushless DC (BLDC) motors, servo motors, and linear actuators, are the most widely used for controlling hand exoskeletons [30].

Linear actuators, in particular, are favored in some applications because they can generate bi-directional forces, enabling them to push or pull the mechanical linkage

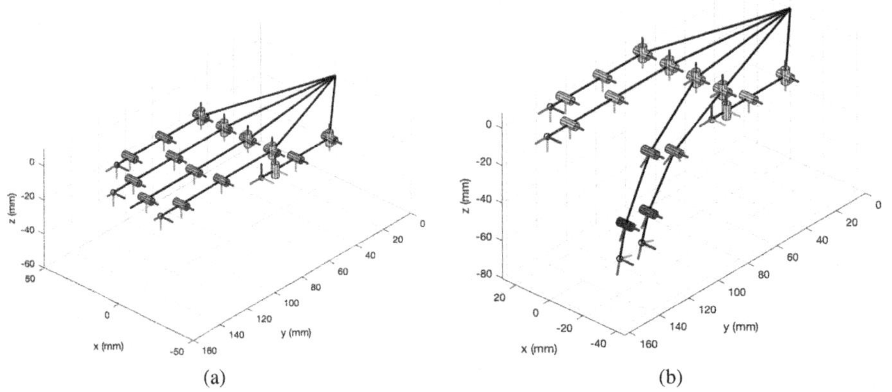

Fig. 2.39 Schematic representation of the human hand 20-DoF model implemented in SynGrasp. **a** The hand in the reference open position. **b** Actuation of the first synergy for the index and middle flexion/extension motions. Copyright © 2022 Dragusanu, Troisi, Villani, Prattichizzo and Malvezzi [72]. This is an distributed under the terms of the Creative Commons Attribution License (CC BY)

system to flex or extend the fingers. Their compact size allows for the installation of one actuator per finger, offering multiple advantages such as the ability to achieve independent finger movements and precise control over finger actions.

However, linear actuators have a finite stroke, which limits the Range Of Motion (ROM) of the fingers. The stroke length of the actuator is inherently linked to the finger's ROM through the kinematics of the exoskeleton [74]. Therefore, both the linear actuator and the dimensions of the linkages in the articulated transmission system must be designed to allow the user to fully flex and extend each finger, a requirement that can result in a bulky and cumbersome solution.

In this context, the miniaturized differential mechanism proposed in this work enables the actuation of two adjacent fingers simultaneously, thereby reducing the number of actuators needed. This not only lessens the weight and complexity of the system but also enhances its wearability. Importantly, the differential mechanism does not rigidly connect the fingers; rather, it keeps them independent. If one branch of the differential mechanism becomes blocked, the other can still move. Notably, when one finger is constrained, the range of motion for the other finger is effectively doubled.

By employing the same mechanical linkage system used for flexing and extending the fingers, the differential mechanism allows for an increased finger ROM compared to what can be achieved without it, where the range is limited by the actuator's stroke.

Differential mechanisms are commonly used in robotics, especially in robotic hands and fingers [75]. For example, planetary gear solutions have been explored in various studies [76–78]. In tendon-based systems, moving pulley differential mechanisms have also been utilized [79]. Research by Zappatore et al. [78] investigated a differential system based on gears for a novel robotic hand architecture, examining the properties of differential mechanisms arranged in cascade through parallel or serial connections. Furthermore, Baril et al. [80] presented an underactuated anthropomorphic gripper for prosthetic applications that featured a mechanical lever within the palm to enhance grasping capabilities and improve force transmission. This mechanism was subsequently developed in Kontoudis et al. [81], incorporating a differential mechanism with locking buttons that allowed users to halt the motion of each finger.

2.5.2 Design and Modeling

On the basis of the requirements described in Sect. 2.5.1, it was designed and modeled the exoskeleton structure using the software Autodesk Fusion 360. The device is designed to ensure that the movements of the exoskeleton match the human hand ones and do not constrain or overload hand joints.

2.5.2.1 Differential Mechanism

As previously mentioned, a gear-based differential mechanism is employed to couple the motion of two adjacent fingers. The CAD model of this differential mechanism is illustrated in Fig. 2.40. The size of the gear-based differential has been minimized to enhance wearability, while the dimensions are carefully balanced to optimize weight, motion smoothness, mechanical resistance, and ease of manufacturing using FDM and SLA (Stereo-Lithography) technologies available in our laboratory. Notably, the gear-based differential mechanism is powered by a single linear actuator, which is entirely housed within the mechanism's enclosure.

The differential mechanism is an epicyclic gear with 2-DoFs, composed of two main parts:

- **The differential gearing** consists of four bevel gears, i.e. two satellites (indicated with B in Fig. 2.40a) gears and two gears joined to the shafts (D), that transmit the motion to the fingers of the exoskeleton by using the differential's branches (G, F).
- **The carrier** is actuated by a rack (H), which is powered by a linear actuator placed in a support base pocket (I). It contains two sites where the satellite gears of the differential gearing are mounted.

The carrier is designed to connect the differential box with the linear actuator. It features a symmetrical structure and incorporates two spur gears on the side (E), which are connected to the crown (C in Fig. 2.40a). Inside the differential box, an epicyclic gear system is housed. This symmetric design is used, as it helps distribute forces and torques uniformly, ensuring mechanical stability.

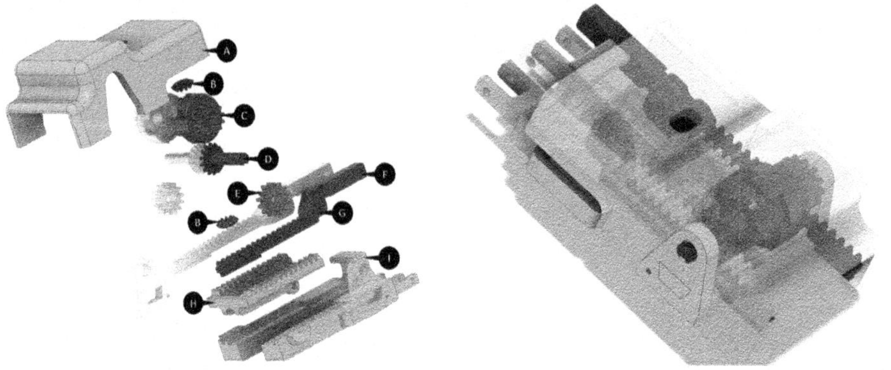

(a) (b)

Fig. 2.40 **a** Exploded CAD view of the differential mechanism. (A) differential mechanism cover box; (I) support for the linear actuator and for the differential mechanism parts. The differential mechanism is composed of: two satellite gears (B), two gears meshed with the shafts (D), two differential's branches (G, F), a rack (H), and two spur gears (E) meshed with two crowns (C). **b** Assembled differential mechanism. Copyright © 2022 Dragusanu, Troisi, Villani, Prattichizzo and Malvezzi [72]. This is an distributed under the terms of the Creative Commons Attribution License (CC BY)

When the actuator is retracted, the hand remains in a rest configuration. Conversely, when the actuator is extended, it moves the rack connected to the differential box, allowing it to rotate freely. If the movement encounters no obstacles, the satellites of the differential mechanism do not rotate about their own axes. Instead, the shafts rotate in unison with the crown at the same angular velocity. The transmission gears, which are keyed to the shafts, actuate two terminal racks connected to the fingers, facilitating the flexion of the hand according to the kinematics of the exoskeleton. If one finger encounters an obstacle, the adjacent finger continues to move at double the velocity, as defined by the relationship governing the differential mechanism:

$$\tau_{l,r} = \frac{\omega_r - \omega_c}{\omega_l - \omega_c} = -1 \Rightarrow \omega_c = \frac{\omega_l + \omega_r}{2} \tag{2.7}$$

where $\tau_{l,r}$ is the transmission ratio of the differential mechanism, according with the Willis equation, ω_r and ω_l are respectively the angular velocities of the right shaft and the left shaft, ω_c is the angular velocity of the carrier. Since the transmission ratio in a rack and pinion system is constant, the above relationship can be easily expressed as a function of linear actuator stroke s and differential output strokes s_i and s_m, as follows:

$$s = \frac{s_i + s_m}{2} \tag{2.8}$$

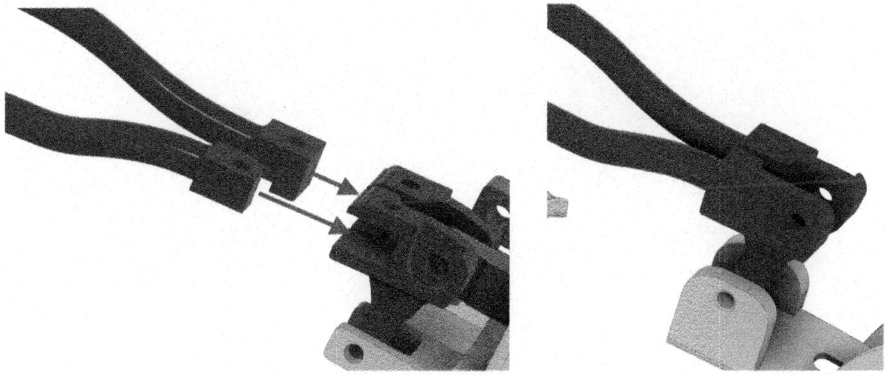

(a) (b)

Fig. 2.41 **a** New finger's module socket. **b** Previous version of finger's module. Copyright © 2022 Dragusanu, Troisi, Villani, Prattichizzo and Malvezzi [72]. This is an distributed under the terms of the Creative Commons Attribution License (CC BY)

In this way the device can move two adjacent fingers with an actuator only and a power source, with the advantage of keeping independent the motion of fingers.

2.5.2.2 Finger Actuation

As discussed in Sect. 2.5.1, user's comfort is a critical requirement for wearable devices, particularly those designed for rehabilitation. To enhance adaptability and wearability, the design of the finger support focuses on ensuring that users can easily and quickly don and doff the device. Additionally, the structure must accommodate users with slightly varying anthropometric measurements.

It is important to note that the developed transmission system is underactuated when worn on the finger, meaning the kinematic structure is effectively closed by the finger itself. This characteristic improves wearability and enhances the adaptability to individual finger dimensions.

The finger module, previously presented, was engineered to meet these wearability and kinematic requirements. However, based on user feedback, several improvements have been made to the finger module. Notably, the new socket design shown in Fig. 2.41a allows for easy assembly and disassembly of the finger modules from the actuator or differential without the need for any tools, in contrast to the version depicted in Fig. 2.41b. The complete CAD model including the modules for the fingers and the differential mechanism is shown in Fig. 2.42.

In particular, Fig. 2.42a shows the solution previously introduced in Sect. 2.3, in which each finger is independently actuated, while Fig. 2.42b shows an upgrade of that version that further simplify the assembly/deassembly of the device and further improve adaptability and wearability, in which fingers are coupled by two differentials and only two actuators are needed. The mechanical transmission between

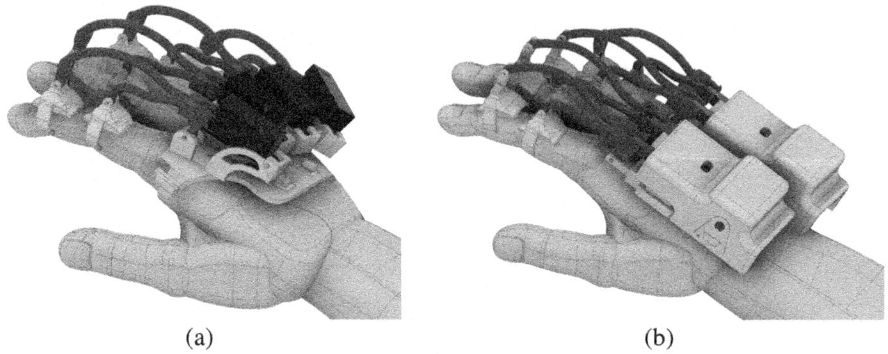

Fig. 2.42 **a** CAD model of the previous version of the exoskeleton worn on the hand. **b** CAD model of the proposed exoskeleton worn on the hand. Copyright © 2022 Dragusanu, Troisi, Villani, Prattichizzo and Malvezzi [72]. This is an distributed under the terms of the Creative Commons Attribution License (CC BY)

differential outputs and finger phalanges has been developed to implement the concept of postural synergies, introduced by the neuroscientific studies summarized in the previous section. In particular, the position and dimension of the exoskeleton linkages have been defined to reproduce the first postural synergy on each finger.

The differential mechanism facilitates independent movement of the fingers. Specifically, the transmission system for each finger is designed to replicate the coordination between the proximal and intermediate interphalangeal joints observed in the first postural synergy, while allowing for independent finger movement.

The finger actuation system is engineered so that, when activated, the flexion and extension motions closely approximate the first postural synergy, as previously mentioned. To demonstrate how the trajectory of the exoskeleton aligns with that of the human hand, a kinematic analysis was conducted [82, 83].

The simplified kinematic model of the transmission is depicted in Fig. 2.43a. From a kinematic perspective, the finger actuation mechanism comprises five rigid links: the actuator (denoted as a) consists of two rigid bodies, links 1 and 2, which actuate the intermediate phalanx, while link 3 actuates the proximal phalanx. It's important to note that element (a) represents the linear actuator for the device, enabling independent actuation of each finger while also functioning as a differential output when the fingers are coupled.

These rigid bodies are interconnected by five revolute (R) joints and one prismatic (P) joint (the actuator itself is not represented in the diagram), resulting in a system with 3-DoF. When the exoskeleton is worn, the kinematic structure of the finger effectively "closes" the mechanism.

Consequently, the resulting kinematic chain consists of seven bodies (the aforementioned links and the proximal and intermediate phalanges of the finger), linked by nine R-joints and one P-joint, yielding one residual DoF. A straightforward kinematic analysis allows the estimation of finger motion as a function of the stroke applied by element (a).

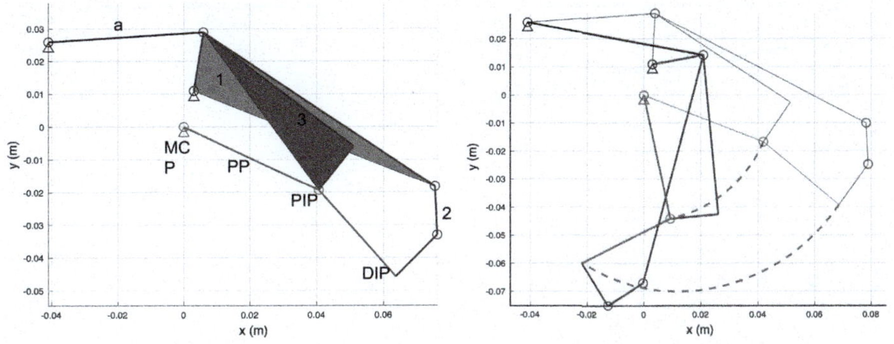

Fig. 2.43 Kinematic scheme of the finger actuation system. **a** Kinematic scheme. The system is composed of an actuator (*a*), two links for intermediate phalange actuation, connected to the finger in correspondence with the DIP joint (elements 1 and 2), and a link for proximal phalanx actuation, connected to the finger in correspondence of the PIP joint. Red links represent the simplified 2-DoFs finger structure. **b** Kinematic simulation. Thin lines represent the reference initial configuration, thick continuous lines represent the final close configuration, red dashed curves represent PIP and DIP point trajectories. Copyright © 2022 Dragusanu, Troisi, Villani, Prattichizzo and Malvezzi [72]. This is an distributed under the terms of the Creative Commons Attribution License (CC BY) (color figure online)

Figure 2.43b shows system initial (thin lines) and final (thick lines), and PIP and DIP point trajectories. Figure 2.44 reports in the upper diagram the variation of index MPC and PIP angles, indicated with $q_{1,i}$ and $q_{2,i}$, respectively, as a function of element (*a*) stroke, indicated with s, while in the lower diagram the ratio $q_{2,i}/q_{1,i}$. It's interesting to notice that both $q_{1,i}$ and $q_{2,i}$ varies almost linearly with respect to s, and that therefore the ratio $q_{2,i}/q_{1,i}$ is almost constant. Such a ratio is very close to the value that can be obtained as $\tau = S_{1,7}/S_{1,6}$ (reported as a red horizontal line in the diagram). This result confirms that the exoskeleton finger actuation couples the MPC and PIP joints so that the finger follows the first postural synergy when its closure motion is guided by the exoskeleton.

Similar results can be obtained for the middle finger, From the above mentioned results, it is possible to directly correlate by means of a linear relationship the synergy inputs for the single fingers $z_{1,i}$ $z_{1,m}$ to differential output strokes s_i, s_m, i.e. it is possible to find four coefficients, a_i, b_i, a_m, b_m, such that

$$s_i = a_i z_{1,i} + b_i, \tag{2.9}$$

$$s_m = a_m z_{1,m} + b_m, \tag{2.10}$$

and, finally, the input stroke provided by the linear actuator is related to s_i and s_m by the differential relationship introduced in Eq. (2.8).

Future improvements of this work will focus on analyzing the sensitivity of the results concerning model uncertainties and individual anthropometric parameters. These investigations will encompass not only finger movements but also more com-

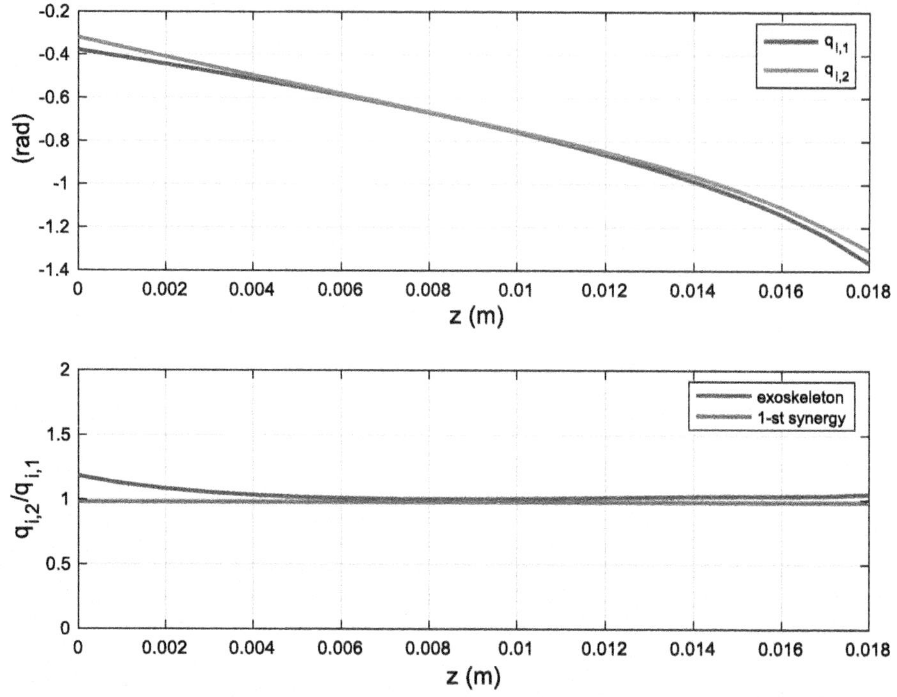

Fig. 2.44 Results of kinematics analysis relative to the index finger module. Upper diagram: MPC and PIP joint rotation angles, $q_{1,i}$ and $q_{2,i}$ as a function of input (actuator or differential) stroke, indicated with z. Lower diagram: ratio between joint rotation angles, $q_{2,i}/q_{1,i}$ as a function of z, compared with the value obtained from the first postural synergy defined in [52].

plex, coordinated tasks such as grasping. To facilitate this, we will explore additional simulation tools, including those proposed in [84].

The link structure has been specifically designed to prevent interference with the finger during the closure motion. After creating the mechanism components using 3D-CAD software, we conducted a straightforward multibody configuration analysis to ensure that the links do not interfere with the subject's phalanges during this motion. The results of this analysis are presented in Fig. 2.45, which illustrates the finger in its final closed configuration, along with the trajectories of the PIP and DIP points.

2.5.2.3 Structural Analysis

This section summarizes the results of a series of basic structural analyses aimed at evaluating the structural resistance of the device and selecting suitable materials for

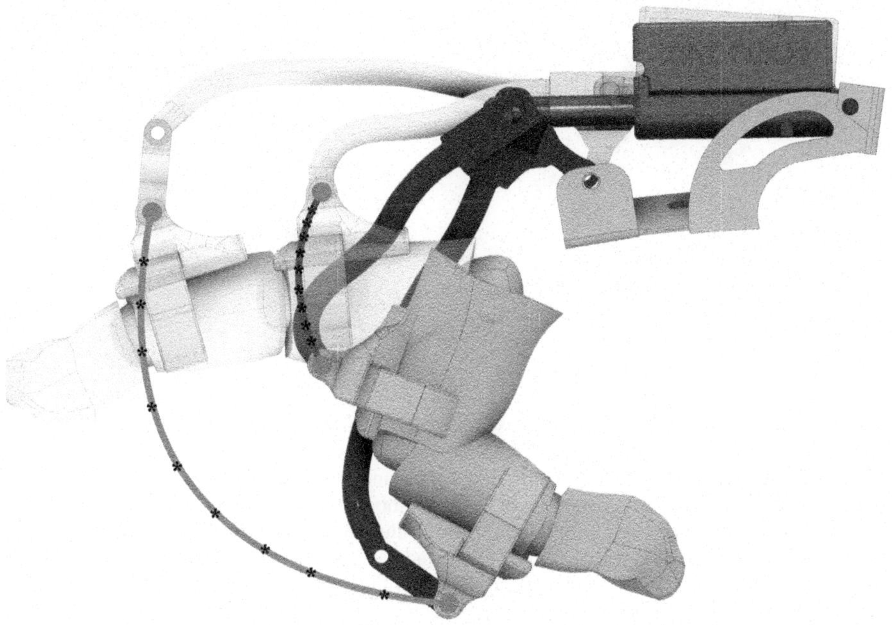

Fig. 2.45 Multibody simulation of the finger exoskeleton worn on the index finger, performed to verify that during closure motion, exoskeleton elements do not interfere with the finger. Copyright © 2022 Dragusanu, Troisi, Villani, Prattichizzo and Malvezzi [72]. This is an distributed under the terms of the Creative Commons Attribution License (CC BY)

the manufacturing phase. The structural analysis focused on both the finger actuation mechanism and the components of the differential mechanism, encompassing the previously introduced exoskeleton structures.

The materials considered for the mechanical structure of the fingers and the differential components included ABS, aluminum, and steel. For the actuator and the differential mechanism supports, ABS was chosen due to its favorable properties. The finger supports for the phalanges were also realised with ABS, while a soft plastic was used for the rings that connect the phalanges to the device. The studies have been realised with FEM analysis using 3D-CAD/CAE Autodesk® Fusion 360 software.

Finger actuation structure The two exoskeleton solutions previously discussed can be used either with the same linear actuator or with the differential mechanism. The primary distinction between them lies in their mechanical structures, which facilitate the assembly and disassembly of the modules. Consequently, for all analyses, the focus is on studying the mechanical structure, while the linear actuator has been disregarded.

To ensure a fair comparison, we focused on the module designed for the index finger across both solutions. The analysis examined various configurations, ranging from fully open to fully closed positions, with the most critical loading condition

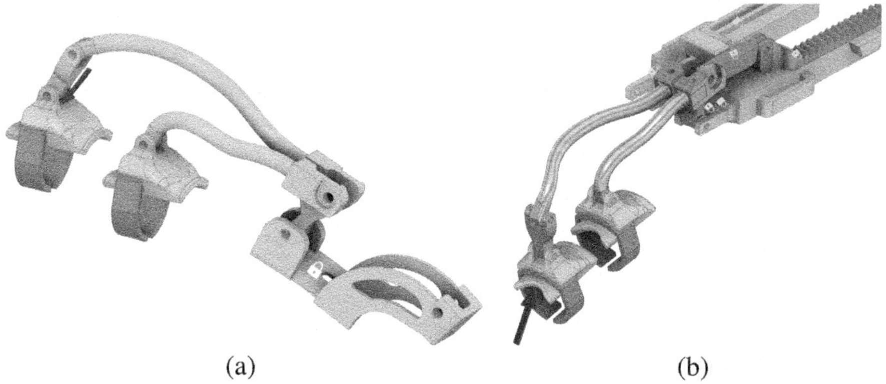

Fig. 2.46 Models of the index module used for FEM analyses. In all the subfigures the finger's support is made with ABS while the ring is composed by soft plastic material. **a** CAD model of the old index finer module solution, where the mechanism and the linear actuator's support are made in ABS. **b** CAD models of the new index finger module solution, where the finger mechanism and the differential mechanism support are made in aluminum. Blue arrows represent the applied forces while the area signed with a white padlock indicates the costrained parts.

occurring in the fully open configuration. For brevity, only the results pertaining to this specific configuration are presented. In Fig. 2.46, both finger actuation structures are illustrated using two of the three materials previously mentioned. The figure highlights the points where forces are applied, indicated by blue arrows, and the constrained areas, marked by white padlocks. Forces are applied at the extremity of the structure, as this area is primarily engaged in the hand rehabilitation process, simulating the physiotherapist's force during finger flexion and extension exercises. The applied force magnitude is set at 20 N, with forces directed both upward (as shown in Fig. 2.46a) and downward (depicted in Fig. 2.46b). The materials evaluated include ABS, steel, and aluminum.

A subset of the performed simulations is presented in Figs. 2.47 and 2.48, while Table 2.5 lists the main findings from all analyses. It is important to note that the maximum stress that standard ABS can withstand is approximately 60 MPa, and none of the models met this constraint when subjected to a force of 20 N. The results indicate that neither solution can be constructed using this material unless the applied forces are reduced or the structure is modified by increasing the thickness, resulting in a bulkier device. In contrast, steel exhibits a much higher resistance, with a maximum allowable stress of up to 500 MPa. The results show that in both solutions, the maximum Von Mises equivalent stress remains below this limit. When using aluminum, which has a maximum yield stress slightly lower than that of steel, the maximum equivalent Von Mises stress values fall within acceptable limits for the material properties. However, because steel and aluminum have different Young's moduli, , i.e., 210 GPa for steel and 75 GPa for aluminum, the maximum displace-

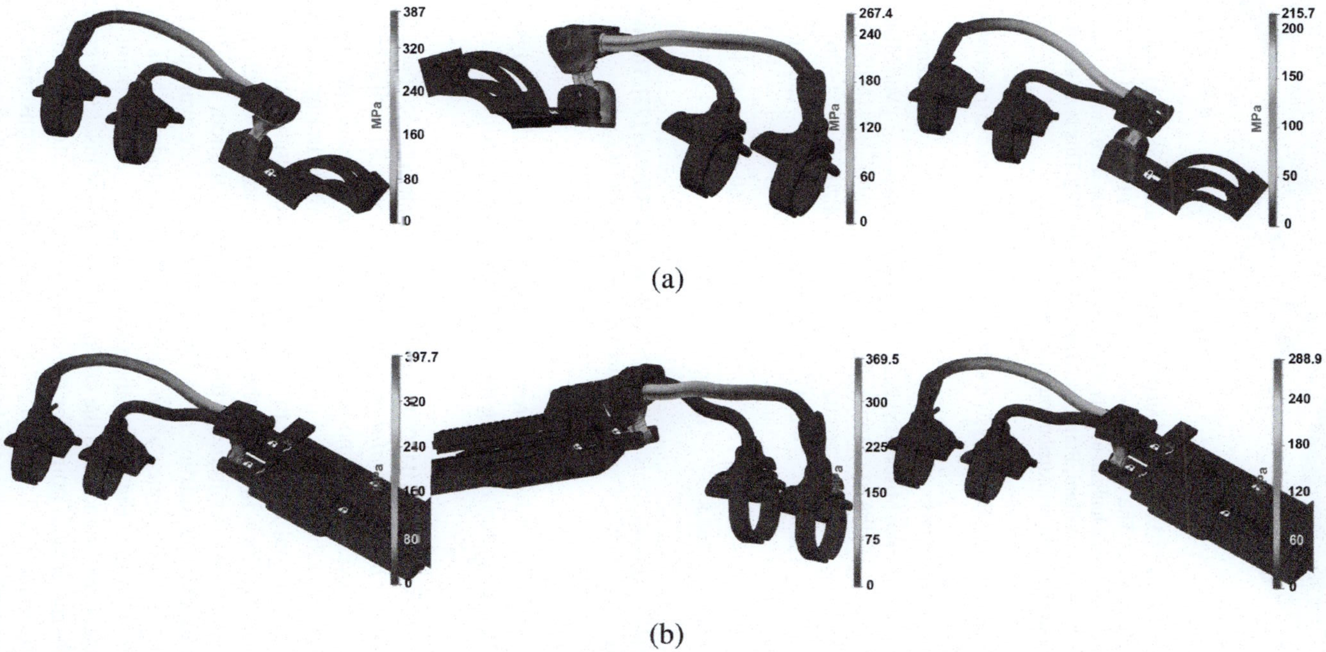

Fig. 2.47 Results of the FEM structural analyses. Equivalent Von Mises stress distributions when a 20 N magnitude force is applied on the distal part. The first row of subfigures **a** reports the results for the previous finger module solution, when the materials used for the finger's links are ABS, aluminum and steel. Subfigures in **b** report the results for the new finger module solution when the materials used for the finger's mechanism are ABS, aluminum and steel, respectively. Copyright © 2022 Dragusanu, Troisi, Villani, Prattichizzo and Malvezzi [72]. This is an distributed under the terms of the Creative Commons Attribution License (CC BY)

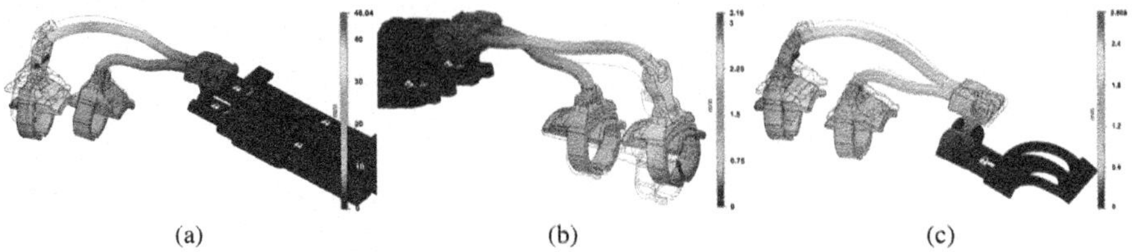

Fig. 2.48 Results of the FEM structural analyses for the new (**a, b**) and old (**c**) index finger module in terms of displacements. The applied force has a magnitude of 20 N in all the cases, while the materials for the finger's mechanism used is ABS in (**a**), aluminum in (**b**) and steel in (**c**). Copyright © 2022 Dragusanu, Troisi, Villani, Prattichizzo and Malvezzi [72]. This is an distributed under the terms of the Creative Commons Attribution License (CC BY)

Table 2.5 Synthesis of the FEM analysis results in terms of stress and displacement with 20 N of applied force magnitude

	Force (N)	ABS		Steel		Aluminum	
		Von Mises (MPA)	Displ. (mm)	Von Mises (MPA)	Displ. (mm)	Von Mises (MPA)	Displ. (mm)
Old finger	20	387.00	63.02	214.50	4.29	215.70	2.87
New finger	20	397.70	46.04	255.10	1.88	288.90	0.70
Old finger	−20	486.20	86.95	267.40	5.60	269.10	3.67
New finger	−20	763.8	74.14	369.50	3.16	429.40	1.28

ments differ, although both values remain limited. Based on this analysis, aluminum emerges as the best material among those evaluated for the structural components of the exoskeleton.

Differential mechanism We have studied the two main assembled parts that compose the differential, i.e. *the differential gearing* and *the carrier*, to verify the overall stress and deformation level and define the best solution in terms of materials to be used for the realization of the proposed differential mechanism. In Fig. 2.49 the two main parts of the differential mechanism with three different combinations of materials are shown. The padlock indicates the parts of the model in which constraints are set, while the blue arrows indicate the forces that are applied. In all the structural analyses, the magnitude and direction of the applied forces are evaluated by analysing the statics of the whole device when a force with magnitude 20 N is applied on the finger. For the carrier, Fig. 2.50a, the force is applied on the point in which the actuator connects to the rack and the constrained parts are inside the crown wheel. In order to study the critical points for the differential gears, forces and constraint are applied as shown in Figs. 2.50b and 2.49c. In particular, the constraints are applied to the satellite gears bases while the forces are applied to create a torque on the shafts.

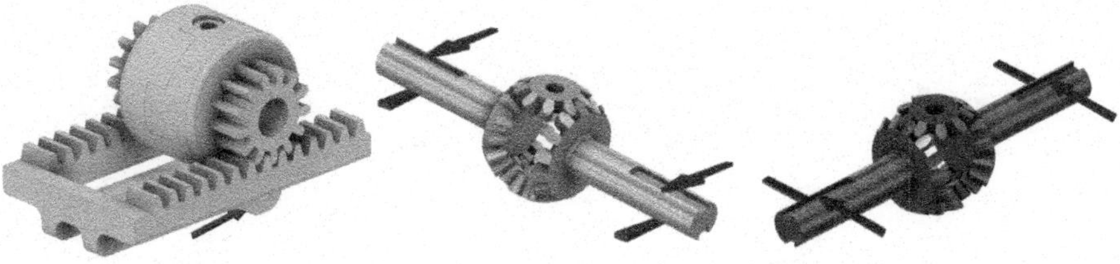

(a) (b) (c)

Fig. 2.49 CAD model of the differential mechanism main parts used for FEM analyses. Blue arrows represent the applied forces while the area signed with a white padlock indicates the constrained parts for the structural analyses. Subfigure **a** shows the carrier made in ABS material while the other two subfigures show the differential gearing made in aluminum (**b**) and steel (**c**). Copyright © 2022 Dragusanu, Troisi, Villani, Prattichizzo and Malvezzi [72]. This is an distributed under the terms of the Creative Commons Attribution License (CC BY)

In Fig. 2.50 simulation results are reported in terms of equivalent Von Mises stress, considering different materials. It can be observed that in all cases the FEM analyses return acceptable Von Mises equivalent stress values. All results are under the maximum stress value of the analysed materials. In this case, therefore, ABS could be a good solution because of its lightness, but on the other hand this material presents some drawbacks in terms of wear and friction, which reduces the effectiveness. Also in this case aluminum results to be the best solutions as it is lighter and more flexible than steel.

Table 2.6 summarizes the weights of both finger module solutions and the two main parts that compose the proposed differential mechanism, based on the material used. Form this table and from the above presented results the outcome is that the best solution, in terms of materials is aluminum for the structural elements of the proposed device.

2.5.3 Prototype

This section presents the exoskeleton prototypes developed using the previously described finger structures and differential mechanism. The exoskeleton is designed to be worn on the back of the hand, assisting the user in flexion and extension motions. Although the analyses presented in the previous section indicate that aluminum is the optimal material for the structural components, the first prototype was constructed using ABS due to the availability of common manufacturing techniques.

All components were manufactured using the FDM technique. The design and development of the exoskeleton followed a specific procedure outlined in [85], which can be summarized as follows: first, CAD modeling was performed using Autodesk Fusion 360; next, the CAD model was converted to an STL file; finally, the STL file was transferred to the 3D printer. The physical realization utilized the *Stratasys*

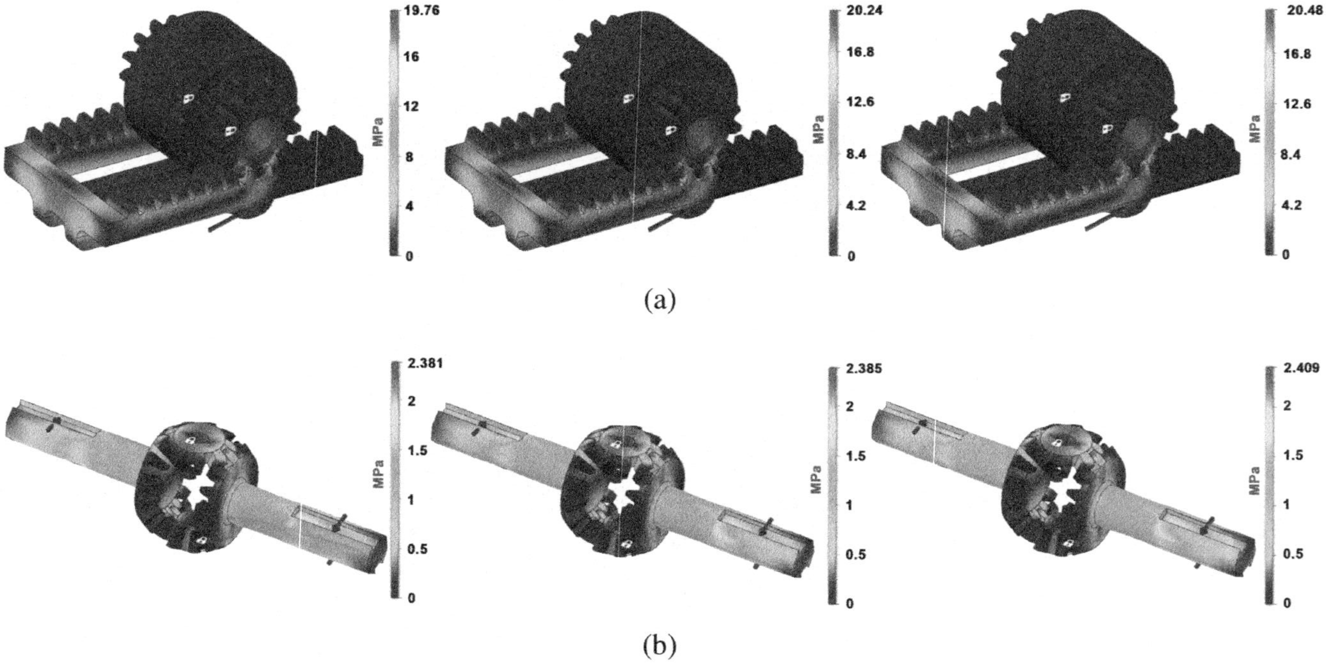

Fig. 2.50 Results of the FEM structural analyses on the differential, equivalent Von Mises stress distributions. The first row of subfigures **a** reports the results, for the carrier, of the FEM analysis when the materials used are ABS (max. Von Mises 19.76 MPa), aluminum (max. Von Mises 20.24 MPa) and steel (max. Von Mises 20.48 MPa). Subfigures in **b** report the results for the differential gearing when the materials are ABS (max. Von Mises 2.38 MPa), aluminum (max. Von Mises 2.39 MPa) and steel (max. Von Mises 2.41 MPa). Copyright © 2022 Dragusanu, Troisi, Villani, Prattichizzo and Malvezzi [72]. This is an distributed under the terms of the Creative Commons Attribution License (CC BY)

Table 2.6 Weights of the main parts of the exoskeleton

	ABS weight (g)	Steel weight (g)	Aluminum weight (g)
Finger module	43.91	99.97	57.45
Differential	1.74	12.88	4.43
Carrier	9.07	67.13	23.09
Total	54.72	179.98	84.97

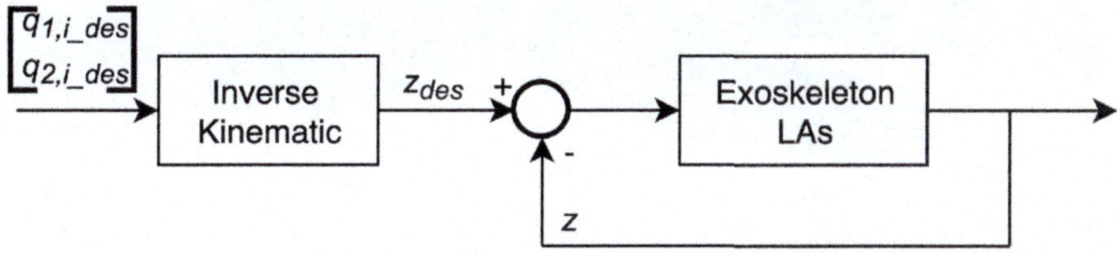

Fig. 2.51 Exoskeleton control scheme. Copyright © 2022 Dragusanu, Troisi, Villani, Prattichizzo and Malvezzi [72]. This is an distributed under the terms of the Creative Commons Attribution License (CC BY)

F123 3D-printer, and the mechanical components were printed using GrabCAD Print software. Components indicated with B, C, D, E, G, H in Fig. 2.40 were printed with a slicing height of 0.18 mm, while the other components, which did not need a high surface precision, were printed with a slicing height of 0.25 mm.

The device is actuated by a linear actuator, which is housed in a pocket between the fingers. The linear actuator used is the Actuonix PQ-12, known for its lightweight design and a stroke length of 20 mm. This actuator is capable of exerting a force that allows the user to apply a maximum equivalent force of 20 N at the fingertip during both flexion and extension. The force is generated by a DC motor connected to a worm gear, enabling the motion of the shaft. The main features of the linear actuator are summarized in Table 2.4. To control the motion of the linear actuator and validate the prototype, an Arduino Uno is employed. The actuator's position is managed according to the scheme presented in Fig. 2.51. For a given desired posture, expressed in terms of index and middle joint rotation angles $\mathbf{q}_{des}$, an inverse kinematic procedure similar to the one presented in [86] is used to estimate the corresponding synergy value z_{des}, that is furthermore converted in actuator desired stroke s_{des}.

A standard PID controller is employed to regulate the linear actuator. The control and electronic components are housed in an armband worn on the forearm, as depicted in Fig. 2.52. The device communicates via Bluetooth with a PC graphical user interface, enabling users to manage and monitor the exoskeleton's movements [68].

Additionally, the hand exoskeleton is part of a more comprehensive device designed to assist individuals with upper limb injuries [68]. This device features a module for wrist rehabilitation, which incorporates a tendon-based transmission

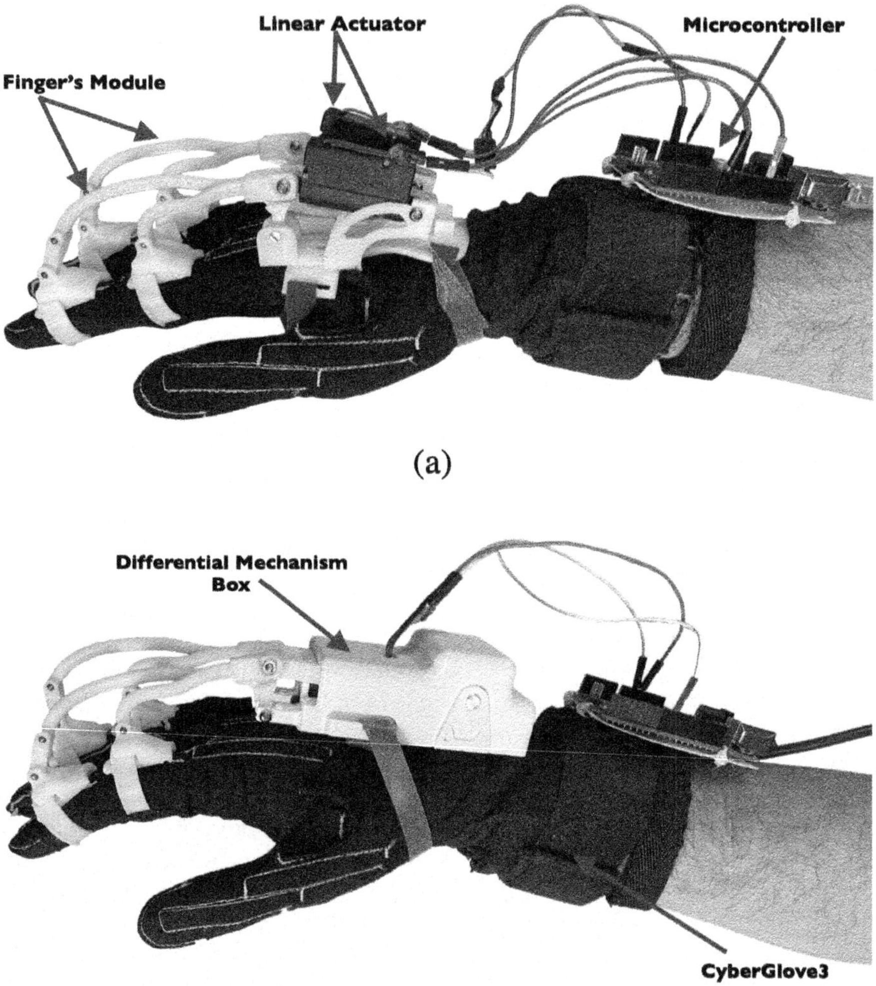

(a)

(b)

Fig. 2.52 Experimental setup for the validation phases using the CyberGlove3. Subfigure **a** shows two previous finger modules while subfigure **b** shows the proposed device, both worn by the user.

system to facilitate wrist movements. Made of thermoplastic materials, the module can be customized to meet the specific needs of each user.

2.5.4 Experimental Validation

The prototypes of the exoskeleton developed in this study were tested and compared with earlier versions. Six participants, aged 24–30 years (4 males and 2 females), first wore a CyberGlove3 (CyberGlove Systems, Inc., US), a commercial hand-tracking system equipped with 22 joint angle sensors. They then wore the third version of the exoskeleton, as described in Sect. 2.3, illustrated in Fig. 2.52a. Each participant completed five repetitions of hand opening and closing with this setup.

Subsequently, the participants performed the same task while wearing the new exoskeleton shown in Fig. 2.52b. In addition, each participant undertook another cycle of five opening and closing movements with one side of the differential mechanism mechanically blocked by the experimenter. All subjects provided written informed consent to participate and were free to withdraw from the study at any time.The experiment protocols followed the declaration of Helsinki, and there was no risk of harmful effects on subjects' health.

Using the CyberGlove3, we recorded the joint angles of the metacarpal and proximal joints of the index and middle fingers for each participant. The range of motion achieved with both versions of the exoskeleton was evaluated by calculating the absolute difference between the mean values of each valley and the mean values of the subsequent peaks.

The experimental results indicate that the new exoskeleton, under free conditions, increases the range of motion of the hand by approximately 10%. When one side of the differential mechanism was mechanically blocked, the range of motion nearly doubled, reaching just under 100%. The data revealed that the metacarpal joints exhibited an increase in movement of $14.02 \pm 6.84\%$ with the free differential mechanism, and $90.02 \pm 8.34\%$ with the blocked mechanism. Similarly, the proximal joints demonstrated an increase in mobility of 13.21 ± 6.67 % in the first scenario and $69.61 \pm 27.03\%$ in the second. An example of one of the experimental trials is presented in Fig. 2.53.

2.5.4.1 Using the Device with Commercial Tracking System

Further tests were conducted to assess the usability of the proposed exoskeleton with a widely used and affordable commercial optical tracking system. This aspect is important for enabling the device to be utilized in real rehabilitation settings outside of research laboratories, where the high costs and complexity of sophisticated tracking systems often pose a barrier. Specifically, we tested the integration of the exoskeleton with the Leap Motion Controller (UltraLeap, Inc., US), as illustrated in Fig. 2.54. The primary metric used to evaluate compatibility with this connection system was

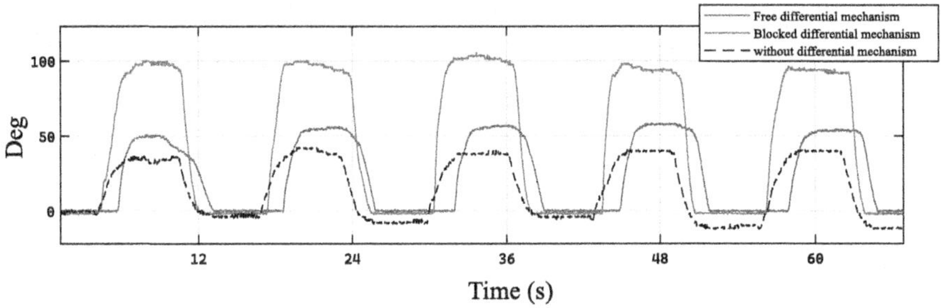

(a)

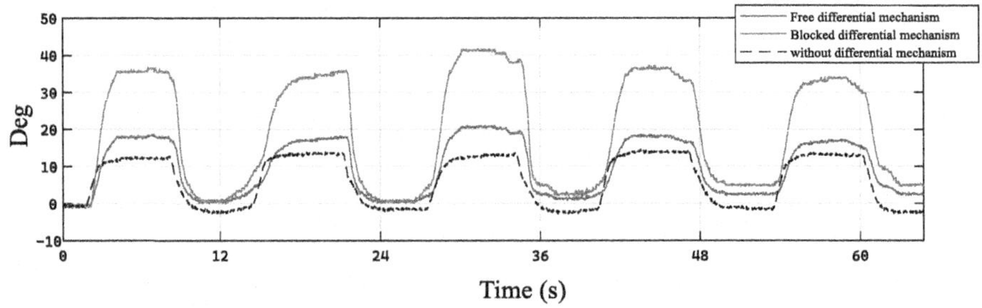

(b)

Fig. 2.53 Joint rotation angles of the **a** metacarpo-phalangeal (MCP) and **b** proximal interphalangeal (PIP) joint of the middle finger recorded by the CyberGlove during a single repetition of the physiotherapy task. Blue curve represents joint angle obtained with the exoskeleton equipped with the differential mechanism, red curve represents the rotation of the same joint when the other finger is blocked, black curve represents joint rotation obtained with the previous version of the exoskeleton. Copyright © 2022 Dragusanu, Troisi, Villani, Prattichizzo and Malvezzi [72]. This is an distributed under the terms of the Creative Commons Attribution License (CC BY)

the average number of disconnections during a bimanual task. We compared the results obtained with and without the exoskeleton to determine its effectiveness in this context.

Six subjects aged between 24 and 30 years, comprising three males and three females, participated in the experimental campaign. Each participant was tasked with completing three test cycles, each consisting of five simultaneous opening and closing movements performed with both hands-the left hand without the exoskeleton and the right hand assisted by the exoskeleton. For this experimental campaign, all subjects provided written informed consent and were informed that they could withdraw from the study at any time. The experiment protocols followed the declaration of Helsinki, and there was no risk of harmful effects on subjects health.

The subjects involved in the experiments were volunteer collaborators from our laboratory, each possessing considerable experience in testing new wearable devices. To ensure safety, several precautions and measures were implemented to minimize risks for everyone involved in the device development. These included: (i) supervision of all experiments by at least one technically skilled supervisor, who could

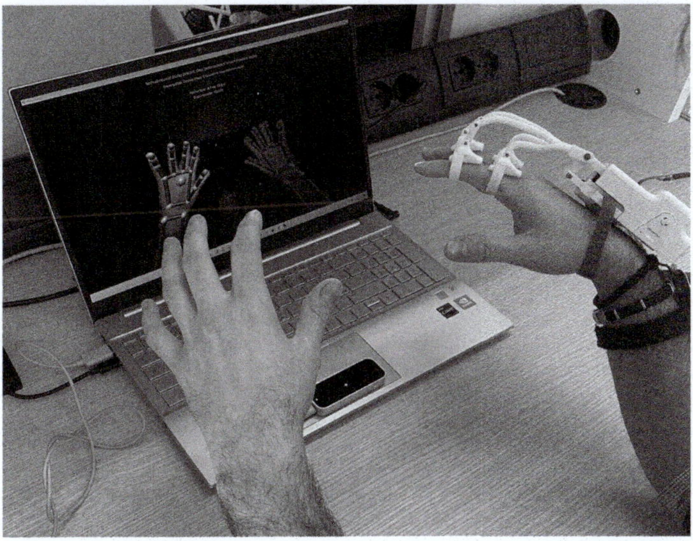

Fig. 2.54 Use of the proposed exoskeleton with the LeapMotion Controller. Copyright © 2022 Dragusanu, Troisi, Villani, Prattichizzo and Malvezzi [72]. This is an distributed under the terms of the Creative Commons Attribution License (CC BY)

Table 2.7 Number of times the hand assisted by the exoskeleton was lost by the LeapMotion Controller tracking system for each individual trial depending on the quality of brightness and cleanliness of the sensor reported by the diagnostics software: G means good, B bad

Trial	1	2	3	4	5	6	7	8	9	10	11	12	13	14	15
Smudge	B	B	G	G	G	G	G	G	G	G	G	G	G	B	B
Lighting	G	G	G	G	G	G	B	B	B	G	G	G	B	B	B
Exos	2	1	1	0	0	2	2	3	1	2	1	0	2	4	3
Free Hand	0	1	0	0	0	1	2	2	1	0	0	0	1	2	2

immediately halt device operation in the event of technical malfunctions or participant discomfort, (ii) software tools designed to detect malfunctions and automatically deactivate the devices when necessary and (iii) physical measures to detach participants from the devices if contact forces exceeded predetermined limits. No personal data related to the subjects were collected during the tests.

The participants' movements were continuously monitored using Leap Motion technology and were mapped joint-to-joint onto two virtual hand avatars displayed on a screen positioned in front of them. The number of hand-lost for both hands and the status of the Tracking system during the experimentation were recorded and the obtained results and reported in Table 2.7.

The results show an inevitable difference in the number of hand-lost between the free hand and the hand assisted by the exoskeleton, the free hand is always tracked

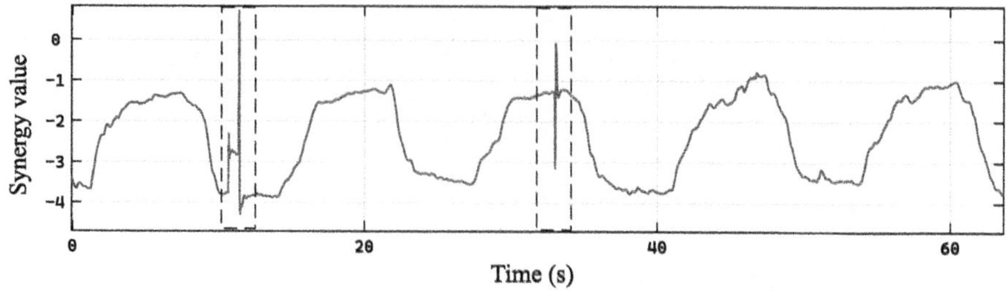

Fig. 2.55 First synergy activation value z estimated during the acquisition of the LeapMotion Controller during a the physiotherapy task. The dotted rectangles highlight the time interval in which the tracking system loose the hand in the frame. Copyright © 2022 Dragusanu, Troisi, Villani, Prattichizzo and Malvezzi [72]. This is an distributed under the terms of the Creative Commons Attribution License (CC BY)

better or equally than the hand assisted by the exoskeleton. The average number of hand-lost in a time interval of about 60 s is equal to 1.44 ± 1.19 for the assisted hand and 0.78 ± 0.88 for the free hand. However, as can be seen from the graph shown in Fig. 2.55, the number of disconnections of the assisted hand and the duration of the same with respect to the length of the task is overall not excessive. These results allow to assert that the the tracking system and the assistive exoskeleton can be jointly used in rehabilitation exercises. The outcome of these tests, therefore, allows us to conclude that the physiotherapy exercises performed with the presented exoskeleton can be recorded and remotely monitored through commercial systems with low economic impact and wide diffusion.

References

1. Bütefisch C, Hummelsheim H, Denzler P, Mauritz K-H (1995) Repetitive training of isolated movements improves the outcome of motor rehabilitation of the centrally paretic hand. J Neurol Sci 130(1):59–68
2. Riener R (2016) The cybathlon promotes the development of assistive technology for people with physical disabilities. J Neuroeng Rehab 13(1):49
3. Krebs HI, Hogan N, Volpe BT, Aisen ML, Edelstein L, Diels C (1999) Overview of clinical trials with mit-manus: a robot-aided neuro-rehabilitation facility. Technol Health Care 7(6):419–423
4. Yue Z, Zhang X, Wang J (2017) Hand rehabilitation robotics on poststroke motor recovery. Behav Neurol
5. Dovat L, Lambercy O, Gassert R, Maeder T, Milner T, Leong TC, Burdet E (2008) Handcare: a cable-actuated rehabilitation system to train hand function after stroke. IEEE Trans Neur Syst Rehab Eng 16(6):582–591
6. Bouzit M, Burdea G, Popescu G, Boian R (2002) The Rutgers master II-new design force-feedback glove. IEEE/ASME Trans Mechatron 7(2):256–263
7. Lambercy O, Dovat L, Gassert R, Burdet E, Teo CL, Milner T (2007) A haptic knob for rehabilitation of hand function. IEEE Trans Neur Syst Rehab Eng 15(3):356–366
8. Wang D, Meng Q, Meng Q, Li X, Yu H (2018) Design and development of a portable exoskeleton for hand rehabilitation. IEEE Trans Neur Syst Rehab Eng 26(12):2376–2386

9. Bianchi M, Cempini M, Conti R, Meli E, Ridolfi A, Vitiello N, Allotta B (2018) Design of a series elastic transmission for hand exoskeletons. Mechatronics 51:8–18
10. Jo I, Park Y, Lee J, Bae J (2019) A portable and spring-guided hand exoskeleton for exercising flexion/extension of the fingers. Mech Mach Theory 135:176–191
11. Bataller A, Cabrera JA, Clavijo M, Castillo JJ (2016) Evolutionary synthesis of mechanisms applied to the design of an exoskeleton for finger rehabilitation. Mech Mach Theory 105:31–43
12. Masia L, Krebs HI, Cappa P, Hogan N (2007) Design and characterization of hand module for whole-arm rehabilitation following stroke. IEEE/ASME Trans Mechatron 12(4):399–407
13. Conti R, Meli E, Ridolfi A, Bianchi M, Governi L, Volpe Y, Allotta B (2017) Kinematic synthesis and testing of a new portable hand exoskeleton. Meccanica 52(11):2873–2897
14. Secciani N, Bianchi M, Meli E, Volpe Y, Ridolfi A (2019) A novel application of a surface electromyography-based control strategy for a hand exoskeleton system: a single-case study. Int J Adv Robot Syst 16(1):1729881419828197
15. Secciani N, Topini A, Ridolfi A, Meli E, Allotta B (2020) A novel point-in-polygon-based SEMG classifier for hand exoskeleton systems. IEEE Trans Neur Syst Rehab Eng 28(12):3158–3166
16. Zhang F, Hua L, Yili F, Chen H, Wang S (2014) Design and development of a hand exoskeleton for rehabilitation of hand injuries. Mech Mach Theory 73:103–116
17. Nycz CJ, Bützer T, Lambercy O, Arata J, Fischer GS, Gassert R (2016) Design and characterization of a lightweight and fully portable remote actuation system for use with a hand exoskeleton. IEEE Robot Autom Lett 1(2):976–983
18. Randazzo L, Iturrate I, Perdikis S, Millán JdR (2017) mano: a wearable hand exoskeleton for activities of daily living and neurorehabilitation. IEEE Robot Autom Lett 3(1):500–507
19. Marconi D, Baldoni A, McKinney Z, Cempini M, Crea S, Vitiello N (2019) A novel hand exoskeleton with series elastic actuation for modulated torque transfer. Mechatronics 61:69–82
20. Popov D, Gaponov I, Ryu J-H (2016) Portable exoskeleton glove with soft structure for hand assistance in activities of daily living. IEEE/ASME Trans Mechatron 22(2):865–875
21. Dragusanu M, Troisi D, Suthar B, Hussain I, Prattichizzo D, Malvezzi M (2024) Mglove-ts: a modular soft glove based on twisted string actuators and flexible structures. Mechatronics 98:103141
22. Dragusanu M, Saeed A, Guinet N, Troisi D, Prattichizzo D, Malvezzi M (2024) Development of the modular finger elements of an actuated glove for hand rehabilitation. In: Quaglia G, Boschetti G, Carbone G (eds) Advances in Italian mechanism science. Springer Nature, Cham, Switzerland, pp 563–570
23. Dragusanu M, Troisi D, Suthar B, Prattichizzo D, Malvezzi M (2024) Development of a soft actuated glove based on twisted string actuators for hand rehabilitation. In: 2024 10th IEEE RAS/EMBS international conference for biomedical robotics and biomechatronics (BioRob), pp 1702–1708
24. Fischer HC, Stubblefield K, Kline T, Luo X, Kenyon RV, Kamper DG (2007) Hand rehabilitation following stroke: a pilot study of assisted finger extension training in a virtual environment. Top Stroke Rehab 14(1):1–12
25. Takahashi CD, Der-Yeghiaian L, Le VH, Cramer SC (2005) A robotic device for hand motor therapy after stroke. In: 9th international conference on rehabilitation robotics, 2005. ICORR 2005. IEEE, pp 17–20
26. Koeneman EJ, Schultz RS, Wolf SL, Herring DE, Koeneman JB (2004) A pneumatic muscle hand therapy device. In: The 26th annual international conference of the IEEE engineering in medicine and biology society, vol 1. IEEE, pp 2711–2713
27. Abdallah IB, Bouteraa Y, Rekik C (2017) Design and development of 3D printed myoelectric robotic exoskeleton for hand rehabilitation. Int J Smart Sens Intell Syst 10(2)
28. Hofmann UAT, Bützer T, Lambercy O, Gassert R (2018) Design and evaluation of a Bowden-Cable-based remote actuation system for wearable robotics. IEEE Robot Autom Lett 3(3):2101–2108

29. Heo P, Gu GM, Lee S-j, Rhee K, Kim J (2012) Current hand exoskeleton technologies for rehabilitation and assistive engineering. Int J Precis Eng Manuf 13(5):807–824
30. du Plessis T, Djouani K, Oosthuizen C (2021) A review of active hand exoskeletons for rehabilitation and assistance. Robotics 10(1):40
31. Shahid T, Gouwanda D, Nurzaman SG, Gopalai AA (2018) Moving toward soft robotics: a decade review of the design of hand exoskeletons. Biomimetics 3(3):17
32. Krebs HI, Volpe BT, Williams D, Celestino J, Charles SK, Lynch D, Hogan N (2007) Robot-aided neurorehabilitation: a robot for wrist rehabilitation. IEEE Trans Neur Syst Rehab Eng 15(3):327–335
33. Gupta A, O'Malley MK, Patoglu V, Burgar C (2008) Design, control and performance of ricewrist: a force feedback wrist exoskeleton for rehabilitation and training. Int J Robot Res 27(2):233–251
34. Cappello L, Elangovan N, Contu S, Khosravani S, Konczak J, Masia L (2015) Robot-aided assessment of wrist proprioception. Front Human Neurosci 9:198
35. Buongiorno D, Sotgiu E, Leonardis D, Marcheschi S, Solazzi M, Frisoli A (2018) WRES a novel 3 dof wrist exoskeleton with tendon-driven differential transmission for neuro-rehabilitation and teleoperation. IEEE Robot Autom Lett 3(3):2152–2159
36. Bartlett NW, Lyau V, Raiford WA, Holland D, Gafford JB, Ellis TD, Walsh CJ (2015) A soft robotic orthosis for wrist rehabilitation. J Med Dev 9(3)
37. Maciejasz P, Eschweiler J, Gerlach-Hahn K, Jansen-Troy A, Leonhardt S (2014) A survey on robotic devices for upper limb rehabilitation. J Neuroeng Rehab 11(1):1–29
38. Perry JC, Rosen J, Burns S (2007) Upper-limb powered exoskeleton design. IEEE/ASME Trans Mech 12(4):408–417
39. Nef T, Guidali M, Riener R (2009) Armin III-arm therapy exoskeleton with an ergonomic shoulder actuation. Appl Bionics Biomech 6(2):127–142
40. Kim B, Deshpande AD (2017) An upper-body rehabilitation exoskeleton harmony with an anatomical shoulder mechanism: design, modeling, control, and performance evaluation. Int J Robot Res 36(4):414–435
41. Qammaz A, Argyros AA (2019) Mocapnet: ensemble of SNN encoders for 3D human pose estimation in RGB images
42. Sabatini AM (2011) Estimating three-dimensional orientation of human body parts by inertial/magnetic sensing. Sensors 11(2):1489–1525
43. Lisini Baldi T, Scheggi S, Meli L, Mohammadi M, Prattichizzo D (2017) GESTO: a glove for enhanced sensing and touching based on inertial and magnetic sensors for hand tracking and cutaneous feedback. IEEE Trans Hum-Mach Syst 47(6):1066–1076
44. Mohammadi M, Baldi TL, Scheggi S, Prattichizzo D (2016) Fingertip force estimation via inertial and magnetic sensors in deformable object manipulation. In: Proceedings IEEE haptics symposium. IEEE, pp 284–289
45. Kim YS, Soh BS, Lee S (2005) A new wearable input device: Scurry. IEEE Trans Ind Electron 52(6):1490–1499
46. Kieliba PJ, Veltink VH, Lisini Baldi T, Prattichizzo D, Santaera G, Bicchi A, Bianchi M, Van Beijnum BJF (2018) Comparison of three hand pose reconstruction algorithms using inertial and magnetic measurement units. In: 2018 IEEE-RAS 18th international conference on humanoid robots (humanoids). IEEE, pp 1–9
47. Jacobsen SC, Ko H, Iversen EK, Davis CC (1989) Antagonistic control of a tendon driven manipulator. In: Proceedings, 1989 international conference on robotics and automation. IEEE, pp 1334–1339
48. Dragusanu M, Baldi TL, Iqbal Z, Prattichizzo D, Malvezzi M (2020) Design, development, and control of a tendon-actuated exoskeleton for wrist rehabilitation and training. In: 2020 IEEE international conference on robotics and automation (ICRA). IEEE, pp 1749–1754
49. Dombroski CE, Balsdon MER, Froats A (2014) The use of a low cost 3D scanning and printing tool in the manufacture of custom-made foot orthoses: a preliminary study. BMC Res Notes 7(1):443

50. Baldi TL, Farina F, Garulli A, Giannitrapani A, Prattichizzo D (2019) Upper body pose estimation using wearable inertial sensors and multiplicative kalman filter. IEEE Sens J
51. Design of a modular hand exoskeleton for rehabilitation and training, Volume 5: Biomedical and biotechnology of ASME international mechanical engineering congress and exposition
52. Santello M, Flanders M, Soechting JF (1998) Postural hand synergies for tool use. J Neurosci 18(23):10105–10115
53. Bicchi A, Gabiccini M, Santello M (2011) Modelling natural and artificial hands with synergies. Philos Trans R Soc B 366(1581):3153–3161
54. Prattichizzo D, Malvezzi M, Gabiccini M, Bicchi A (2013) On motion and force controllability of precision grasps with hands actuated by soft synergies. IEEE Trans Robot 29(6):1440–1456
55. Catalano MG, Grioli G, Farnioli E, Serio A, Piazza C, Bicchi A (2014) Adaptive synergies for the design and control of the Pisa/IIT softhand. Int J Robot Res 33(5):768–782
56. Gioioso G, Salvietti G, Malvezzi M, Prattichizzo D (2013) Mapping synergies from human to robotic hands with dissimilar kinematics: an approach in the object domain. IEEE Trans Robot 29(4):825–837
57. Malvezzi M, Lisini Baldi T, Villani A, Ciccarese F, Prattichizzo D (2020) Design, development, and preliminary evaluation of a highly wearable exoskeleton. In: Proceedings of the IEEE international symposium in robot and human interactive communication, Napoli, IT, September 2020
58. Malvezzi M, Gioioso G, Salvietti G, Prattichizzo D (2015) Syngrasp: a matlab toolbox for underactuated and compliant hands. IEEE Robot Autom Mag 22(4):52–68
59. Bianchi M, Liarokapis MV (2013) Handcorpus, a new open-access repository for sharing experimental data and results on human and artificial hands. In: IEEE world haptics conference (WHC)
60. Achilli GM, Amici C, Dragusanu M, Gobbo M, Logozzo S, Malvezzi M, Tiboni M, Valigi MC (2023) Soft, rigid, and hybrid robotic exoskeletons for hand rehabilitation: roadmap with impairment-oriented rationale for devices design and selection. Appl Sci 13(20)
61. Nycz CJ, Meier TB, Carvalho T, Meier G, Fischer GS (2018) Design criteria for hand exoskeletons: measurement of forces needed to assist finger extension in traumatic brain injury patients. IEEE Robot Autom Lett 3(4):3285–3292
62. Boser QA, Dawson MR, Schofield JS, Dziwenko GY, Hebert JS (2021) Defining the design requirements for an assistive powered hand exoskeleton: a pilot explorative interview study and case series. Prosthet Orthot Int 45(2):161–169
63. Lee J, Kunii TL (1995) Model-based analysis of hand posture. IEEE Comput Graph Appl 15(5):77–86
64. In H, Kang BB, Sin MK, Cho K-Y (2015) Exo-glove: a wearable robot for the hand with a soft tendon routing system. IEEE Robot Autom Mag 22(1):97–105
65. Li M, He B, Liang Z, Zhao C-G, Chen J, Zhuo Y, Guanghua X, Xie J, Althoefer K (2019) An attention-controlled hand exoskeleton for the rehabilitation of finger extension and flexion using a rigid-soft combined mechanism. Front Neurorobot 13:34
66. Borboni A, Mor M, Faglia R (2016) Gloreha-hand robotic rehabilitation: design, mechanical model, and experiments. J Dyn Syst Measur Control 138(11)
67. Dragusanu M, Iqbal MZ, Baldi TL, Prattichizzo D, Malvezzi M (2022) Design, development, and control of a hand/wrist exoskeleton for rehabilitation and training. IEEE Trans Robot 38(3):1472–1488
68. Dragusanu M, Lisini Baldi T, Iqbal Z, Prattichizzo D, Malvezzi M (2020) Design, development and control of a tendon-actuated exoskeleton for wrist rehabilitation and training. In: Proceedings of the IEEE international conference on robotics and automation, Paris, FR, June 2020
69. Valero-Cuevas FJ, Elise Johanson M, Towles JD (2003) Towards a realistic biomechanical model of the thumb: the choice of kinematic description may be more critical than the solution method or the variability/uncertainty of musculoskeletal parameters. J Biomech 36(7):1019–1030

70. Kratochwill TR, Hitchcock J, Horner RH, Levin JR, Odom SL, Rindskopf DM, Shadish WR (2010) Single-case designs technical documentation. What works clearinghouse
71. Ao D, Song R, Gao J (2016) Movement performance of human-robot cooperation control based on EMG-driven hill-type and proportional models for an ankle power-assist exoskeleton robot. IEEE Trans Neur Syst Rehab Eng 25(8):1125–1134
72. Dragusanu M, Troisi D, Villani A, Prattichizzo D, Malvezzi M (2022) Design and prototyping of an underactuated hand exoskeleton with fingers coupled by a gear-based differential. Front Robot AI 9
73. Cobos S, Ferre M, Sánchez-Urán MA, Ortego J (2007) Constraints for realistic hand manipulation. Proc Presence, 369–370
74. Malvezzi D, Baldi TL, Villani A, Ciccarese F, Prattichizzo D (2020) Design, development, and preliminary evaluation of a highly wearable exoskeleton. In: 2020 29th IEEE international conference on robot and human interactive communication (RO-MAN). IEEE, pp 1055–1062
75. Birglen L, Gosselin CM (2006) Force analysis of connected differential mechanisms: application to grasping. Int J Robot Res 25(10):1033–1046
76. Birglen L, Gosselin CM (2003) On the force capability of underactuated fingers. In: 2003 IEEE international conference on robotics and automation (Cat. No. 03CH37422), vol 1. IEEE, pp 1139–1145
77. Fukaya N, Toyama S, Asfour T, Dillmann R (2000) Design of the tuat/karlsruhe humanoid hand. In: Proceedings. 2000 IEEE/RSJ international conference on intelligent robots and systems (IROS 2000) (Cat. No. 00CH37113), vol 3. IEEE, pp 1754–1759
78. Zappatore GA, Reina G, Messina A (2017) Analysis of a highly underactuated robotic hand. Int J Mech Control 18(4):17–23
79. Massa B, Roccella S, Carrozza MC, Dario P (2002) Design and development of an underactuated prosthetic hand. In: Proceedings 2002 IEEE international conference on robotics and automation (Cat. No. 02CH37292), vol 4. IEEE, pp 3374–3379
80. Baril M, Laliberté T, Gosselin C, Routhier F (2013) On the design of a mechanically programmable underactuated anthropomorphic prosthetic gripper. J Mech Des 135(12):121008
81. Kontoudis GP, Liarokapis MV, Zisimatos AG, Mavrogiannis CI, Kyriakopoulos KJ (2015) Open-source, anthropomorphic, underactuated robot hands with a selectively lockable differential mechanism: Towards affordable prostheses. In: 2015 IEEE/RSJ international conference on intelligent robots and systems (IROS). IEEE, pp 5857–5862
82. Carbone G, Gerding EC, Corves B, Cafolla D, Russo M, Ceccarelli M (2020) Design of a two-dofs driving mechanism for a motion-assisted finger exoskeleton. Appl Sci 10(7)
83. Cafolla D, Carbone G (2014) A study of feasibility of a human finger exoskeleton. In: Service orientation in holonic and multi-agent manufacturing and robotics. Springer, pp 355–364
84. Zappatore GA, Reina G, Messina A (2019) A toolbox for the analysis of the grasp stability of underactuated fingers. Robotics 8(2):26
85. Cafolla D, Ceccarelli M, Wang MF, Carbone G (2016) 3D printing for feasibility check of mechanism design. Int J Mech Control 17(1):3–12
86. Mulatto S, Formaglio A, Malvezzi M, Prattichizzo D (2012) Using postural synergies to animate a low-dimensional hand avatar in haptic simulation. IEEE Trans Haptics 6(1):106–116

Chapter 3
Design of Haptic Devices for Rehabilitive/Assistive Applications

Technology is becoming an integral part of our daily lives, with emerging innovations focused on replicating tactile, kinesthetic, and skin sensations gaining attention across various fields. These advancements allow enriching human sensory experiences, particularly in virtual environments, augmented or mixed reality, and teleoperation tasks. Research shows that tactile technologies not only improve user engagement in teleoperation but also boost accuracy and performance [1, 2]. Notably, haptic technologies are finding valuable applications in telemedicine and telerehabilitation. The use of haptic robotic devices in rehabilitation is growing rapidly. According to *Mordor Intelligence*, the rehabilitation robotics market is projected to achieve a compound annual growth rate of approximately 26% between 2021 and 2026. Several factors drive this trend, including the complexity and long-term nature of medical rehabilitation for injury sufferers, which often involves both psychological and physical challenges with uncertain outcomes. Robotic rehabilitation therapy can provide high-intensity training without the constant need for direct physical interaction from physiotherapists.

These applications have gained particular importance since the onset of the COVID-19 pandemic, when maintaining social distance and minimizing physical human contact, such as handshakes and holding hands, became essential [3]. The pandemic made personal computers, tablets, and smartphones our primary means of staying connected to society, enabling active and effective communication with family, friends, and colleagues. This disruption in affective communication was especially profound for critically ill patients, who were isolated in hospital beds, unable to interact with their loved ones. Another crucial concern was the heightened risk of contagion for healthcare workers, such as doctors, nurses, and hospital staff, during patient interactions, necessitating that physical contact be restricted to only essential tasks [4]. Beyond the physical suffering caused by the illness, both patients and healthcare workers experienced significant psychological and emotional distress [5, 6]. A portion of this non-physical pain could be alleviated if some form of contact with family and friends were restored. Innovative solutions, such as

M. Dragusanu, *Design of Soft–Rigid Devices for Rehabilitative and Assistive Robotics*, Springer Theses, https://doi.org/10.1007/978-3-031-84823-0_3

autonomous mobile robots equipped with tablets to facilitate video calls for patients, have recently been proposed to address this need [7].

The goal of this thesis chapter is to explore how haptic robotics can offer innovative solutions for remote assistance, allowing the transmission of tactile sensations between individuals and enabling remote rehabilitation, with a particular focus on hand-based interactions, as discussed in the introductory chapter.

3.1 State of the Art

The hand serves as one of the primary interfaces through which humans interact with their environment and is a key focus in the development of haptic technologies. Most haptic devices designed for tactile stimulation are concentrated on the fingers or wrist, with fewer targeting the palm specifically [8]. However, as noted by Klatzky and Lederman, tactile sensations in the palm significantly influence hand-closing movements [9]. The biomechanical structure of the palm-comprising bones, muscles, and ligaments-enables complex movements such as radial abduction, ulnar adduction, palmar flexion/dorsiflexion, and thumb opposition/apposition. During apposition, the thumb's side contacts other fingers, while during opposition, the thumb's distal pulp touches the fingertips of other digits [10].

Unfortunately, the hand can be affected by various traumas, fractures, sprains, tissue pathologies, and chronic pain conditions. Many of these issues are treated using Manual Therapy (MT), which involves joint mobilization, rhythmic stimulation, and targeted force applications. MT is also a common alternative treatment for musculoskeletal conditions like Complex Regional Pain Syndrome Type-I (CRPS-I), a chronic pain disorder characterized by altered sensation [11]. Other hand conditions, such as carpal tunnel syndrome, stenosing tenosynovitis (trigger finger), and De Quervain's tenosynovitis, are also commonly treated with MT. These conditions cause pain, tingling, numbness, and restricted movement in the hands, often impacting daily function.

Treatment for hand conditions typically follows two main paths: conservative clinical therapy or, in severe cases, surgical intervention. Conservative therapy includes patient education on pain management, desensitization techniques, gradual strength and flexibility exercises, and manual therapy. Research has shown that MT can reduce pain and improve hand functionality [12, 13]. Preliminary studies suggest that MT also has analgesic effects by activating the enzymatic antioxidative system, reducing oxidative stress, which is responsible for triggering inflammatory events and thereby alleviating pain [14–16].

Haptic technologies have become increasingly integrated into both preclinical research and therapeutic applications. For instance, research has demonstrated that haptic devices can aid in the occupational therapy of children with autism spectrum disorder by facilitating smoother transitions during treatment [17]. Similarly, in [18], the authors support the potential for haptic-based mechanical therapy to improve cardiovascular autonomic control in patients with Parkinson's disease.

Research in the field of haptics has provided valuable clinical tools for the rehabilitation and treatment of hand issues, including joint, ligament, and skin conditions. As highlighted by Choukou et al. [19], various haptic technologies, often integrated with robotic systems [20–23], Virtual Reality (VR) environments, and gaming platforms [24–26], or a combination of both [27, 28], have been utilized for rehabilitating the paretic upper limbs of stroke patients.

Haptic devices designed for the palm of the hand can be broadly categorized into two types: **desktop-grounded** devices, which are anchored to an external base, and **wearable** devices. Regarding grounded devices, Iwata et al. [29] introduced a system that alters the shape of the surface in contact with the hand through the vertical movement of pistons, while Borst et al. [30] developed an actuator array that provides vibrotactile stimuli to the user's palm. Bouri et al. [31] presented an innovative haptic device specifically designed for rehabilitating hemiplegic children, which activates hand joints in a manner similar to manual therapy (MT).

In [32, 33], the authors explored novel haptic technologies to address graphomotor difficulties in handwriting and drawing, designing tools and protocols for eye-hand coordination assessment and therapy. Additionally, Ferre et al. [34] developed a haptic framework that replicates manual therapy techniques using a multifinger device. In another study, Martínez et al. [35] created a planar grounded device that uses ultrasound technology to deliver haptic feedback to the user's palm without physical contact, allowing the hand to move freely within a larger workspace.

However, no current devices are capable of delivering precise, controlled forces or vibrations to specific points on the palm. This gap in the literature makes the basis for my research on desktop-grounded devices.

In this chapter, as outlined in Sect. 3.2, is introduced a novel haptic device. This device is for preclinical investigations into the correlation between symptom reduction in Complex Regional Pain Syndrome Type-I (CRPS-I) and MT, as well as for the clinical treatment of CRPS-I and other conditions affecting the carpus and metacarpus. The device mimics traditional mechanical and rhythmic stimulations characteristic of manual therapy.

However, research in this area is increasingly shifting toward wearable devices to fully liberate users and expand their workspace flexibility. Wearability has now become a critical requirement for haptic devices. In this context, a trade-off is often necessary between the size of the palm area that can be stimulated and the number of actuators used [8]. Most devices in this field rely on localized, fixed contact points on the palm. These can be broadly categorized into two types: vibrotactile actuators and mechanical actuators. Mechanical actuators typically use tightening bands to apply normal pressure to the palm, as demonstrated in [36], but this technology limits the sensations users can experience to predetermined and basic stimuli. Similarly, Minamizawa et al. [37] introduced a band with a mobile contact surface for the palm, while Achibet et al. [38] developed a passive device using an elastic band to provide haptic feedback related to hand-body distance.

In [39, 40], two haptic gloves with multiple mechanical actuation points were designed: the first used small rigid links, and the second relied on tendon-based actuation. However, these devices face the challenge of requiring a high number of actuators to cover the large surface area of the palm, which increases complexity. To mitigate this, some researchers, such as those in [41–43], opted for vibrotactile matrices in contact with the palm, reducing the number of mechanical actuators. This approach simplifies the design but diminishes the realism of the transmitted stimuli. A combination of mechanical and vibrotactile stimuli was explored by Kovacs et al. [44], where a mobile mass touches the palm when a hand avatar in virtual reality collides with objects in the virtual environment. Pneumatic solutions were proposed by Kajimoto et al. [45] and by Zubrycki and Grzegorz [46], providing another alternative for haptic feedback. Additionally, the authors in [47] introduced a wearable haptic interface for natural object manipulation in virtual reality, using a sensorized mobile mass grounded on the wrist to render contact forces.

Haptic devices with mobile and orientable contact areas, such as those presented by Trinitatova et al. in [48, 49], share similarities with the design proposed in this thesis. However, the focus of this work is on exploring ways to minimize the device's footprint on the palm and reduce the overall mechanical load on the hand by using cable-driven force transmission.

The device introduced in this thesis stimulates a large area of the palm with only three actuators, ensuring both effective force application and improved wearability. The details of this device, which applies force to the palm, are discussed in Sect. 3.4. An enhanced version of its end-effector, capable of delivering both force and vibration for rehabilitative purposes, is presented in Sect. 3.6.

A device designed for both assistance and rehabilitation is presented in Sect. 3.3. However, the primary focus of this work is on enhancing social and emotional interactions, specifically through handshaking and holding hands, which play crucial roles in our interpersonal relationships. The goal is to introduce an additional sensory channel to these interactions, allowing the tactile sensation of holding hands to be transmitted between people who are physically apart. Human-robot handshakes have been explored in the literature from various perspectives, with the aim of enabling robots to perform handshakes that feel human-like, conveying emotional and affective content, as well as serving rehabilitative purposes. A comprehensive review of the current state of the art was recently presented in [50].

For instance, in [51], researchers conducted experiments with humanoid robots to examine how haptic interaction and facial expression can convey emotions during a handshake. Beaudoin et al. [52] developed a haptic device to reproduce a realistic human-robot handshake, featuring an anthropomorphic design with a focus on replicating the compliance of the human hand, particularly the palm. In [53], Vigni et al. investigated the importance of feedback in handshake behavior by comparing open-loop and closed-loop force control systems. Their experiments, conducted with a soft, underactuated anthropomorphic robot hand equipped with pressure sensors, demonstrated the critical role of haptic feedback and closed-loop control in creating a more natural handshake. However, such systems tend to be complex and costly, making them impractical for widespread use outside of laboratory settings.

Meanwhile, the field of wearable haptics is rapidly advancing, offering compact and lightweight devices that can not only render forces [54] and simulate contact with angled surfaces [55] on the fingertips and palm, but also provide haptic feedback as a social cue during remote communication [56]. An example is the work by Teh et al. [57], who introduced a mobile, wearable interaction system allowing users to send and receive touch and hug sensations.

In this thesis, it is proposed a novel haptic system capable of both sensing and applying the tactile pressure experienced when two people hold hands. While initially focused on interpersonal communication, the system is designed with future potential applications in clinical research and investigation.

Desktop-Grounded

3.2 HAPP

In this section, leveraging our expertise in hand stimulation by haptic devices described in the following on this chapter and robotic systems for rehabilitation described in Chap. 2, here it is presented HAPP (see Fig. 3.1), a haptic device for preclinical investigation on correlation between CRPS-I symptoms reduction and MT, and also for clinical treatment of CRPS-I and other diseases of carpus and metacarpus, by mimicking traditional mechanical and rhythmic stimulations proper of manual treatments. The haptic device is designed as a parallel kinematic structure with 3-DoFs, enabling planar movement and orientation of its interchangeable end-effector beneath the patient's palm. This allows the device to deliver targeted

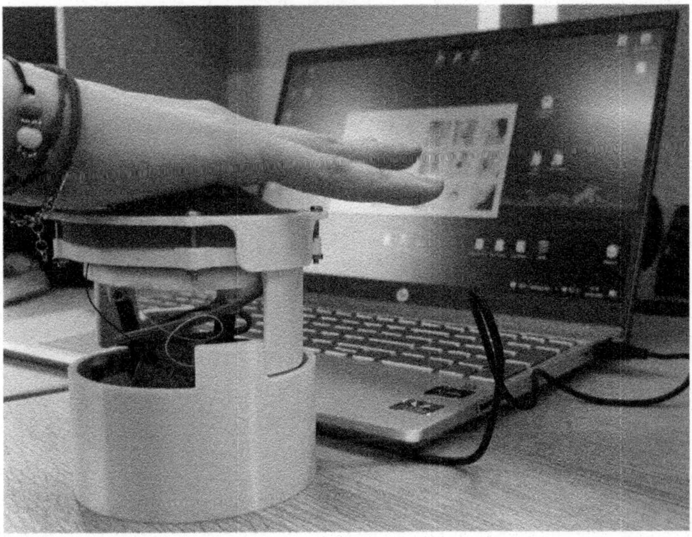

Fig. 3.1 HAPP prototype during preliminary investigation. Reproduced from [58] with permission from IEEE. © IEEE 2022

mechanical stimulation tailored to the researcher's specific needs and objectives. In the current prototype, the end-effector is designed to apply controlled forces to stimulate predefined areas of the palm. To ensure sterility, a silicone rubber pad is placed between the patient's palm and the end-effector. While silicone facilitates sterilization, it does affect the transmission of forces to the patient. Consequently, theoretical studies and practical tests have been conducted to account for these variations and accurately assess the forces applied by the device.

3.2.1 Device Description

In this section, it is detailed the HAPP design and hardware components. The CAD model, shown in Fig. 3.2. All components were 3D-printed using ABS via FDM technology. The device is composed of two main parts: a fixed section, referred to as the *bottom part*, and an interchangeable section, known as the *top part*. The *bottom*

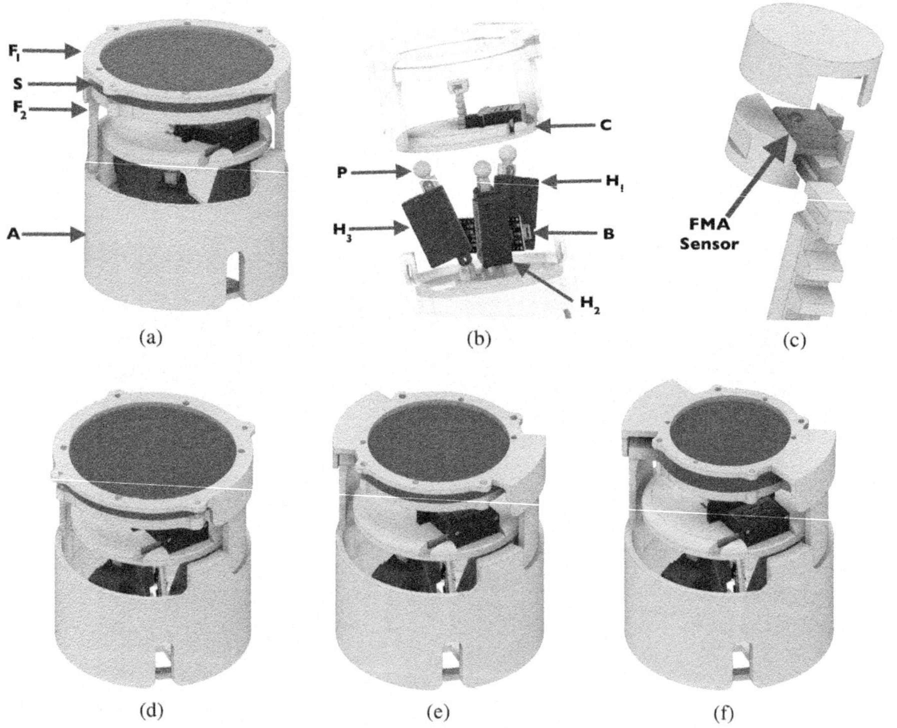

Fig. 3.2 HAPP main features. **a** HAPP external CAD model. **b** HAPP internal CAD model. **c** CAD model for the FMA sensor housing. **d–f** CAD model of the top part with different sizes, i.e. large (**a**), medium (**b**) and small (**c**). Reproduced from [58] with permission from IEEE. © IEEE 2022

part houses the electronic components, the actuation module, and a circular plate containing the device's end-effector, denoted as **B**, $\mathbf{H}_i$, and **C** in Fig. 3.2b. The *top part* is designed to contact the user's palm and can be easily attached to the support base (**A** in Fig. 3.2a) using a simple twisting motion.

The device allows for the interchangeability of various support structures to accommodate users with different hand sizes. Specifically, the *top part* is available in small, medium, and large sizes, as shown in Fig. 3.2d–f. The end-effector, identified as part **C**, contains a housing for a servomotor that drives a rack-and-pinion mechanism. The servomotor used is the Kuman MG90S (Kuman Trade Shenzhen Co., Ltd., US), which provides a stall torque of 25 N cm at 6 V. The motor shaft enables HAPP to exert the necessary force on targeted areas of the *top part*. To offer various tactile stimuli on the user's palm, the head of the shaft is designed to be interchangeable. The CAD model of the force sensor is illustrated in Fig. 3.2c. The sensor employed is the FMA MicroForce Sensor FMAMSDXX025WCSC3 (Honeywell, North Carolina), a piezoresistive-based force sensor that outputs a digital signal proportional to the applied force. The chosen model has a force range of 25 N, with an accuracy of 0.5 N, and is interfaced via the SPI protocol. It operates at a maximum clock frequency of 800 kHz and is powered with a 3.3 V supply. Part **C** also plays a crucial role in the orientation of the end-effector, as its lower section houses spherical joints connecting the actuation module $\mathbf{H}_i$ to part **C**. These spherical housings, arranged in a Y-shape, align with the actuators. The device uses Actuonix PQ12-P linear actuators, which have a maximum stroke of 20 mm and can exert forces up to 45 N. The main specifications of these actuators are summarized in Table 2.4. Three actuators control the movement and orientation of plate **C**, connected via rigid spherical links, denoted as **P**. The actuators are inclined at 45° relative to the plate to ensure device stability, structural integrity, and compactness. The entire system is managed using an Arduino Nano 3.0. To prevent direct contact between the motor shaft and the user's palm, the *top part* of the device is divided into two sections: **F1** and **F2**. These sections accommodate a soft, sterilizable material (**S**). **F1** is attached to the *bottom part*, while **F2** is fixed to **F1**. The inserted material is a silicone rubber pad made from Eco-flex 00-30 (Smooth-On, Inc., US), a bi-component silicone rubber with a platinum catalyst that allows for a hardness range of [0−30] on the Shore A scale (ASTM D-412). The pad is created through molding and cured for four hours. The mold, 3D-printed in ABS, is coated with Easy Release 200 (Mann Release Technologies, Inc., US) to facilitate pad removal after curing. The chemical properties of the silicone rubber allow for sterilization, either by cleaning with 70 % ethanol (CH_3CH_2OH) or autoclaving, as the silicone maintains its elasticity up to 230°C, well above the standard autoclaving temperature of 180 °C.

3.2.2 Mathematical Model

3.2.2.1 Configuration Analysis

From the kinematics point of view, HAPP is a 3-RPS (Revolute-Prismatic-Spherical), 3-DoFs parallel mechanism. Let us indicate with B_i, $i = 1, 2, 3$ the centers of the spherical joints on the *end effector* **C**, with O_1 the center of the circle passing through them, and with b its radius. Let us also indicate with $S_1 = \langle O_1, x_1, y_1, z_1 \rangle$ a reference frame in which the x_1 axis is parallel to $\overrightarrow{O_1 B_1}$, z_1 is orthogonal to the plane defined by the B_i points, and y_1 is consequently defined. We assume that B_i points form an equilateral triangle, the coordinates of each vertex B_i, expressed in the S_1 reference frame are collected in the three-dimensional vectors $\mathbf{b}_i^1 = [b_{ix}^1, b_{iy}^1, b_{iz}^1]^\mathrm{T}$.

Each leg is composed of two links: the first is connected to the fixed base trough a revolute joint, the second one is connected to the end effector through a spherical joint. The links are connected to each other through a prismatic joint. Let us indicate with $\mathbf{u}_i$ the unit vector identifying, for each leg, the direction of the revolute joint axes. We can then define the plane π_i passing through B_i and perpendicular to $\mathbf{u}_i$. The revolute joint axes intersect this plane in A_i points.

On the *bottom part*, we define O_0 as the center of the circle passing through A_i, and with a its radius. Let $S_0 = \langle O_0, x, y, z \rangle$ be a reference frame on the *bottom part*, with origin in O_0, x axis parallel to the $\overrightarrow{O_0 A_1}$ vector, z axis orthogonal to the plane defined by A_i points, and y consequently defined. Also in this case we assume that A_i points define a equilateral triangle.

The movement of the end-effector relative to the *bottom part* is governed by the displacement imposed by the linear actuators and the kinematic constraints of the mechanical structure. Specifically, each leg moves within a plane, meaning that the points B_i are constrained to move within the planes, that were defined earlier, π_i.

To express this mathematically, let i_*, j_*, k_*, where $* = x, y, z$, represent the unit vector components corresponding to the axes x_1, y_1, and z_1, respectively, as expressed in the reference frame S_0. Using these components, the rotation matrix **R** can be defined to describe the transformation between frames S_1 and S_0.

The coordinates of B_i w.r.t. S_0, collected in the three dimensional-vectors $\mathbf{b}_i = [b_{i,x}, b_{i,y}, b_{i,z}]^\mathrm{T}$, can be evaluated as

$$\mathbf{b}_i = \mathbf{p} + \mathbf{R}\mathbf{b}_i^1, \tag{3.1}$$

where $\mathbf{p} = [p_1, p_2, p_3]^\mathrm{T}$ is the three dimensional vector containing the coordinates of O_1 w.r.t. S_0.

Since B_i move on the three fixed planes π_i, the following constraint equations hold

$$b_{1,y} = 0, \quad b_{2,x} = \frac{1}{\sqrt{3}} b_{2,y}, \quad b_{3,x} = -\frac{1}{\sqrt{3}} b_{3,y}. \tag{3.2}$$

Equation (3.2) introduces three constraints that limit the generic six-dimensional motion of the mobile platform. In particular, since three independent costraints have been introduced, the mobile platform has 3-DoFs.

The position and orientation of the end effector can be defined by the position and orientation of O_1 w.r.t. S_0, described through its coordinates $\mathbf{p} = [p_x, p_y, p_z]^T$ and Roll (α)-Pitch (β)-Yaw (ϕ) (RPY) angles $\boldsymbol{\varphi} = [\alpha, \beta, \phi]^T$, respectively. Since the platform has 3-DoF, it can be selected three of these six variables and evaluate the remaining ones. A convenient choice for the *independent* variables includes the displacement in the z direction, p_z, and the roll (α) and pitch (β) angles. Let us collect those variables in the vector $\boldsymbol{\xi} = [p_z, \alpha, \beta]^T$. Recalling the rotation matrix expression as a function of RPY angles, and the constraints in Eq. (3.2), it can be evaluated the other variables as

$$\phi = \arctan\left(\frac{\sin\beta\sin\alpha}{\cos\beta + \cos\alpha}\right), \tag{3.3}$$

$$p_x = \frac{b}{2}\left(\cos\phi\cos\beta - \sin\phi\sin\beta\sin\alpha - \cos\phi\cos\alpha\right), \tag{3.4}$$

$$p_y = -b\sin\phi\cos\beta. \tag{3.5}$$

To complete the preliminary analysis of the mechanism, let us analyse the position of the pin on the mobile platform, represented by point R. Its coordinates in S_1 frame are:

$$\mathbf{r}^1 = [0, 0, h]^T, \tag{3.6}$$

using the above mentioned relationships, it is possible to evaluate its coordinates with respect to S_0 frame. Finally, using the relationships in Eqs. (3.3)–(3.5) it's possible to express pin position as a function of the independent variables, i.e. $\mathbf{r}(\boldsymbol{\xi})$.

3.2.2.2 Inverse Kinematics

In the inverse kinematics problem, the independent variables $\boldsymbol{\xi} = [p_z, \alpha, \beta]^T$ are defined, and we want to evaluate the corresponding displacements $\mathbf{q} = [q_1, q_2, q_3]^T$ of the linear actuators. For a given $\boldsymbol{\xi}$, Eqs. (3.3)–(3.5) allow to define the vector $\mathbf{p}$ and the rotation matrix $\mathbf{R}$, completing the representation of the mobile platform configuration. Then, from Eq. (3.1), it is possible to evaluate the coordinates of B_i w.r.t. S_0. The actuator displacements q_i can be then evaluated as

$$q_i = s_i - l_0, \tag{3.7}$$

where $s_i = |\mathbf{b}_i - \mathbf{a}_i|$ and l_0 is the actuator length in its reference configuration.

The previously described relationships were utilized to evaluate the device's workspace, which represents the range of positions that point R can reach, based

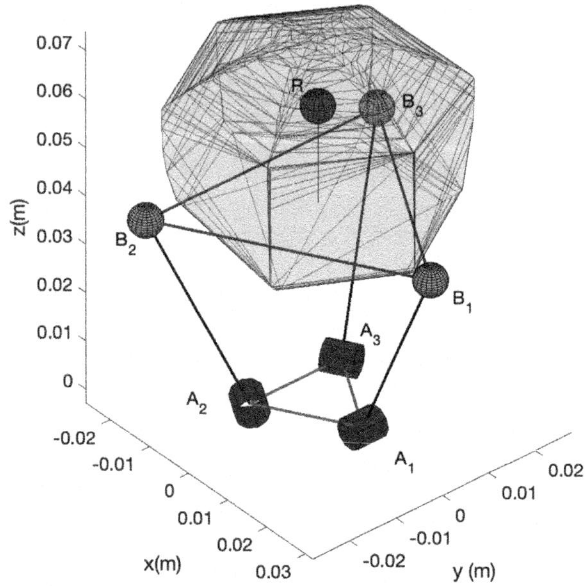

Fig. 3.3 HAPP kinematic scheme and and workspace evaluation (cyan solid). The workspace is represented as the set of possible positions that R point can assume, considering actuators' strokes and device kinematic constraints. Reproduced from [58] with permission from IEEE. © IEEE 2022

on the device's kinematic structure and the actuator stroke. The resulting workspace, calculated using a Matlab script, is illustrated in Fig. 3.3.

A theoretical analysis and experimental investigation were conducted to assess the force that HAPP can apply to a patient's palm. The net theoretical force, $\boldsymbol{f}_n$, depends on the end-effector's orientation angles α and β relative to the normal vector of the silicone rubber plane. In this evaluation, the yaw angle ϕ was disregarded as its value remains limited across all configurations considered.

$$\mathbf{f}_n(t) = |\mathbf{f}_b| \cos(\alpha) \cos(\beta), \tag{3.8}$$

where $|\boldsymbol{f}_b|$ is modulus of the normal force in *bottom part* reference frame evaluated as effect of the end-effector indentation in silicone rubber pad:

$$|\mathbf{f}_b| = \frac{l_2 - l_1}{l_1} \pi \rho_{EE}^2 E,$$

with $\frac{l_2-l_1}{l_1}$ is the material deformation (l_1 and l_2 are the thins of pad before and after indentation), ρ_{EE} is the radius of the end-effector contact area, and E is the approximated Young modulus of neo-Hookean material, evaluated starting from its hardness on Shore A scale σ_A, according to conversion function presented in [59]:

$$\log_{10}(E) = 0.0235\sigma_A - 0.6403.$$

In accordance with Eq. (3.8), the theoretical maximum forces is function of the end-effector orientation angles (Fig. 3.4a) that can be evaluated starting from pin position:

$$\alpha = \arctan\left(\frac{r_z}{r_y}\right), \text{ and } \beta = \arctan\left(\frac{r_z}{r_x}\right).$$

3.2.3 *Force Evaluation*

On the other hand, several tests were conducted on four discrete points on the pad to determine the actual maximum forces that HAPP can exert. These tests examined the forces at four specific points, as outlined in Table 3.1 and illustrated in Fig. 3.4b, within one quadrant of the pad's circumference. Due to the central symmetry of the pad's geometry, the results can be extrapolated to the entire surface. The testing procedure involved ten repetitions of end-effector indentations to apply maximum forces on the user's hand. The force data were recorded using a high-precision ATI force sensor (ATI Industrial Automation Inc., US), placed between pad and human hand by means of glove pocket. A single participant was involved in the force testing, having provided written informed consent, with the option to withdraw from the experiment at any time. The experimental protocols adhered to the Declaration of Helsinki, ensuring no risk of harmful effects to the participant's health. Data were acquired at a frequency of 1 kHz, with each pressure peak being maintained and then released after a duration of $\delta t = 8.0$ s. The recorded forces $\tilde{f}(t)$ were analyzed to extract information about the net forces applied by HAPP, $\tilde{f}_n$, as:

$$\tilde{\mathbf{f}}_n = \frac{1}{2N\delta t}\sum_{n=0}^{N}\left|\sum_{t=n\delta t}^{(n+1)\delta t}\tilde{\mathbf{f}}(t) - \sum_{t=(n+1)\delta t}^{(n+2)\delta t}\tilde{\mathbf{f}}(t)\right|.$$

To reconstruct the force distribution on the pad surface, interpolation was performed on the collected data. Among various mathematical 3D interpolation functions, a thin-plate spline model was selected, achieving a goodness of fit of $R^2 = 0.97$. The

Table 3.1 Joint extensions and relative orientation angles of end-effector to reach the four selected points for maximum net force distribution reconstruction

Point	p_{H1} (mm)	p_{H2} (mm)	p_{H3} (mm)	α (°)	β (°)
1	20.0	0.0	20.0	−50.0	50.0
2	20.0	0.0	0.0	0.0	50.0
3	0.0	10.0	20.0	−25.6	25.6
4	20.0	20.0	20.0	0.0	0.0

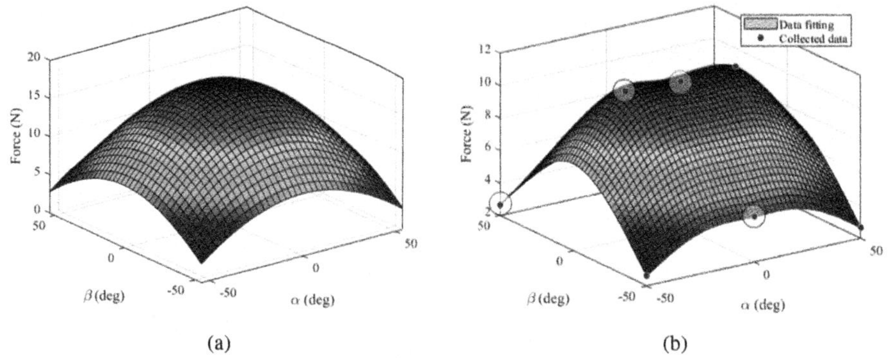

Fig. 3.4 In **a**, the theoretical net force distribution through HAPP silicon pad depending on end-effector orientation angles α and β, in **b** the experimentally estimated net forces reconstructed for symmetry and interpolation by means of repeated force measures in four notable points (circled blue dots). Reproduced from [58] with permission from IEEE. © IEEE 2022

experimental results, graphically represented in Fig. 3.4b, showed generally lower maximum forces compared to theoretical estimations. Additionally, the tests indicated that the user began to lift their hand from the pad once the applied force exceeded 10 N.

3.2.4 Demonstrative Scenario

HAPP was designed to enable researchers and doctors to set up and control the device by using their laptop. Specifically, they can select the desired position, force, and other stimuli references as well as initial information about the discrete anthropometric dimensions that are then sent to the device via USB cable. To facilitate this, the operator has access to a graphical user interface (GUI) that enables easy configuration of stimuli via percentage bars and allows the placement of the piston in one of nine discrete areas on the patient's palm (see Fig. 3.5). This graphical interface is highly modular and easily expandable, enabling users to modify and increase the contact areas at the request of the researcher, as well as integrate future end-effector modules for additional types of stimulation.

A serial connection between the laptop and the device facilitates data exchange in both directions, allowing users to view and record information provided by the device, such as the force measured by the force sensor, for retrospective analysis. The communication protocol is optimized to ensure prompt responsiveness; references are transmitted only when modified by the user. The data sent consists of two bytes: the first carries a modified reference ID, while the second conveys the value within a specified range, as detailed in Table 3.2. Figure 3.6 illustrates the positions that HAPP can reach using the aforementioned GUI.

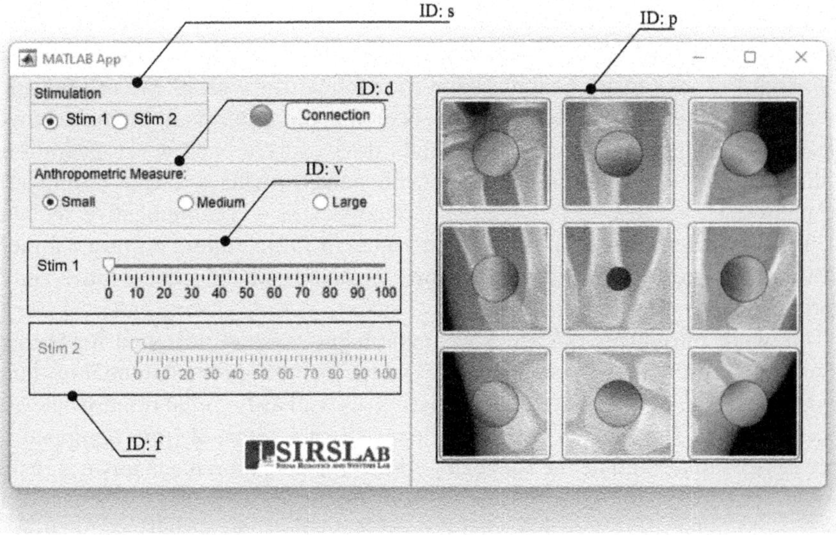

Fig. 3.5 Graphical user interface for HAPP. Reproduced from [58] with permission from IEEE. © IEEE 2022

Table 3.2 ID signals and their values sent from graphic user interface to microcontroller for HAPP setting, regulation, actuation, and control

Reference signal	ID	Values
Stimualtion type	s	$[s, v]$
Anthropometric dimensions	d	$[L, M, S]$
Stimulation 1	v	[0–255]
Stimulation 2	f	[0–255]
Desired position	p	[1–9]

Reproduced from [58] with permission from IEEE. © IEEE 2022

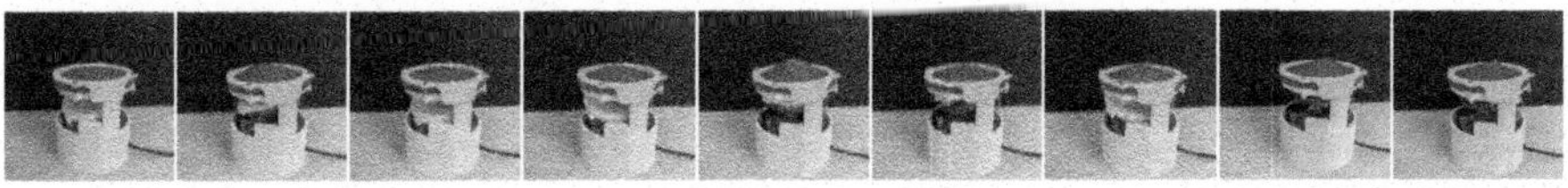

Fig. 3.6 From left to right, the nine discrete positions reached by the haptic device. Reproduced from [58] with permission from IEEE. © IEEE 2022

Wearable

3.3 HANS

While the studies briefly discussed here have provided fundamental insights into the handshaking task from physical, psychological, and emotional perspectives, a significant limitation of these research efforts is that the devices used for perceiving and executing artificial were grounded rather than wearable. Such systems tend to be complex and costly, making them impractical for widespread use outside of laboratory settings. In parallel, there has been notable progress in the field of wearable haptics [60]. Compact and lightweight devices have been developed not only to simulate forces [54] and interactions with slanted surfaces [55] at the fingertips and palm [61], but also to provide haptic feedback as a communicative social cue during remote conversations [56]. For instance, in [57], authors proposed a mobile and wearable interaction system that allows users to send and receive touch and hug interactions.

This work introduces HANS, a wearable haptic system designed for both perceiving and reproducing the contact between hands during remote human-to-human handshakes (e.g. , in teleconference scenarios) as well as for rehabilitation and assistance purposes. The sensing component consists of a series of rings equipped with force sensors that estimate the squeezing force. The actuation mechanism is realized through an active band worn on the palm of the hand. This band is actuated by a motorized tendon-driven system that reduces its length, handshakessimulating the squeezing force on the palm, similar to the h-bracelet presented in [63]. The overall system concept is visually summarized in Fig. 3.7.

3.3.1 Design Requirements

A handshake is a task in which the hand simultaneously perceives and applies a grasping force. Therefore, a haptic system designed to replicate this stimulus must encompass both aspects. In this study, both elements are intended to be rendered in devices worn by the user. Another important consideration in a handshake is that the entire hand is involved, by means actively as an actuator and passively as a sensing system. Designing a device that integrates both functionalities in a single unit is technologically challenging. To enhance versatility for various use cases, the sensing and actuation modules are conceptualized as independent devices: an actuation bracelet and a set of sensing rings. This allows users the flexibility to choose whether to wear one or both devices.

As a first step toward the development of HANS, the study utilizes the findings from [64] to identify the key contact areas involved in the handshake gesture. These areas include the concave space between the thumb and index finger, the lateral side near the little finger, the hand palm.

The fingers are primarily responsible for applying the handshake force through their closure, while the palm predominantly senses this force. Based on these considerations, a set of three rings equipped with force sensors was designed and developed for the proximal phalanges of the thumb, index, and middle fingers to measure the handshake force. The choice of three rings represents a balance between measurement reliability, system wearability, overall complexity, and weight.

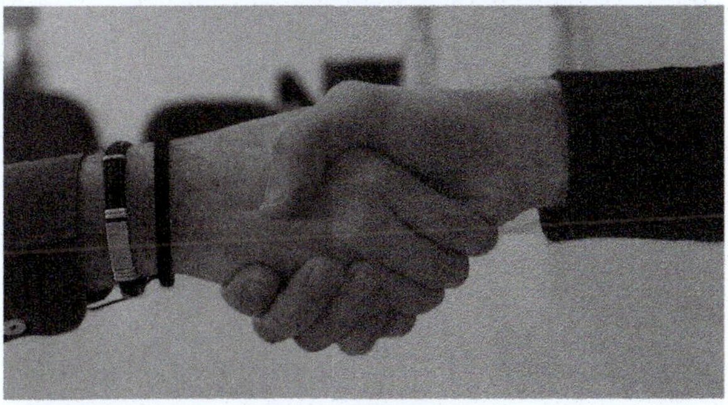

(a)

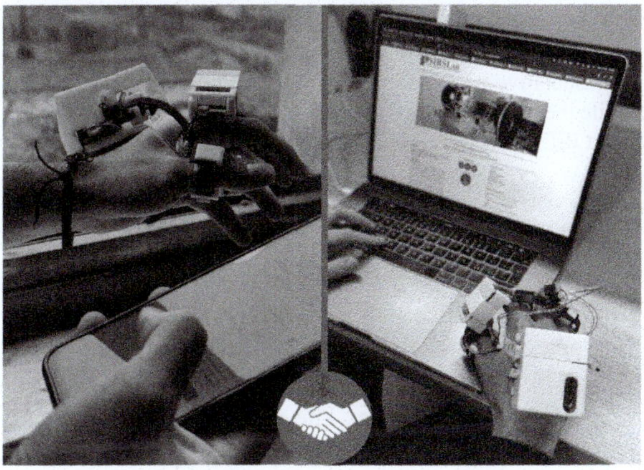

(b)

Fig. 3.7 HANS concept. In **a**, a real handshake. In **b**, a remote handshake realised with HANS. Reproduced from [62] with permission from IEEE. © IEEE 2022

For the actuation part, a bracelet was designed to apply forces to the palm. A preliminary literature review was conducted to determine appropriate force values. The available data vary widely, ranging from a maximum of 6 N in [65] to 40 N in [52], and a mean value of 67 N in [64]. Additionally, handshake force results from a complex, non-homogeneous pressure distribution, and its quantification is highly dependent on the measurement setup.

To quantify the force exerted during the handshake interaction, an ad hoc measuring setup was created using a 3D-printed dummy hand made of ABS, covered with a glove, and equipped with two OptoForce 3D force sensors OMD-20-SE-40N (OptoForce Ltd., Budapest), as illustrated in Fig. 3.8a. These sensors measure three-dimensional force, with a maximum capacity of 40 N along the principal axis (denoted as z) and a resolution of 2.5 mN. They can also measure up to 20 N in the secondary directions (denoted as x and y) with a resolution of 2 mN. Since the focus was on measuring the force normal to the contact point, the sensors were mounted with the z-axis perpendicular to the surface, and only data along this axis were collected.

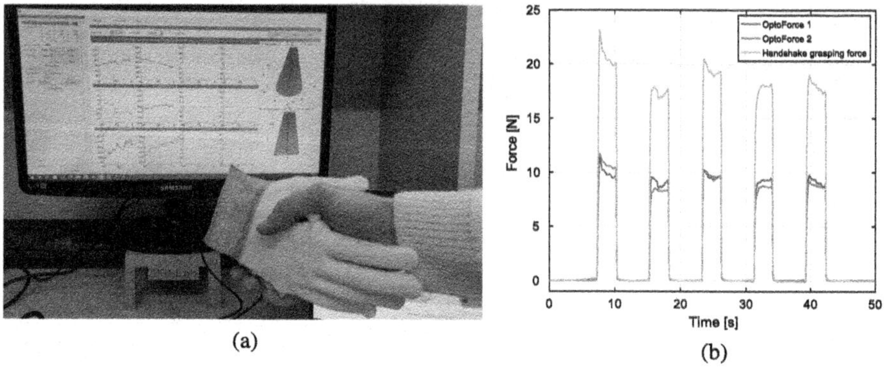

Fig. 3.8 Preliminary experiment for handshake grasping force measurement. In **a**, a user is asked to squeeze the dummy hand and the force applied on the sensors is acquired. In **b**, results of a representative trial. Blue and red lines report force measurements along the z-axis of each sensor, while the total grasping force is depicted in yellow. HANS. Reproduced from [62] with permission from IEEE. © IEEE 2022

Twelve participants (8 males and 4 females, aged 27–54, all right-handed) took part in a preliminary experiment. Each session consisted of three trials, with each trial including five handshakes performed at five-second intervals. Participants were instructed to shake the dummy hand naturally for a duration of three seconds (as shown in Fig. 3.8a). A beep signal was used to cue participants when to initiate and release each handshake. The grasping force was calculated by summing the forces recorded by the sensors. The average grasping force across participants (calculated as the mean of fifteen squeezes for all twelve subjects) was found to be 17.37 ± 5.08 N. A representative trial is reported in Fig. 3.8b.

3.3.2 *The Haptic System*

HANS is composed of two independent modules: one concerning the sensing part used to record the contact forces during the remote handshake while the other concerns the cutaneous device part used to apply those forces based on where it is wearing (i.e. , at the user's palm, forearm or arm).

3.3.2.1 Feeling the Handshake: The Sensing Rings

The device in charge of measuring the handshake force consists of three rings, a flexible support connecting them, and a control box, as depicted in Fig. 3.9a.

The three rings are designed to be worn on the ring finger, index finger, and thumb. They share a common design, with the CAD model shown in Fig. 3.9b. Each

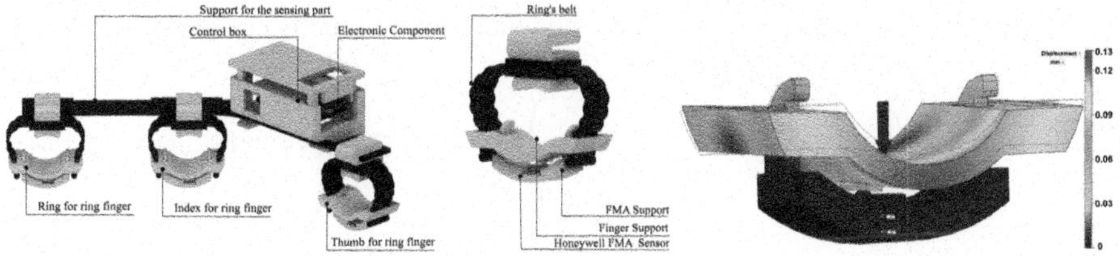

Fig. 3.9 HANS sensing rings. In **a**, the complete CAD model of the sensing device is reported. It consists of three rings, a flexible support connecting them, and a control box containing electronic circuitry and battery. In **b**, the CAD model of a single sensing ring is detailed. In **c**, the results of the FEM structural analysis performed on a single ring simulating the force applied by the finger during the handshake. The padlocks indicate the parts of the model in which constraints are set in the simulation, while the blue arrow indicates the force applied with a magnitude of 10 N. The transparent wireframe CAD model is the reference model, while the coloured surface corresponds to a 1X deformation. HANS. Reproduced from [62] with permission from IEEE. © IEEE 2022 (color figure online)

ring consists of four components: a support for the force sensor, a finger support, a flexible belt, and a mechanism for attaching the ring to the sensing device. The force sensor support, finger support, and attachment mechanism were fabricated using ABS material via FDM. To accommodate different anthropometric characteristics and enhance user comfort, the flexible belt was made using NinjaFlex material, a thermoplastic polyurethane that allows easy wearing while ensuring a secure fit on the proximal phalanx.

Each ring is equipped with an FMA MicroForce Sensor FMAMSDXX025WCSC3 (Honeywell, North Carolina), a piezoresistive force sensor that provides a digital output proportional to the applied force. Known for its small size and high accuracy, this sensor model was selected based on the handshake force measurements described in Sect. 3.3.1. The chosen FMA version has a force range of 25 N and an accuracy of 0.5 N. The sensors communicate using the SPI protocol with a maximum digital clock frequency of 800 kHz, and they are powered with an operating voltage of 3.3 V.

The finger support was specifically designed to ensure effective pressure is applied to the top of the force sensor during finger closure in grasping tasks. FEM analyses were performed during the design phase to verify that the sensor would be properly pressed during use. The control box contains the electronic circuitry and the battery for standalone operation. An Arduino Pro Mini (5 V, 16 MHz) serves as the main control unit, receiving force measurements from the three rings, processing them, and sending the corresponding handshake force data to the actuation bracelet. A Bluetooth RN42-i/rm module is integrated for communication, and the entire sensing device is powered by a 3.7 V Li-Ion battery.

When the sensing device is worn and activated, the user is instructed to keep open the hand while the rings acquire force samples at a frequency of 1 kHz for five seconds. This process is required for calibration, as the average value of the samples is used to establish a zero-force reference, accounting for any bias δ from the ring's positioning on the finger. After calibration, each force value is computed as:

$$FMA_i = \beta_i \left(\frac{1}{20} \sum_{j}^{20} \gamma_{j,i} - \delta_i \right) \quad \forall i \in \{1, 2, 3\}, \forall j \in [1, 20]$$

where δ_i is the offset of the *i-th* FMA force sensor, $\gamma_{j,i}$ is the j-th sample acquired by the i-th force sensor, and β_i is the gain associated to the i-th FMA force sensor, calculated as reported in Sect. 3.3.2.4. The force value is averaged each 20 samples to remove possible unwanted noise. As soon as a new force value is available for all the three sensors, data are packed and sent to the actuation bracelet.

3.3.2.2 Applying the Handshake: The Actuation Bracelet

The proposed actuation bracelet features a flexible structure that wraps around the palm of the hand, while a compact box housing the electronics and motors is positioned on the back of the hand. This design ensures that the actuating mechanism remains unobtrusive, providing a comfortable fit while delivering the necessary force for haptic feedback. The flexible structure conforms to the hand's natural shape, enhancing both comfort and functionality during use, see Fig. 3.10. The hand band is composed of two parts, i.e. one reproducing four fingers close together, and one simulating the thumb.

The outer layer of the hand band is constructed using a flexible material, specifically Flex-45 thermoplastic co-polyurethane, while the inner layer combines various silicone rubbers. To replicate the handshake contact area as reported in [64], the stiffness of specific sections of the hand band was enhanced by incorporating thicker finger pads. Additionally, to make the device's contact feel more human-like, the finger pads were covered with a combination of silicone rubber and ethylene-vinyl acetate (EVA) foam. A Velcro strap connects the two sections, securing the actuation bracelet to the user's hand. The casing on the back of the hand is made of ABS material and houses the key hardware components: an Arduino Pro Mini (5 V, 16 MHz), a Bluetooth RN42-i/rm module, and three Kuman MG90S servo motors (Kuman Trade Shenzhen Co., Ltd., US). Each motor has a stall torque of 25 N cm at 6 V, sufficient for recreating handshake forces according to initial design specifications. To convert the motor's torque into a force applied to the palm, a tendon-driven actuation system was developed. Tendons were connected to each contact area on the palm: four finger pads on one side and a flexible thumb pad on the opposite side. The finger tendons were grouped into two pairs-index/middle and ring/little-and each pair was driven by one motor. The thumb tendon had a dedicated motor. Internal pathways were integrated into the support structure to guide the tendons from the motors to the contact points. Each motor was fitted with a pulley of radius $r = 5$ mm, translating motor rotation θ into tendon displacement d, as per the relation $d = r\theta$. Two pulley types were designed: one with a single groove for the thumb tendon and two double-groove pulleys for the finger tendons.

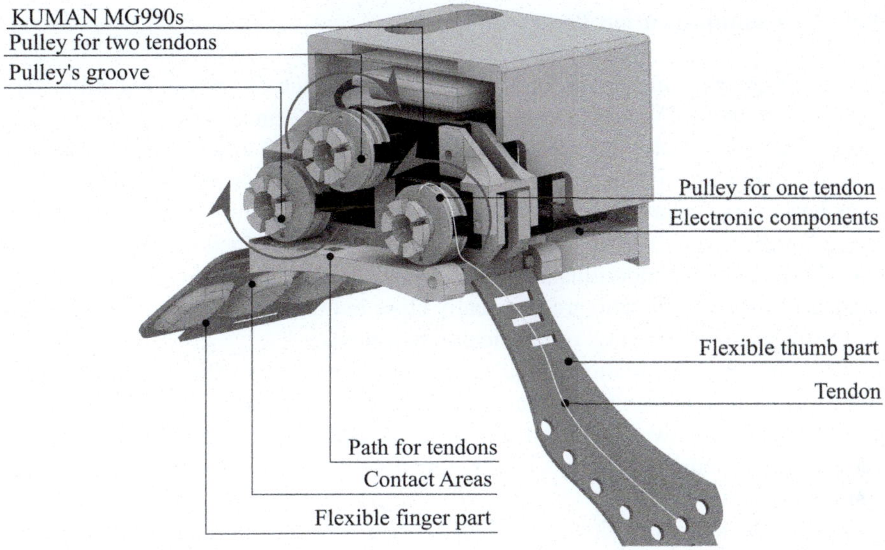

Fig. 3.10 CAD model of HANS actuation bracelet. It consists of a flexible structure designed to wrap the palm of the hand, and a box placed on the hand back containing the electronics and the motors. The hand band is composed of two parts, i.e. one reproducing four fingers close together, and one simulating the thumb. HANS. Reproduced from [62] with permission from IEEE. © IEEE 2022

The bracelet is powered by a 3.7 V Li-Ion battery, with a step-up booster providing 6 V to the servo motors. Both the Velcro strap and the tendons are adjustable, allowing the actuation bracelet to be customized to the user's hand dimensions. When the device is worn and powered on, the motors return to their initial position, and the tendon lengths can be fine-tuned using the additional grooves on the pulleys.

Each motor applies the force measured by its corresponding sensing ring: the thumb motor works with the thumb ring, the index/middle motor with the index ring, and the ring/little motor with the remaining ring. To ensure the applied squeezing force is proportional to the measured force, human hand stiffness data from [66] was used. Specifically, data for the handshake-involved areas, by means *medial and proximal palm* and *rest of distal palm*, were extracted. Since hand stiffness changes with applied force, stiffness values were interpolated to fit the elastic response of the human hand under varying loads. A power-law distribution was used, yielding an adjusted R-squared of 0.79, and the tendon displacement d was calculated as $d = \frac{F}{k(F)}$, where $k(F) = aF^b$ represents stiffness at force F, with parameters $a = 0.76$ and $b = 0.43$ derived from the fit. Given that the FMA force sensors have a full-scale output of 25 N, the maximum tendon displacement is $d_{max} = 8.2$ mm, corresponding to a motor rotation $\theta_{max} \approx 100$ deg, well within the servo motors' range.

3.3.2.3 Communication Protocol

The data transmission system for HANS relies on Bluetooth communication, serving a dual purpose. First, Bluetooth offers a practical balance between rapid system prototyping and developing wireless capabilities. Once the system's functionality is validated, the built-in Bluetooth interface allows for seamless integration with common devices like smartphones and computers, facilitating long-distance connections through web-based applications. Second, the system is designed not only to transmit handshakes between individuals in different locations but also to enable contactless handshakes for people who are physically close but unable to touch due to hygiene protocols, social distancing, or physical impairments.

The sensing and actuation modules communicate via two Bluetooth RN42-i/rm modules, capable of transmitting and receiving data at a frequency of 50 Hz. When both devices are powered on, an initialization phase is triggered, which includes calibrating the sensing rings and setting the motors of the actuation bracelet to their resting position.

The two Bluetooth modules establish a connection and initiate the data exchange process. During the handshake, the sensing device gathers information from the three sensing rings and transmits it to the actuation bracelet. These data are then used to control the handshake force applied by the actuation bracelet. Specifically, the communication protocol is designed such that the actuation device continuously requests updates from the sensing device. The sensing device processes the data from the three FMA force sensors, formats the information into a data packet, and includes start and end markers to frame the data clearly. Upon receiving the data packet, the actuation bracelet converts the sensor readings into digital signals that control the three servo motors, ensuring they replicate the handshake force detected by the sensors.

Figure 3.11 illustrates the communication flow of the wearable haptic system used for the remote handshake interaction.

3.3.2.4 System Calibration and Validation

A preliminary stationary structural FEM analysis was performed on the CAD model of one of the rings to assess the stress and deformation distribution when a force is applied by the finger's proximal phalanx during a handshake. Figure 3.9c presents the results for an applied force of 10 N. The analysis revealed how the force is distributed across the two key components of the ring: the finger support and the sensor support. Specifically, the results demonstrate that the force is effectively concentrated on the sensor, aided by the design of the finger support. This outcome was used to fine-tune the calibration process for each ring after fabrication. Each ring underwent three calibration trials, in which an orthogonal force was applied in a decreasing pattern from 20 to 0 N. The applied and measured forces were simultaneously sampled at 400 Hz using a dual-range Vernier dynamometer (Vernier Software & Technology, US) with an accuracy of 0.05 N, alongside the ring's sensor readings. The dynamometer

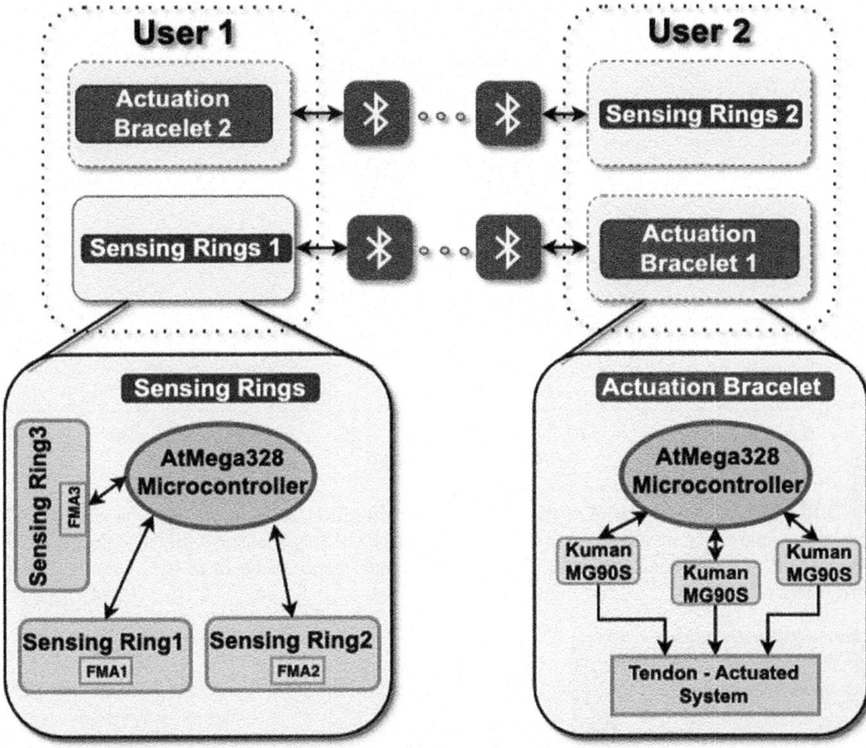

Fig. 3.11 Block diagram representing HANS's functioning. Reproduced from [62] with permission from IEEE. © IEEE 2022

was routed normally to the sensor through a specially designed 3D-printed guide. A systematic error between force exerted and force measured was detected for each ring.

The calibration process involved evaluating and applying a multiplicative gain β, calculated as the mean of the ratio between the applied force and the measured value. This approach aimed to minimize measurement errors for each sensor. Following calibration, the root mean squared error (RMSE) between the applied and measured force profiles was recorded as 0.54 N, 0.75 N, and 0.45 N for the three rings, respectively. These values align well with the sensors' specified accuracy. A representative trial from the calibration procedure is illustrated in Fig. 3.12.

Regarding the actuation bracelet, it was placed on the sensorized dummy hand used in the preliminary experiments (see Sect. 3.3.1) to assess the maximum force exerted by the motors, ensuring safety and facilitating device force analysis (see Fig. 3.13a). Although each motor can produce a maximum torque of 25 N cm, factors such as non-ideal mechanical coupling and friction between components may reduce effective force application.

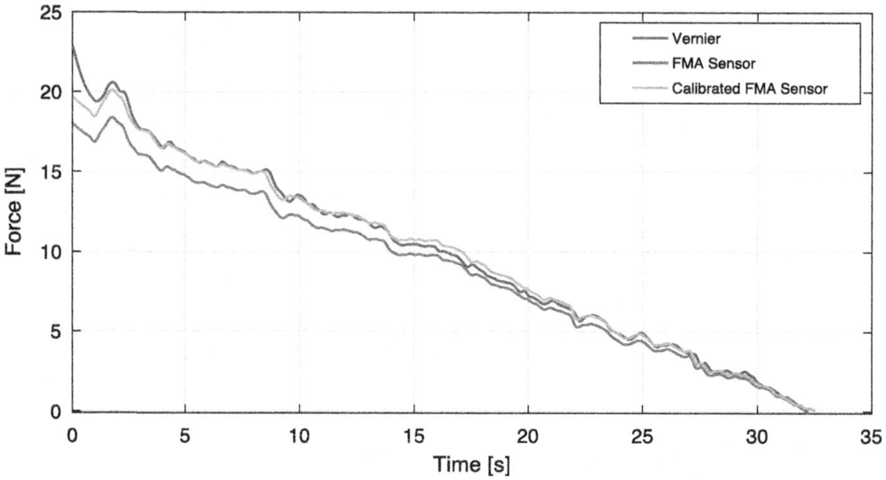

Fig. 3.12 A representative trial of the sensing ring calibration. In blue, the force acquired by the Vernier dynamometer, in red the force values read by the FMA force sensor, while in yellow the FMA force sensor measurement corrected with the gain factor. Reproduced from [62] with permission from IEEE. © IEEE 2022

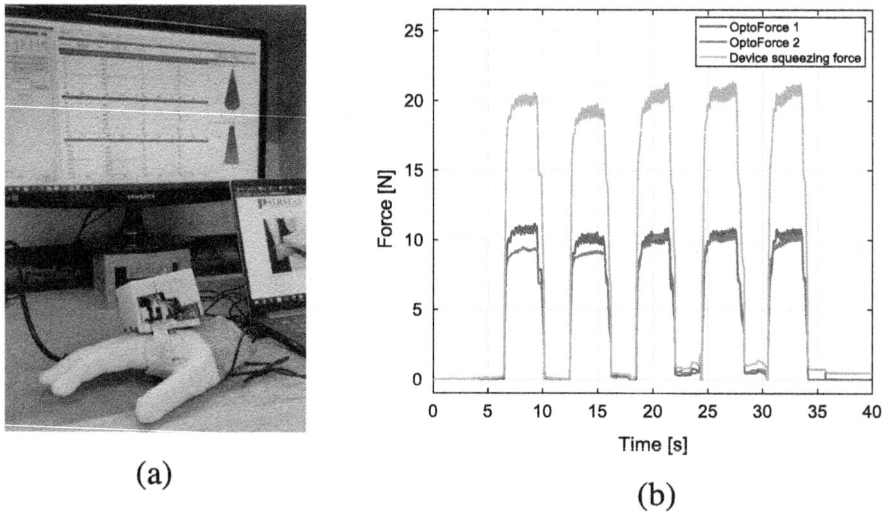

Fig. 3.13 HANS actuation bracelet validation. In **a**, the measurement setup. In **b**, the grasping force acquired in a representative trial. Blue and red lines report force measurements along the z-axis of each dummy hand's sensor, while the total grasping force is depicted in yellow. Each motor is driven until the stall is reached, as it can be seen looking at the distinctive noisy profile presented by the sensors measurements at about 10N. Reproduced from [62] with permission from IEEE. © IEEE 2022

To evaluate the device's performance, a profile encompassing the servo motors' range of motion was simulated using Matlab and transmitted to the actuation bracelet via Bluetooth communication at a sample rate of 50 Hz. The experiment involved a total of fifteen squeezes, each lasting three seconds with five-second intervals between them. The average force during these squeezes was 20.11 N, with a standard deviation of 0.57 N, indicating a reasonable outcome when compared to the average grasping force computed in Sect. 3.3.1. The grasping force data from a representative trial is depicted in Fig. 3.13b.

3.3.3 User Studies

This section presents an investigation into user opinions regarding the wearable haptic system designed for remote handshakes.

The study involved twelve participants (6 males and 6 females, aged 24–59, all right-handed), none of whom had prior experience in haptics or robotics. Each participant provided written informed consent to take part in the study and was informed of their right to withdraw from the experiment at any time. The experimental evaluation protocol followed the declaration of Helsinki, and there was no risk of harmful effects on subjects' health.

Each participant was asked to shake hands with one of the two investigators of their choice in order to standardize all tests of the experimental campaign.

The designated investigator demonstrated how to properly wear the actuation bracelet and sensing rings by first donning the equipment himself. After this demonstration, participants were instructed to follow suit, allowing them to experience the complete haptic system for remote handshaking. Each participant engaged in three remote handshakes with the experimenter, with a rest period of two minutes between each handshake. For each trial, the experimenter randomly selected a different object from a range of options: a 3D-printed model of a human hand used in preliminary experiments, a tennis ball, and a bottle. These objects were specifically chosen for their varying levels of abstraction from the human hand and their commonality in domestic and office settings, allowing us to assess the system's feasibility in transmitting a handshake while interacting with familiar, everyday items. Therefore, each participant was asked whether he/she perceived differences between the three handshakes, and then was asked to complete a survey. The evaluation questionnaire developed to collect users' opinions and feedback was defined by elaborating the Technology Assessment Model [67, 68]. In particular, the survey was divided into three topics: (i) perceived usefulness (Us), (ii) characteristics of the equipment (Eq), and (iii) perceived ease of use (Ea). Each topic consisted of four to six sentences for a total of 15 statements, reported in Table 3.3.

The judgements were expressed in the form of a Mean Opinion Score (MOS), a standardize policy to evaluate the Quality of Experience according to [69]. The user opinion scale ranged from 0 to 5, where 0 indicates "*Strongly Disagree*", and 5

Table 3.3 Survey statements arranged by topic of investigation

Perceived usefulness	
Us.1	*I think using the device is an effective way to feel the handshake with a distant friend/relative*
Us.2	*I would feel embarrassed to wear the device in my everyday life*
Us.3	*I find that the tactile information provided by the handshake device are insightful*
Us.4	*I find human-like the handshake perception*
Us.5	*I find pleasant the handshake perception provided by the device*
Us.6	*I found that the device is useful*
Quality of equipment	
Eq.1	*I feel safe while wearing the device*
Eq.2	*I was concerned that the device is not securely attached to me*
Eq.3	*I would be able to perform my daily tasks as usual while wearing the device*
Eq.4	*I find the device comfortable*
Ease of use	
Ea.1	*I find the device easy to use*
Ea.2	*I was able to wear the device easily without help from another person*
Ea.3	*I was able to remove the device easily without help from another person*
Ea.4	*I was able to put the device on in a reasonable time*
Ea.5	*I have the knowledge necessary to use the device*

means "*Strongly Agree*". It is denote with $s_{i.j|k}$ the score assigned to the j-th sentence of the i-th topic ($i \in \{Us, Eq, Ea\}$) by the k-th participant.

3.3.3.1 Results

The initial findings indicated that none of the participants perceived any differences in the handshakes conducted by the experimenter while grasping the three different objects. Each handshake was experienced as similar to both the preceding and following ones.

Survey results qualitatively revealed a generally positive sentiment across all areas of investigation. To quantify and mathematically analyze the results, the complement to the five-point scale was calculated for the scores assigned by each participant to statements Us.2 and Eq.2:. $s_{Us.2|k} = 5 - s_{Us.2|k}$ and $s_{Eq.2|k} = 5 - s_{Eq.2|k}$ $\forall k \in [1, 12]$. This adjustment was made because Us.2 and Eq.2 were the only statements with a negative connotation among all the questions posed.

The scores assigned by each participant to each statement are visually represented in Fig. 3.15 for every section of the survey. Additionally, Fig. 3.14 provides histograms of the scores for each question, organized by topic, to enhance clarity and comprehensiveness.

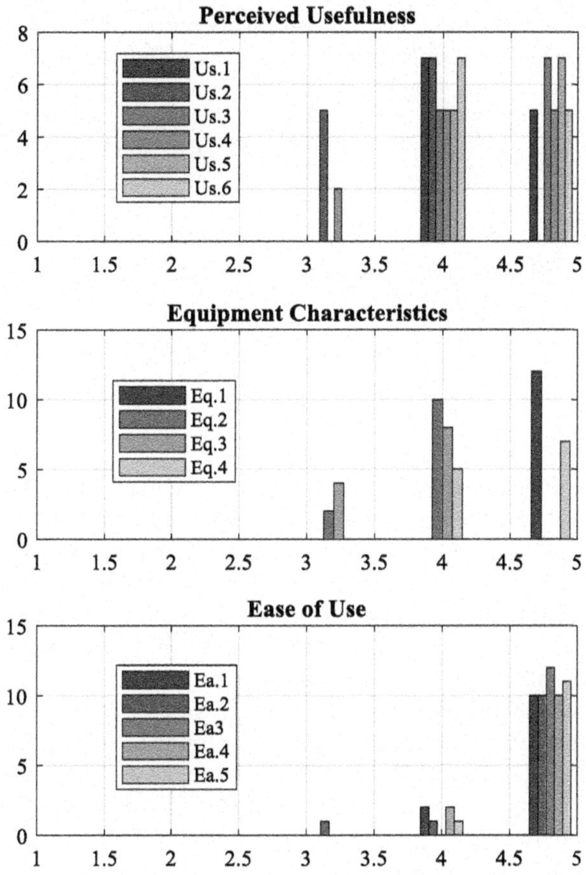

Fig. 3.14 The occurrence of the same opinions expressed as a numerical score are reported from top to bottom in the form of histograms for each sentence for the three survey topics. Reproduced from [62] with permission from IEEE. © IEEE 2022

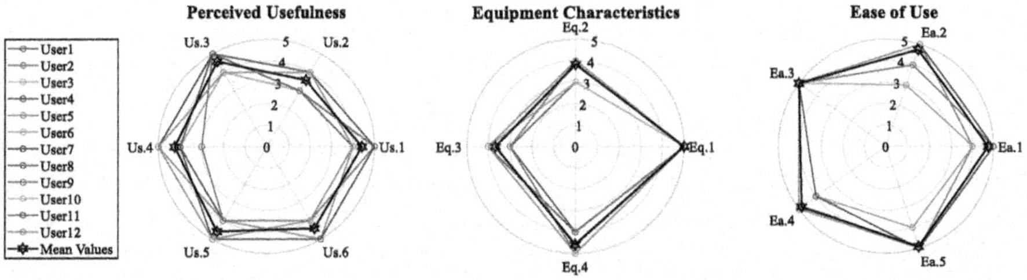

Fig. 3.15 The scores equivalent to the users' opinions about each sentence are reported from right to left for perceived usefulness, equipment characteristics, and ease of use, respectively. The user opinion scale ranges from 0 to 5, where 0 indicates "*Strongly Disagree*", and 5 means "*Strongly Agree*". The users' average score is depicted in black for each topic. Reproduced from [62] with permission from IEEE. © IEEE 2022

The average user's opinion per topic of investigation was defined as the average of the scores assigned to each statement of the same topic, that is

$$\overline{s}_{j|k} = \frac{1}{N_j}\sum_{i}^{N_j} s_{i.j|k} \quad \forall j \in \{Us, Eq, Ea\} \text{ and } \forall k \in [1, 12]$$

where N_j is the number of sentences used to investigate the topic j. Accordingly, it was defined a general opinion score (GOS) $\overline{\overline{s}}_j$ for the *i-th* topic as the average on the users of the $\overline{s}_{j|k}$ values, i.e.

$$\overline{\overline{s}}_j = \frac{1}{12}\sum_{k}^{12} \overline{s}_{j|k} \quad \forall j \in \{Us, Eq, Ea\}$$

The General Opinion Score (GOS) regarding the perceived utility was $\overline{\overline{s}}_{Us} = 4.31 \pm 0.31$, while the characteristics of equipments have achieved a GOS equal to $\overline{\overline{s}}_{Eq} = 4.27 \pm 0.22$. Finally, the results of the survey have reported that users were extremely satisfied about the ease of use, with a value of GOS equal to $\overline{\overline{s}}_{Ea} = 4.87 \pm 0.29$.

A further analysis of the symmetry in the distribution of scores assigned to the statements revealed that the average scores $\overline{s}_{Eq|k}$ and $\overline{s}_{Ea|k}$ were typically lower than both the median and mode. The skewness values μ_i were calculated as $\mu_{Eq} = -0.55$ for equipment characteristics and $\mu_{Ea} = -2.39$ for ease of use. For completeness, the skewness value for perceived usefulness was found to be $\mu_{Us} \approx 0$. This analysis indicates that the sample population rated the system's usefulness, equipment characteristics, and ease of use within a range between "Good" and "Excellent," with a slight inclination toward more favorable opinions.

3.4 HapticPalm

The device described in this study effectively stimulates a wide area of the palm using only three actuators, ensuring excellent wearability. To accomplish this, a parallel mechanism was designed in which the mobile platform (end-effector) features interchangeable contact interfaces. These diverse contact interfaces, each with distinct shapes, can be easily attached or detached from the device, allowing for the reproduction of tactile sensations that closely resemble the desired stimulus across various tasks.

Inspired by a family of wearable devices developed for fingertip stimulation [70, 71], the mobile platform of this device features a "Y" shape and is actuated by three servomotors located on the back of the hand, utilizing tendons to transmit motion. While the kinematic structure of this device shares some similarities with those designed for fingertip stimulation, stimulating the palm of the hand introduces

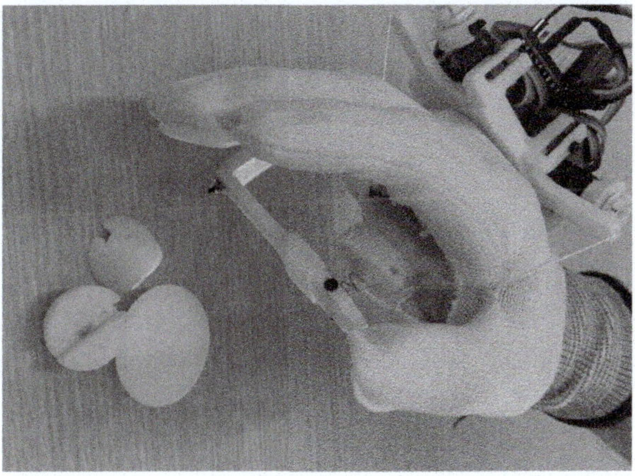

Fig. 3.16 Prototype of the wearable haptic defice for hand palm stimulationworn by a usef. Copyright © 2021 Dragusanu, Villani, Prattichizzo and Malvezzi [61]. This is an open-access article distributed under the terms of the Creative Commons Attribution License (CC BY)

distinct challenges due to differences in size, kinematic structure, form factor, and required force levels.

To enhance user comfort and minimize continuous contact with the palm, we incorporated an elastic element at the base of the platform. This combination of tendons and springs enables the reproduction of cutaneous stimuli in both static and dynamic conditions. The use of three actuators allows for the simulation of both normal and tangential components of contact force, which are essential for replicating shear forces, as well as for interacting with virtual or remote surfaces at varying orientations, such as those found on curved surfaces.

The wearable haptic device designed for palm stimulation is illustrated in Fig. 3.16. Additionally, to summarize and clarify the existing solutions in the literature, Table 3.4 provides details on the implementation and electronics of the devices referenced in the state of the art, along with the device presented in this section.

3.4.1 Biomechanics and Perceptive Receptor of Palm

The design of the wearable haptic device began with an analysis of the hand's palm, focusing on its biomechanical structure and the characteristics of the stimuli to be rendered. This analysis informs both the requirements and constraints of the device. Anatomically, the palm is the ventral (or anterior) region of the hand, where the fingers converge when punching.

The back of the hand is located opposite the palm. The bones in the palm can be categorized into two groups: carpals and metacarpals. The metacarpus consists of five long bones that connect the carpus to the phalanges, numbered from 1 to 5, starting from the thumb to the little finger. The carpus, made up of eight short bones, is organized into two rows, i.e., proximal and distal, and connects the radius to the metacarpus.

Table 3.4 Comparison between the proposed haptic device (indicated as HaptiPalm, last row) and other solutions available in the literature

Name	Type of actuation	Contact area	Form factor of Electronics
Ghostglove [36, 37]	Sqeezing band	Fixed and extended	On board
Achibet et al. [38]	Passive elastic band	Fixed and pont-like	–
Son et al. [39]	4 pressure points	Fixed and point-like	On arm
Son et al. [40]	10 pressure points tendon drive	Fixed and point-like	Delocalized
Gollner et al. [41]	35 vibrating motors	Fixed and point-like	On arm
Martınez et al. [42]	6 vibrating motors	Fixed and point-like	Delocalized
Borja et al. [43]	5 vibrating motors	Fixed and point-like	On arm
Haptic pivot [44]	Mobile vibrating mass	Fixed and extended	On arm
Zubrycki et al. [46]	10 pneumatic pad	Fixed and extended	Delocalized
Weatavix [47]	Mobile mass	Fixed and extended	On arm
Deltatouch [48, 49]	3D Mobile platform	Mobile and point-like	Delocalized
HapticPalm –	3D Mobile platform tendon drive	Mobile and interchangable	On board

The proximal row includes the scaphoid, lunate, triquetrum, and pisiform bones, while the distal row comprises the trapezium, trapezoid, capitate, and hamate bones. The biomechanical structure of the palm, including its bones, muscles, and ligaments, facilitates various movements: radial abduction, ulnar adduction, palmar flexion, and dorsiflexion, as depicted in Fig. 3.17. According to [72], palmar flexion refers to bending the wrist toward the palm and ventral side of the forearm, while dorsiflexion denotes hyperextension of the wrist joint toward the dorsal side. Radial abduction involves pulling a structure away from the midline of the wrist, whereas ulnar adduction draws the hand toward the midline. Additional key movements include the opposition and apposition of the thumb: in apposition, the side of the thumb touches other fingers, while during opposition, the pulp of the thumb's distal end contacts the fingertips of other digits [10].

The contact surface of the developed haptic device has been carefully sized and positioned according to the biomechanics of the palm to avoid overcrowding and preserve the mobility of the carpus. The mobile platform must not restrict the aforementioned motions; it should be situated beneath the metacarpal bones, extending from the upper boundary of the first row of carpal bones to the transverse metacarpal ligament.

The articulation of the carpal bones creates a cavity on the palmar side known as the carpal tunnel. This tunnel runs through the wrist and houses the superficial and deep flexor muscles of the fingers, as well as the long flexor of the thumb. The median nerve also traverses the carpal tunnel; its palmar branches, known as digital cutaneous

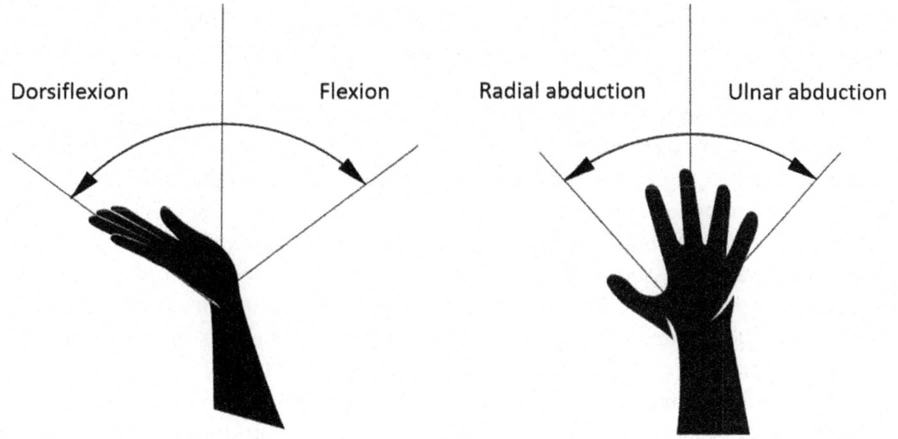

Fig. 3.17 Primary hand movements due to the biomechanical structure of the carpus: palmarflexion/dorsiflexion (left) and radial abduction/ulnar adduction (right). Copyright © 2021 Dragusanu, Villani, Prattichizzo and Malvezzi [61]. This is an open-access article distributed under the terms of the Creative Commons Attribution License (CC BY)

branches or cutaneous digital nerves, supply sensation to the skin of the first three fingers (thumb, index finger, and middle finger). The palm, much like the fingertips, is one of the densest regions of mechanoreceptors in the human body. Consequently, the channel for haptic stimulus transmission is similar for both the palm and fingertips. However, the biomechanics of the palm are more complex than those of the fingers. Differences in geometry, anatomical constraints, and mechanical compliance [73] contribute to this complexity. The extended design of the device results in greater structural fragility, while the higher forces required to simulate sensations in the palm increase the structural stress on the device.

3.4.2 Haptic Stimulus of Hand Palm: Design Principles and Modeling

The proposed device is able to both push the end-effector towards the palm and to differentiate applied force direction and contact location and orientation, ensuring robustness, ergonomics and low weight. To meet the design requirements, the end-effector is supported passively by a spring connected to a C-shaped structure that is fixed to the back of the hand. Movement of the end-effector is achieved through three tendons, each actuated by motors located on the back of the hand. Both the fixed component on the hand and the active end-effector are shaped like a "Y," with their vertices interconnected by the three tendons. This configuration allows for a broad range of movements, enabling effective interaction with most of the palm surface.

In the following section, it will be introduced a simplified mathematical model that relates the forces applied to the palm to the forces exerted by the motors through the tendons.

The study of cable-driven parallel mechanisms is a fascinating area of research within robotics. Using cables and tendons for motion transmission allows designers to create compact, lightweight devices, minimizing the weight and inertial effects of mechanical components. Research has explored various aspects of this topic, such as the direct geometric-static problem of three cable-driven parallel robots using interval analysis, as discussed in [74]. Additionally, the direct geometric-static analysis of an underconstrained four-cable parallel robot is presented in [75]. The differential kinematics relevant for calibration and system analysis is examined in [76]. Dynamic modeling of cable-driven parallel robots is also addressed, focusing on fully constrained planar cases in [77] and underconstrained spatial cases in [78].

Solving the forward kinematics problem involves determining the relationship between cable lengths and the posture of the moving platform, which is crucial for device control. However, this problem can be challenging in parallel mechanisms. Conversely, the inverse kinematics problem assesses the lengths of the cables that correspond to a specific platform posture. Static analysis establishes the relationship between cable tensions and the resultant forces exerted on the palm.

To characterize the device as a cable-driven parallel robot, we will define two coordinate frames. The first one $\mathscr{A} = \{O_A, \mathbf{u}_1, \mathbf{u}_2, \mathbf{u}_3\}$ is fixed on the device body on the hand back, while the second one $\mathscr{B} = \{O_B, \mathbf{v}_1, \mathbf{v}_2, \mathbf{v}_3\}$ is fixed on the mobile platform in contact with hand palm, as shown in Fig. 3.18. In the following, to simplify the notation, if quantities are expressed in $\mathscr{A}$ frame, superscript $\mathscr{A}$ is omitted.

On the device body we define three connection points A_1, A_2, A_3, representing the points where the tendons pass through in the device fixed part; assuming they define an equilateral triangle, their coordinates are:

$$\mathbf{a}_1 = \left[\frac{\sqrt{3}d_u}{-6}, \frac{d_u}{-2}, 0\right]^{\mathrm{T}} \mathbf{a}_2 = \left[\frac{\sqrt{3}d_u}{-6}, \frac{d_u}{2}, 0\right]^{\mathrm{T}} \mathbf{a}_3 = \left[\frac{\sqrt{3}d_u}{3}, 0, 0\right]^{\mathrm{T}} \tag{3.9}$$

where d_u is the upper triangle side length. The wires are connected to the mobile platform in three points B_1, B_2, B_3, defining an equilateral triangle with center O_B, their coordinates in $\mathscr{B}$ frame are:

$$\mathbf{b}_1^{\mathscr{B}} = \left[\frac{\sqrt{3}d_l}{-6}, \frac{d_l}{-2}, 0\right]^{\mathrm{T}} \mathbf{b}_2^{\mathscr{B}} = \left[\frac{\sqrt{3}d_l}{-6}, \frac{d_l}{2}, 0\right]^{\mathrm{T}} \mathbf{b}_3^{\mathscr{B}} = \left[\frac{\sqrt{3}d_l}{3}, 0, 0\right]^{\mathrm{T}} \tag{3.10}$$

where, d_l is the length side of lower triangular plate, while their coordinates in $\mathscr{A}$ reference frame are indicated as:

$$\mathbf{b}_1 = [x_1, y_1, z_1]^{\mathrm{T}}, \mathbf{b}_2 = [x_2, y_2, z_2]^{\mathrm{T}}, \mathbf{b}_3 = [x_3, y_3, z_3]^{\mathrm{T}},$$

and vary according to the platform motion. The coordinates of O_B point, expressed in $\mathscr{A}$ frame, are defined by the vector $\mathbf{o}_B = [x, y, z]^{\mathrm{T}}$.

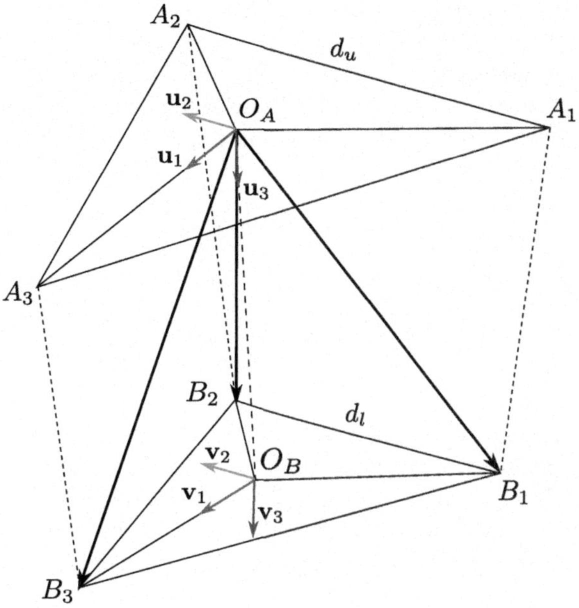

Fig. 3.18 Main points and coordinate frames for the analysis of the wearable haptic device. Copyright © 2021 Dragusanu, Villani, Prattichizzo and Malvezzi [61]. This is an open-access article distributed under the terms of the Creative Commons Attribution License (CC BY)

Let us define a rotation matrix $\mathbf{R}(\eta) = \mathbf{R}_z(\phi)\mathbf{R}_y(\theta)\mathbf{R}_x(\psi)$ representing the orientation of $\mathscr{B}$ frame w.r.t. $\mathscr{A}$ frame. We indicate with $\boldsymbol{\eta} = \left[\psi, \theta, \phi\right]^{\mathrm{T}}$ a vector containing roll, pitch, and yaw angles, respectively.

3.4.2.1 Inverse Kinematics

The inverse kinematic problem consists in finding the values of cable lengths l_i for a given position $\mathbf{o}_B$ and orientation $\mathbf{R}$. The geometric constraints of the parallel structure relates the length of the cables to the norm of the geometric vectors connecting B_i to A_i, i.e. ,

$$\|\mathbf{b}_i - \mathbf{a}_i\| = l_i \quad i = 1, 2, 3 \tag{3.11}$$

where l_i is the length of cable i, that can be controlled by the motors. The coordinates of the mobile platform connection points can be evaluated as

$$\mathbf{b}_i = \mathbf{o}_B + \mathbf{R}\mathbf{b}_i^{\mathscr{B}} \quad i = 1, 2, 3 \tag{3.12}$$

By substituting (3.12) in the cable constraint relationship (3.11), we can easily evaluate l_i as a function of $\mathbf{o}_B$ and $\mathbf{R}$.

3.4.2.2 Statics

In stationary conditions, the sum of the forces and torques (wrench) applied to the platform through the wires is balanced by the forces and torques (wrench) due to the physical contact with the finger pad as follows:

$$\sum_{i=1}^{3} \mathbf{f}_i + \mathbf{f}_{O_B} + \mathbf{f}_s = 0 \tag{3.13a}$$

$$\sum_{i=1}^{3} \boldsymbol{\tau}_i + \boldsymbol{\tau}_{O_B} + \boldsymbol{\tau}_s = 0 \tag{3.13b}$$

we indicate with $\mathbf{f}_i \in \mathbb{R}^3$ the forces applied by the cables, with $\boldsymbol{\tau}_i \in \mathbb{R}^3$ the corresponding momentum, with $\mathbf{f}_{O_B} \in \mathbb{R}^3$ the reaction force applied by the hand palm to the platform, with $\mathbf{f}_s \in \mathbb{R}^3$ the force due to spring deformation, with $\boldsymbol{\tau}_{O_B} \in \mathbb{R}^3$ the reaction torque and with $\boldsymbol{\tau}_s \in \mathbb{R}^3$ the torque due to spring deformation, both expressed w.r.t. O_B point. Expanding the equilibrium equations (3.13a) and (3.13b) we get:

$$\sum_{i=1}^{3} \rho_i \mathbf{u}_{\mathbf{f}_i} + \mathbf{f}_{O_B} + \mathbf{f}_s = 0 \tag{3.14a}$$

$$\sum_{i=1}^{3} \rho_i \mathbf{b}_i \times \mathbf{u}_{\mathbf{f}_i} + \boldsymbol{\tau}_{O_B} + \boldsymbol{\tau}_s = 0 \tag{3.14b}$$

where ρ_i is the tension cable i, and $\mathbf{u}_{\mathbf{f}_i}$ is the unit vector representing the cable direction, and can be evaluated as:

$$\mathbf{u}_{\mathbf{f}_i} = \frac{\mathbf{b}_i - \mathbf{a}_i}{l_i} \tag{3.15}$$

From (3.14a) and (3.14b), and (3.15), we can express (3.13a) and (3.13b) in the matrix form:

$$\begin{bmatrix} \mathbf{u}_{\mathbf{f}_1} & \mathbf{u}_{\mathbf{f}_2} & \mathbf{u}_{\mathbf{f}_3} \\ \mathbf{b}_1 \times \mathbf{u}_{\mathbf{f}_1} & \mathbf{b}_2 \times \mathbf{u}_{\mathbf{f}_2} & \mathbf{b}_3 \times \mathbf{u}_{\mathbf{f}_3} \end{bmatrix} \begin{bmatrix} \rho_1 \\ \rho_2 \\ \rho_3 \end{bmatrix} + \begin{bmatrix} \mathbf{f}_{O_B} + \mathbf{f}_s \\ \boldsymbol{\tau}_{O_B} + \boldsymbol{\tau}_s \end{bmatrix} = 0 \tag{3.16}$$

which is well-known as geometric-statics equation of cable driven parallel robots [74].

3.4.3 *Design and Analysis*

The device presented in this work strikes a balance between wearability, weight, and resistance to mechanical stress. The symmetrical geometry of the supports on the back of the hand and beneath the palm facilitates a uniform distribution of forces applied by the motors and transmitted through the tendons.

A notable challenge of tendon-actuated devices is the necessity for the end-effector to maintain constant contact with the hand while keeping the tendons under tension. To address this issue and enable the device to engage and disengage contact with the palm, the end-effector is connected to a C-shaped fixed element via an elastic component.

In the following it is described with more details the device from the design point of view, the interchangeable end-effector's modules that are in contact with the palm, and it is shown some results of a structural mechanical analysis.

3.4.3.1 HapticPalm

The device features a parallel structure composed of two primary components: one positioned on the back of the hand and the other situated beneath the palm, referred to as the end-effector.

The back component serves as a mechanical support for the force actuation and transmission system, as well as housing the microcontroller and power supply (indicated as A in Fig. 3.19).

Three tendons are routed through extruded paths from this support, arranged at 120 °C from one another to form an equilateral "Y-shape." These tendons transmit the forces applied by the motors through pulleys, transferring them from the back of the hand to the end-effector (B) and subsequently to the palm. This actuation method enhances wearability and mitigates the issues associated with parallel mechanisms reliant on rigid links, which tend to be heavier and less adaptable, often requiring complex adjustments to suit different users and needs [79].

The end-effector comprises two platforms, labeled (C) and (D). The first platform connects to the actuation system via the tendons, while the second platform is directly linked to the back component through a "C"-shaped rigid link (E). An elastic element, specifically a spring (I), connects the two platforms, facilitating disconnection between the tip and palm when no contact or force is needed. The connection points between the tendons and the platform are designed in a "Y-shape," mirroring the support structure on the back of the hand.

Additionally, a magnetic "T-shape" interlocking mechanism is integrated into the first platform, allowing for easy interchange of various end-effector modules (H) designed to replicate different types of cutaneous stimuli.

The rigid link connecting the two main components (G, F, E) features an adjustable telescopic height, enabling the device to accommodate users with diverse hand anthropometry. Furthermore, it can rotate through two revolute joints (J1, J2), ensur-

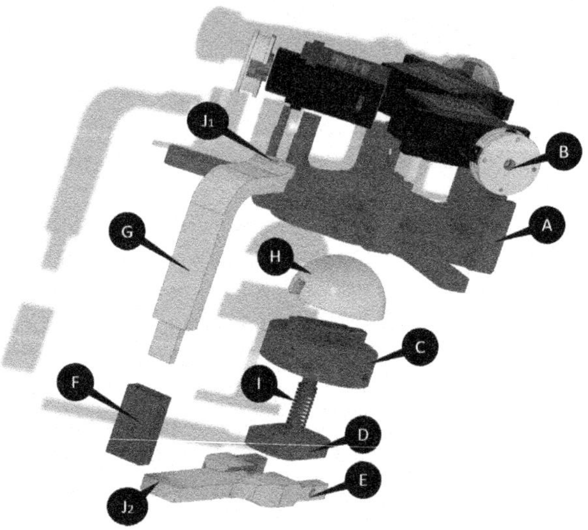

Fig. 3.19 Exploded CAD view of the device. The end-effector of the device is composed of the components indicated with (C), (I), (D). (H) indicates the end-effector's module while the "Y-shape" platform is indicated with (A) and the pulleys are indicated with (B). (E), (F) and (G) are the elements that realize the link between the two platforms. (J_1) and (J_2) are the two joints that allow to rotate the end-effector.

ing ergonomic adaptability for multiple users and allowing temporary repositioning of the end-effector away from the palm without requiring the removal of the device.

3.4.3.2 Modules

As mentioned before the end-effector modules of the device are manually interchangeable.

The modules are secured to the device using a "T-shape" interlocking system, allowing for easy connection and disconnection from the end-effector platform. Each module features a magnet that ensures precise alignment at the center of the "Y-shape" platform and maintains stability during force rendering. To effectively convey the sensation of touching various objects and surfaces relevant to haptic applications, four distinct end-effector modules have been developed. The primary goal is to enable users to experience common shapes such as spheres, corners, edges, and flat surfaces. Specifically, two spherical modules with differing radii of curvature have been designed to replicate curved surfaces (H1, H4 in Fig. 3.20), along with a rectangular-shaped module and a flat module to simulate contact with edges and flat surfaces, respectively (H2, H3).

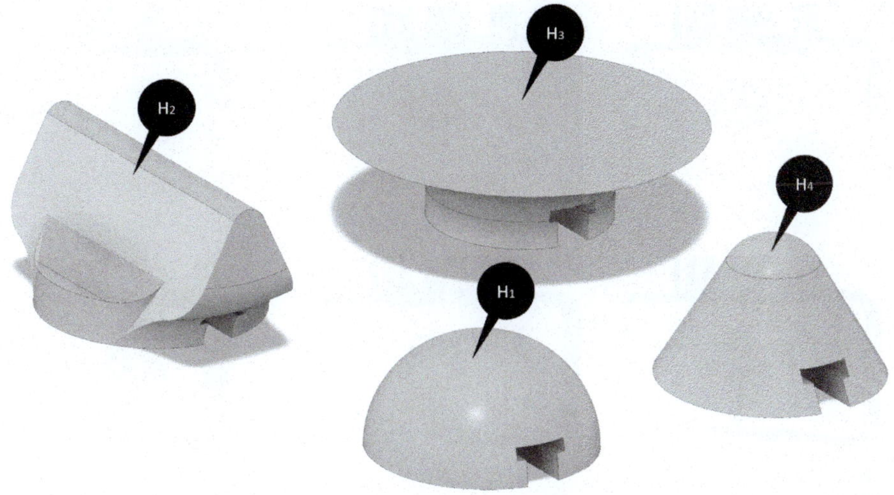

Fig. 3.20 CAD models of the end-effector' modules. (H_1) and (H_4) indicate the spherical modules with different radii of curvature while (H_2) and (H_3) are respectively the rectangular-shaped module and the plane-shaped module.

3.4.3.3 FEM Analysis

While the basic structure of this device is similar to that developed for fingertip stimulation, as described in [70], its larger dimensions and the magnitude of the applied forces present significant mechanical challenges. To evaluate the overall stress and deformation of the device under various operational conditions, a structural stationary finite element method (FEM) analysis was conducted, examining four distinct loading scenarios. Three of these scenarios analyzed the device's behavior when a set of forces, defined according to the previously described model, were applied. The fourth scenario investigated the device's response when skin elasticity becomes saturated, simulating a fixed end-effector.

The analysis was performed using the 3D-CAD/CAE software Fusion 360 (Autodesk Inc., US). For this assessment, all components of the device were constructed from ABS plastic, except for the spring, which was made of steel.

The device's behavior was analyzed under the application of forces indicated by blue arrows in Fig. 3.21, which were applied to the three vertices of both platforms. A fixed constraint was implemented at the bottom of the back hand's platform to simulate contact with the hand. Six forces were applied to the fixed and movable "Y" vertices, with their directions selected to represent the actions of the tendons. The magnitudes of these forces were determined based on the overall interaction force that needed to be simulated.

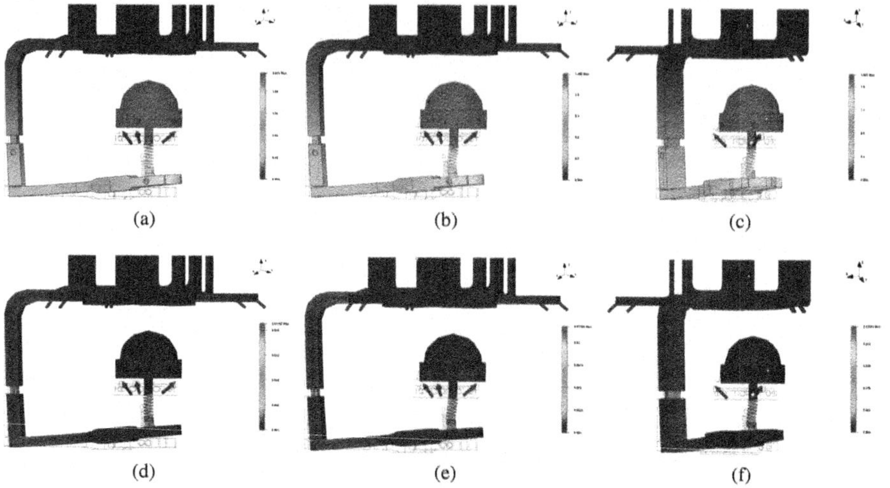

Fig. 3.21 Results of the FEM structural analysis. The blue arrows indicate the forces applied in the simulations, the wireframe transparent CAD model represents the undeformed model, while a 1X deformation of the device is represented in the colored surfaces. **a** The displacements when a force with only z-component is applied, **b** and **c** show respectively the results of the displacements when a force with z-component and x-component or y-component is applied, subfigures **d–f** on the right side report the results of the deformation for the same loading cases. Copyright © 2021 Dragusanu, Villani, Prattichizzo and Malvezzi [61]. This is an open-access article distributed under the terms of the Creative Commons Attribution License (CC BY)(color figure online)

Figure 3.21 presents the results of the FEM analysis across three axes. The subfigures at the top display the results in terms of displacements, while those at the bottom illustrate the results in terms of deformations.

In Figs. 3.21a and d, the results corresponding to an overall force acting along the z direction are shown, with each simulated tendon experiencing an equal force magnitude of 1 N. The corresponding displacement in Fig. 3.21d indicates that, as anticipated, the primary movement occurs predominantly along the$z$ axis.

Figure 3.21b and e illustrate the outcomes of a simulation involving an overall force with components along both the z and y directions. In this case, four forces were symmetrically adjusted, with their magnitudes reduced to 0.5 N.

Finally, Fig. 3.21c and f report the results when an equivalent force is applied with components along the x and z directions. Similarly, these forces were symmetrically modified.

Additionally, the response of the device was assessed when skin elasticity becomes saturated to evaluate the resistance of the platform on the back of the hand. In this scenario, all forces were applied with the same direction and intensity of 5 N, while two fixed constraints were established: one on the end-effector module and the other on the bottom part of the back hand's platform (see Fig. 3.22).

Overall, the FEM analysis results demonstrate that the mechanical structure of the device can withstand the forces encountered in haptic applications. As anticipated,

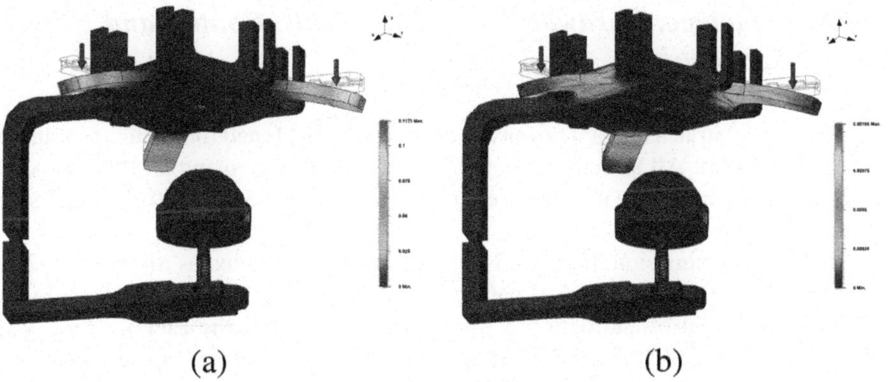

Fig. 3.22 Results of the FEM analysis for the platform of the back of the hand under the action of an overall 15 N force (5 N for each side of the "Y-shape"). Blue arrows indicate the forces applied while the transparent wireframe CAD model, is the reference undeformed model, while the colored surface corresponds to a 1X deformation of the haptic palm device. Subfigure **a** shows the displacement of the platform and the Subfigure **b** reports the deformation of the platform. Copyright © 2021 Dragusanu, Villani, Prattichizzo and Malvezzi [61]. This is an open-access article distributed under the terms of the Creative Commons Attribution License (CC BY) (color figure online)

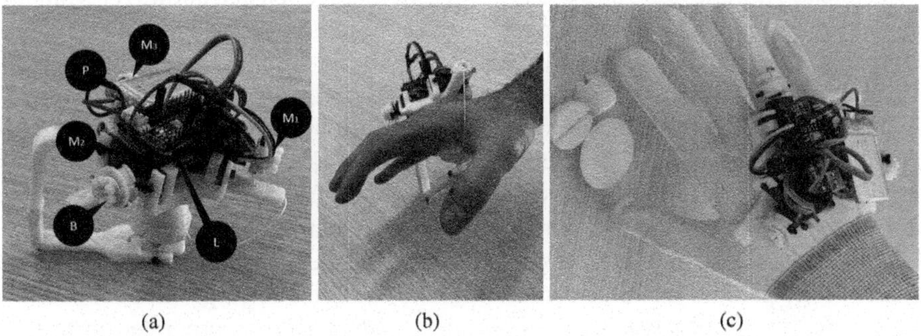

Fig. 3.23 Prototype of the device presented in this thesis part. Subfigure **a** shows the device from a hardware point of view. Subfigure **b** report the device worn by a hand's user. Subfigure **c** shows the final Prototype worn by the user together with the different modules. Copyright © 2021 Dragusanu, Villani, Prattichizzo and Malvezzi [61]. This is an open-access article distributed under the terms of the Creative Commons Attribution License (CC BY)

the primary critical points of the structure are located at the rigid link and the base of the spring. Furthermore, the selection of the spring is a crucial aspect to ensure the device's robustness and functionality.

3.4.4 Prototype, Hardware and Components, Control and Application

Figure 3.23 illustrates the first prototype of the device designed for haptic stimulation of the hand palm. All structural components are fabricated using an FDM process with ABS material, while the elastic element consists of a standard off-the-shelf steel spring.

For force transmission, three MG-90S microservos (denoted as M_i in Fig. 3.23b) are employed, powered by a 5 V battery (P). Each microservo has a stall torque of 20 N cm. The control and data processing are managed by the Elegoo Nano V3+ microcontroller (ELEGOO Inc., CHN) (L), with communication between the device and the virtual environment facilitated via serial communication.

As mentioned earlier, the force rendering on the hand palm utilizes a tendon-based transmission system. The tendons are anchored at one end to the motor pulleys mounted on the "Y-shape" platform (A) at the back of the hand and at the other end to the "Y-arranged" connectors of the end-effector. The minimum length of each tendon is determined by the thread required to maintain tension between the end-effector platform and the "Y-shape" platform on the back of the hand. To facilitate length adjustment, the pulleys are designed with an external section that allows for wrapping any excess tendon. The initial version of the pulleys is depicted in the CAD model (B in Fig. 3.19), while an updated version can be seen in the prototype in Fig. 3.23a (B).

Figure 3.23b shows the first prototype being worn by a user. Initial user feedback indicated that the "bare" device was not intuitive to wear due to uncertainties regarding its orientation, caused by its symmetrical shape. To address this ambiguity and assist users in properly positioning their hands within the tendons, the device has been integrated into a glove. This glove features a specially shaped opening in the center of the palm to facilitate contact with the end-effector (Fig. 3.23c).

As previously mentioned, an elastic element has been incorporated to provide passive support for the end-effector when it is not in contact with the palm. On one hand, the spring must be sufficiently stiff to maintain the end-effector in an upright position, even when the tendons are not engaged. On the other hand, it must also be soft enough to prevent overloading the motors, allowing them to allocate part of their torque to generating the required haptic force while reserving some for spring deformation, as discussed in Sect. 3.4.2.2.

To achieve this balance, a spring with a stiffness coefficient of 6.7 N/mm was selected. Additionally, a short spring measuring 7 mm in length was chosen to keep the end-effector as compact as possible. This design choice resulted in symmetric behavior of the spring in both axial and radial directions during testing.

Table 3.5 summarizes the main characteristics of the developed prototype. The maximum and minimum theoretical forces that can be applied to the palm are evaluated based on the model presented in Sect. 3.4.2.2.

Table 3.5 Haptic palm device prototype main hardware/software details and technical specifications

	Technical specifics
Weight	89.92 g
Dimensions $L \times l \times (h \pm \Delta h)$	$104 \times 81 \times 97$ mm
Degrees of freedom	3
Microprocessor	ATmega328
Clock speed of microcontroller	16 MHz
Computer interface	Serial COM
Input Voltage	5.0 V
Battery life	$\approx$ 5 h
Maximum speed	9.5 rad/s
Maximum resisting force	60.0 N
Maximum theoretical force on palm	29.5 N
Minimum theoretical force on palm	0.81 N
Maximum recall force	30.5 N
Maximum contact surface	$\approx$ 7.06 cm^2
Cost	$\approx$ \$50

The dimensions of device are measured without the glove, the value of Δh is equal the capability to extend and shorten the rigid link F respect G link.

3.4.4.1 An Example of VR Application

We have developed a virtual reality scenario to showcase the functionality of the device in various extended contact situations. This scenario was created using CoppeliaSim (Coppelia Robotics AG, CHE) and simulates a typical office workstation.

Within the simulated environment, users can interact with a variety of objects on a desk, each specifically designed to test different end-effectors of the haptic device. For instance, module H2 is tailored for exploring laptop frames (Fig. 3.24b), while the circular module H1 is intended for interaction with the paperweight (Fig. 3.24a). Modules H3 and H4 are designed for engaging with the desk surface and stacked books, respectively (Fig. 3.24c and d).

Interactions with these objects are facilitated through a hand avatar, which is equipped with sensors in the palm and controlled by a LeapMotion controller (Ultraleap Inc., US), a camera-based hand-tracking system. In future developments, we plan to integrate an IMU-based tracking system with the haptic device.

The forces generated during interactions are estimated using a triaxial virtual sensor, which simulates collisions between the hand model and the objects. Collision forces are processed through the Bullet 2.78 physics engine. During navigation, these contact forces are transmitted to the device, and it is also possible to generate on-demand signals from recorded force profiles obtained during previous explorations.

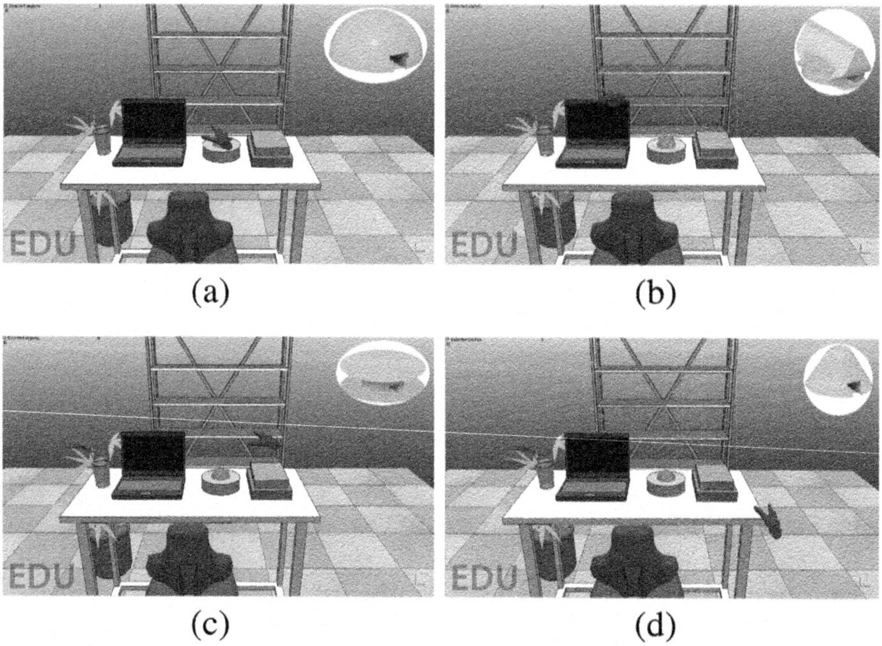

Fig. 3.24 The testing virtual scenario is composed by a rack and a plant in vase in background and a office station in the foreground. The interaction is provided by a red avatar of hand and the objects in foreground are chosen to use all modules: paperweight for H1 module (**a**); laptop frames for H2 module (**b**); cover of book and surface of desk for H3 module (**c**); desk, laptop and book peaks for H4 module (**d**).

Communication between the device and the virtual environment is established via a serial port.

3.5 HapticPalm: Validation and Usability Assessment

In this chapter three section a set of experimental tests to asses the functionality and usability of the HapticPalm are presented. In addition a validation on the force exerted by the device, comparing it with the theoretical values estimated in the design phase, presented in the section before.

With respect to the version presented in Sect. 3.4, the rigid link has been structurally modified in order to increase its strength and stiffness. The parts (D) and (C) of the end-effector, visibile in Fig. 3.26, have been also modified to allow an easy connection of the spring and tendons. The end-effector module has different contact interfaces manually interchangeable and easily connected to the device by means of a magnetic clip and a "T-shape" socket.

As mentioned before the HapticPalm design started from the analysis of the hand palm biomechanical structure and the features of the stimuli to be rendered, that defined the design requirements and the constraints. With the aim of avoiding cluttering of palm and the reduction of carpus mobility, the contact surface of the developed haptic device has been dimensioned and placed according with biomechanics features of the palm. Furthermore, the end-effector has been placed under metacarpal bone situ and extended from upper bound of first row of carpal bone to transverse metacarpal ligament to avoid interference with finger motions.

3.5.1 Experimental Evaluation

3.5.1.1 Force Validation

To evaluate the capability of the HapticPalm in following a specified force profile, a series of tests were conducted. The validation process involved repeatedly recording predefined forces exerted by the device, which were measured using a high-precision ATI force sensor (ATI Industrial Automation Inc., US).

During the tests, a user donned the HapticPalm and positioned the ATI sensor within a textile pocket placed between the end-effector module (H_2) and the palm of their hand. The haptic device then performed a stepwise force profile in the normal direction. The force range tested was from [0, 50] N with increments of 10 N. Each force measurement was repeated ten times and recorded in a text format.

The results from one of the repetitions are illustrated in Fig. 3.25a. All data collected from the ATI sensor were utilized to create a lookup table of effective forces exerted by the HapticPalm. This data was then compared with the theoretical forces calculated from the static formulations presented in Sect. 3.4.2.2.

The interpolated results of the measurements and the theoretical evolution are displayed in Fig. 3.25b. Based on preliminary observations of the data obtained, various logistic functions were tested to interpolate the curves representing the force measurements. The most effective interpolating curve was found to be an unbiased and scaled hyperbolic tangent function, expressed as:

$$F_s = \alpha + \beta \tanh\left(\gamma \sum_{i=1}^{3} n_{f,i}\right)$$

With $\alpha = 27.46$, $\beta = -0.77$, and $\gamma = 0.044$, while $n_{f,i}$ indicates the normal force component due the tensions of i-th tendon.

In the force range from 0 to 25 N, the measured forces exhibit a nearly linear trend, with a mean error of 0.87 ± 0.22 N. compared to theoretical evaluations. Additionally, in the saturation zone, the mean error in steady-state conditions relative

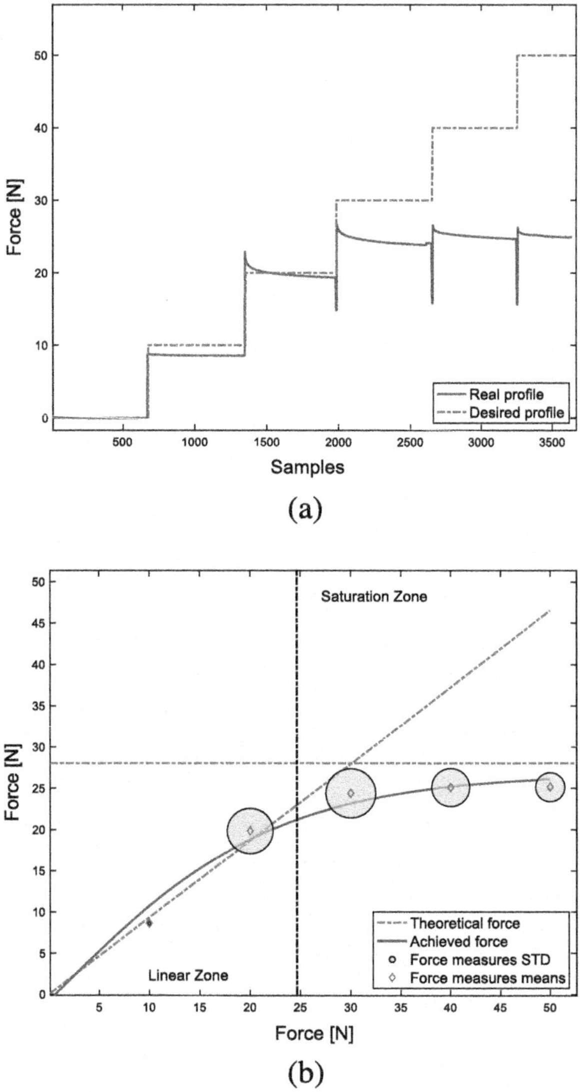

Fig. 3.25 Validation of the HapticPalm. **a** Results of force profile chase: orange dash-dot curve represents the theoretical reference force profile, blue curve is the real profile with obtained the HapticPalm. **b** Characterization function of the device: red curve represents the device's real behavior, generated by interpolating the force measures means points at each step of 10 N in the range [0, 50] N while in blue the theoretical behaviour obtained exploiting the formulation described in 3.4.2.2. The horizontal blue line corresponding to 28 N, that is is the maximum theoretical force [61], while the black vertical line is the threshold between the linear zone and nonlinear zone of the real device characterization function. Reproduced from [80] with permission from IEEE.

to the theoretical limit value estimated by [61] is 3.14 ± 0.95 N. This steady-state error in the saturation zone is approximately 10 % of the theoretical threshold value proposed in [61]. While this error is not negligible, it can be attributed to uncertainties in the dynamic mass-spring-friction model of the user's hand, which affects the parameters σ and k. For this study, these parameters were set to$k = 500$ N/m and $\sigma \approx 0$, following the guidelines established by [81].

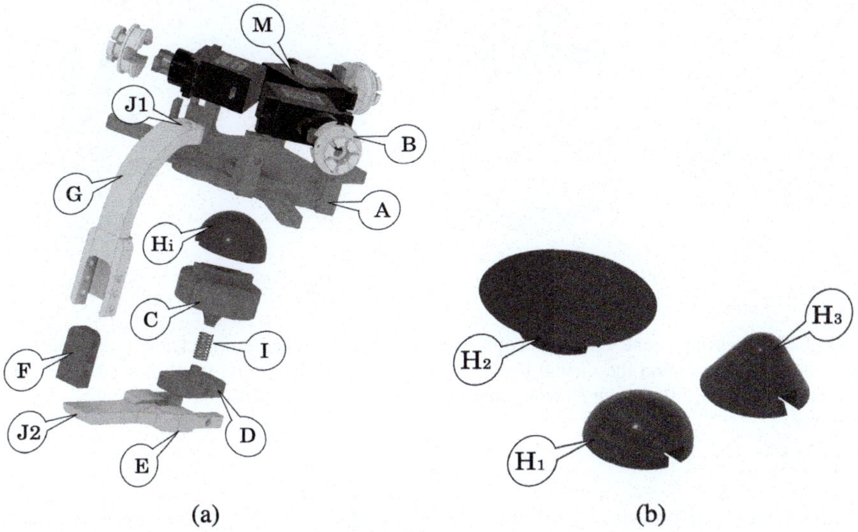

Fig. 3.26 In **a** the exploded CAD model of the HapticPalm. The end-effector consists in (C), (I), (D) parts. (H_i) is one of the end-effector's modules, (A) is the "Y-shape" platform and the pulleys are indicated with (B). (E), (F), (G), (J1) and (J2) are rigid link components. In **b** end effector interchangeable modules: H_1—shere surface, H_2—flat surface, H_3—cone surface. Reproduced from [80] with permission from IEEE. © IEEE 2024

Moreover, the structural compliance of the Y-arranged guides used for routing the tendons introduces additional uncertainties in the force saturation zone, particularly when the elasticity of the palm's skin is saturated.

3.5.1.2 Users Studies

To assess usability based on the device's design specifications and functionality, four key criteria were established: (i) realism, (ii) interchangeability of modules H_i, (iii) carpal cluttering, and (iv) overall opinions regarding wearability. A user study was conducted to evaluate these factors. Ten participants (4 females and 6 males), all right-handed and aged between 25 and 39 years, took part in the trial. Each participant provided written informed consent and was free to withdraw from the study at any time. The experimental protocols adhered to the Declaration of Helsinki, ensuring that there were no risks of harm to the participants' health. The experiments took place in a virtual environment, as depicted in Fig. 3.27a, which included three geometrically regular virtual objects: a cylinder, a cone, and a hemisphere. Participants interacted with these objects using a virtual hand avatar equipped with a three-axial force sensor in the palm (Fig. 3.27b). The movements of the participant's hand, while wearing the device, guided the avatar's interactions. The virtual environment was created using CoppeliaSim v4.2 (Coppelia Robotics, Ltd., CHE),

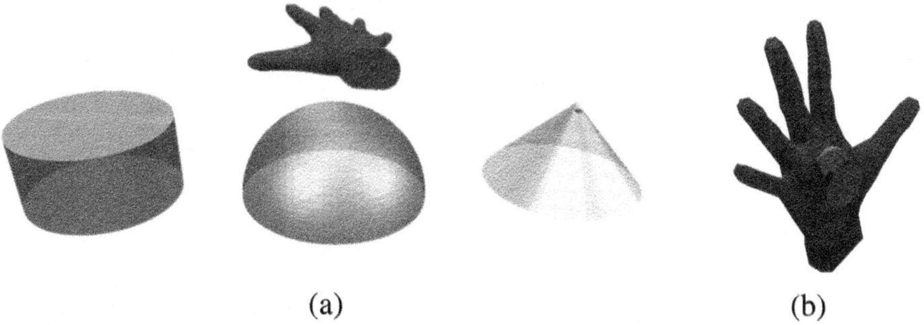

Fig. 3.27 **a** Virtual scene elements consists of the three touchable object: the cone, the cylinder and the half sphere, and the virtual hand. **b** Hand avatar details: hand (red), force sensor (green), contact area (blue). Reproduced from [80] with permission from IEEE. © IEEE 2024 (color figure online)

with interaction physics simulated using the Bullet 2.78 physics engine at a time step of 10 ms. The participants' hand movements were tracked using a LeapMotion controller (Ultraleap, Inc., US), allowing their actions to be accurately reflected in the movements of the virtual hand avatar. Participants viewed the simulation through a display positioned in front of them. The communication between tracker system and virtual environment was provided by the Robotics Operating System (ROS). A experimental protocol was designed for the usability validation testing, composed of 13 steps:

S.0 Participant sits in front of the desktop and s/he gets acquainted with tracker system and virtual scene;
S.1 The experimenter explain the protocol to the participant;
S.2 The participant wears the HapticPalm;
S.3 The participant chooses an end-effector module on table and connects its to the device;
S.4 The experimenter shows the finger position to test the carpus cluttering state;
S.5 The participant mimes the the experimenter to the best of her/his possibility;
S.6 The experimenter records the mobility score.
S.7 The participant interacts with one of three objects;
S.8 The experimenter submits the realism survey to the participant and records the statement;
S.9 Experimenter and participant repeat S.7 and S.8 for each object in the scene;
S.10 Participant detaches the end-effector module from device and put it in a box under the table;
S.11 Experimenter and participant repeat all step since S.3, until all end-effector modules are in the box;
S.12 Experimenter submits the surveys about interchangeability and records the participant statement;

S.13 Experimenter submits the surveys about general opinion to the participant and records the participant statement.

(S.4–S.6) Cluttering testing At the beginning of each experiments the participants verified their residual carpal mobility as to estimate the cluttering state of the palm. Wearing the current end–effector module, they performed the Kapandji test for the mobility of the metacarpal carpal joint that, according to [82], consists in reaching with the thumb, in order, ten predefined sites:

(1) Radial side of the proximal phalanx of the index finger;
(2) Radial side of the middle phalanx of the index finger;
(3) Tip of the index finger;
(4) Tip of the middle finger;
(5) Tip of the ring finger;
(6) Tip of the little finger;
(7) Distal interphalangeal joint crease of the little finger;
(8) Proximal interphalangeal joint crease of the little finger;
(9) Metacarpophalangeal joint crease of the little finger:
(10) Distal palmar crease.

The test stopped at the first unreachable site and returns a score equal to the number of sites successfully reached.

(S.7–S.9) Realism investigation In accordance with the device features described in Sect. 3.4, it is investigated about perceived realism during interaction with virtual objects. In order to investigate this hypothesis, all the users were asked to inspect the 3 tangible virtual objects in sequence. At each single identification for nine total identifications the participant was asked to express the perceived realism measured by MOS on a scale of 5 where 1 means "bad" while 5 "excellent". The MOS is a standardize policy to evaluate the quality of experience according to [69].

(S.12) Interchangeability survey At the end of the experiment, each user was asked to evaluate the perceived load during the fulfillment of the task of changing the end-effector modules. We used the NASA task load index (NASA TLx) to measure the task load ([83, 84]). The questionnaire collects six factors, i) Mental Demand (MD), ii) Physical Demand (PD), iii) Temporal Demand (TD), iv) Performance (PR), v) Effort (EF) and vi) Frustration (FR), through the following questions:

- MD: "*How mentally demanding was the task?*"
- PD: "*How physically demanding was the task?*"
- TD: "*How hurried or rushed was the pace of the task?*"
- PR: "*How successful were you in accomplishing what you were asked to do?*"
- EF: "*How hard did you have to work to accomplish your level of performance?*"
- FR: "*How insecure, discouraged, irritated, stressed, and annoyed were you?*"

Each of the six questions has a scale of 7 levels, considering 1 as "very low" and 7 as "very high" , except for the performance opinions where the scale is reversed (1 as "very high" and 7 as "very low").

Table 3.6 Questions for the CRSs evaluation

Index	Questions
e1	*I feel worried and embarrassed*
e2	*I feel tense*
e3	*I would wear the device if it was invisible*
a1	*feel the device on the body*
a2	*I feel the device moving*
a3	*I was not able to move as usual*
a4	*I have difficult in putting on the device*
h1	*The attached device causes me some kind of harm*
pc1	*I feel more bulky*
pc2	*I feel change in the way people look at me*
m1	*The device obstructs my movements*
an1	*I do not feel secure with the device*
an2	*I feel that I do not have the device properly attached*
an3	*I feel that the device is not working properly*

In accordance with the guidelines of the NASA TLx questionnaire, the weights of the individual questions, ω_i with $i \in \{MD, PD, TD, PR, EF, FR\}$, were chosen to obtain a final estimate of the task load TLx and therefore of module interchangeability. All load factors were pair-wised compared and the most relevant was chosen from time to time. The weight of each factor is therefore equal to the times in which it has been chosen as more relevant than another.

Ultimately the weights obtained following the protocol are the: $\omega_{MD} = 0, \omega_{PD} = 4, \omega_{TD} = 5, \omega_{PR} = 1, \omega_{EF} = 3, \omega_{FR} = 2$ The MD is deprecated with zero weight due the extreme intuitiveness of the requested task.

(S.13) General opinion survey Furthermore, the completion of the experiment was followed by the compilation of a survey based on the Comfort Rating Scales (CRSs) presented in [85]. Through the CRSs questions, reported in Table 3.6, it is aimed at evaluating the perceived comfort in the use of the device by measuring (i) Emotion (e), (ii) Attachment (a), (iii) Harm (h), (iv) Perceived chang (pc), (v) Movement (m), and (vi) Anxiety (an).

In particular, the harm is the physical sensation of conveying pain, and the movement is the awareness of modification to posture or movement due to direct impedance or inhibition by the device. The perceived change is the non-harmful indirect physical sensation making the wearer feel different overall with perceptions such as being awkward or uncoordinated, may result in making conscious compensations to movement or actions.

The CRSs uses for each questions a 21-point scale, from 0 to 20, anchored at each end with the labels "low" and "high", To calculate the average CRS score the scale

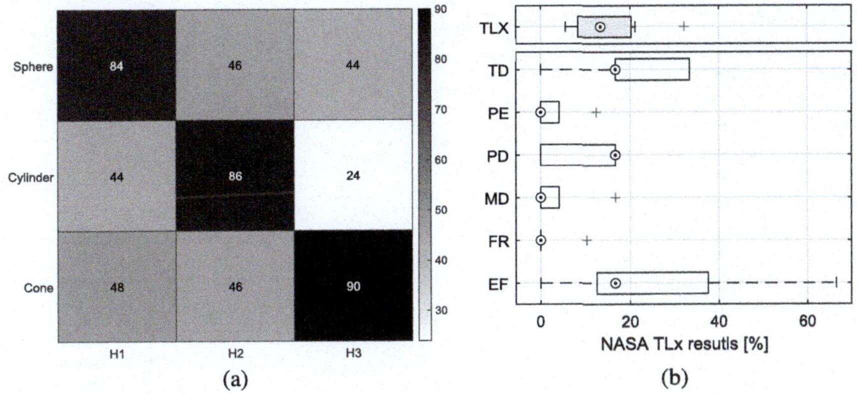

Fig. 3.28 **a** Perceived realism matrix, on principal diagonal are reported the results of most similar couple sof virtual contact surfaces and modules. **b** Evaluation of the participants' experience detaching and attaching the end-effector modules through NASA TLx in the form of a 7-point Likert scale. Reproduced from [80] with permission from IEEE. © IEEE 2024

of e3 was mirrored, making the e3 score homogeneous with all the other comfort values, where the lowest the value the better in terms of wearability.

3.5.1.3 Discussion

An analysis of the data regarding perceived realism reveals that the perceived realism increases with the similarity between the touched object and the module shape. To illustrate this relationship clearly, we organized the average user ratings on realism into a 3×3 heat-map (Fig. 3.28a), which compares the touched objects with the corresponding end-effector modules.

While the average score generally exceeds the *Poor* threshold, a significant increase is observed along the principal diagonal of the heat map, where the average perceived realism values align with the similarity between tactile modules and touched surfaces.

This finding supports the hypothesis that perceived realism enhances as the likeness between the real and virtual surfaces in contact with the palm increases. Therefore, the design of a haptic device, such as the HapticPalm, should incorporate a strategy for adapting contact areas to align with the virtual surfaces the user interacts with, ensuring a more immersive experience.

One potential approach to enhance realism is to enable the interchangeability of touch sensors. However, this must be balanced to avoid increasing the user's cognitive load or making the experience more time-consuming and frustrating.

Analysis of the additional load associated with connecting and disconnecting the modules, assessed using the NASA TLX questionnaire, indicated that the total extra load is under 20%.

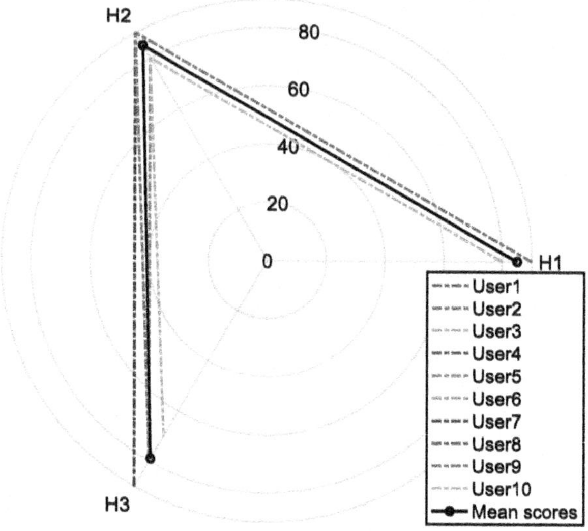

Fig. 3.29 Results of Kapandji test for the three end-effector modules H_1 (half sphere), H_2 (flat), H_3 (cone), the dashed lines correspond to individual participant's result, while the continuous black one is the mean score. Reproduced from [80] with permission from IEEE. © IEEE 2024

Figure 3.28b illustrates that the factors contributing most to the overall task load are the time requirements and effort involved. The time requirement is unavoidable, as users must pause their primary task to replace the touch sensor. In contrast, the effort is a time-dependent factor that decreases as users gain experience with the device, becoming inversely proportional to their familiarity.

Additionally, the device does not significantly impede mobility in the palm. Results from the Kapandji test, shown in Fig. 3.29, indicate that the average residual mobility while wearing the device ranges from 79% with the end-effector module H_2 to 85% with the other two modules. The general opinions collected by CRSs survey are graphically reported for each questions in Fig. 3.30. Generally the emotion load of experience is equal to 0.9 ± 0.85 while the attachment, mobility and perceived change are equal to 1.25 ± 2.41, 0.1 ± 0.1, and 0.9 ± 1.8, respectively. The harm is usually equal to 1.2 ± 0.17 and the score of anxiety is 0.3 ± 0.2. It's worth to notice that the attachment parameter is not very significant for the nature of the device itself whose purpose is to generate contact perception and must therefore be perceptible on the body.

3.6 HapticPalm for Haptics and Rehabilitative Hand Treatments

This section presents enhancements to the HapticPalm device, initially introduced in Sect. 3.6, focusing on its application in rehabilitation as a motivational tool for individuals experiencing hand pain or impairments. Specifically, we introduce an improved version of the HapticPalm end-effector and the design of new interchange-

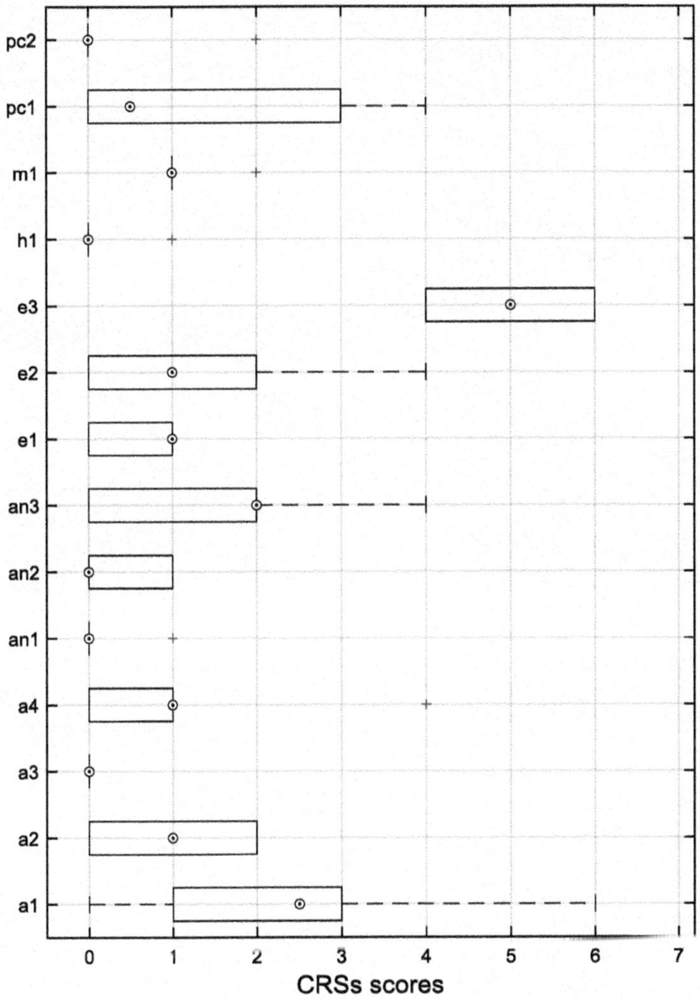

Fig. 3.30 Evaluation of the participant's complete experience through CRSs scores in the form of a 5-point Likert scale for each survey question. Reproduced from [80] with permission from IEEE. © IEEE 2024

able modules that provide compliant and vibrational stimulation to the palm, as suggested in studies by [87, 88]. The system and the upgraded wearable haptic device are depicted in Fig. 3.31.

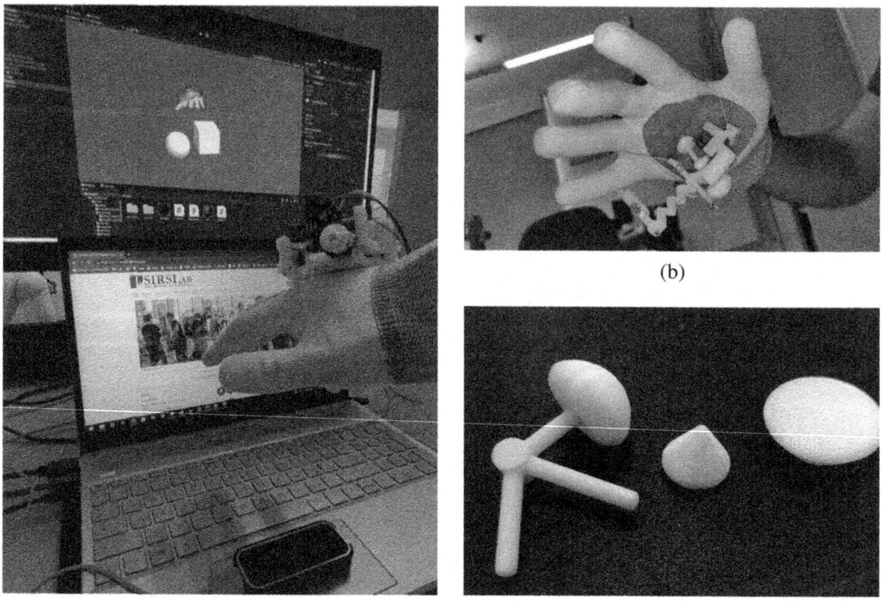

(a) (b) (c)

Fig. 3.31 New HapticPalm prototype for rehabilitation in virtual reality. In **a** the complete system. **b** Bottom view of the new prototype while in **c** the new new interchangeable modules. Copyright © 2022 Troisi et al. [86]

3.6.1 Design of the End-Effector with Interchangeable Modules

The end-effector features a "wave" shaped compliant link, inspired by the work in Sect. 4.2 and [89, 90], which supports the contact modules. It incorporates three elements that facilitate easy connection and disconnection of the tendons, along with a new interchangeable module mechanism (see Fig. 3.32b). One element connects directly to the back of the device using a previously described "C" shaped rigid link, while the other components link to the actuation system via the tendons. In comparison to the previous version presented in Sect. 3.4, this compliant mechanism allows for tip-palm disconnection when there are no contacts or forces to be rendered on the palm. The connection points between the tendons and the HapticPalm end-effector are structured in a triangular configuration, comprising three links and an ad hoc locking system for the cables, as highlighted by the green circles in Fig. 3.32b.

The new end-effector design includes a shaft connected directly to a micro servo, enabling rotation to change modules (see Fig. 3.32b). This shaft accommodates three different modules, arranged such that a 65° clockwise or counter-clockwise rotation of the micro servo allows for a total range of 130°.

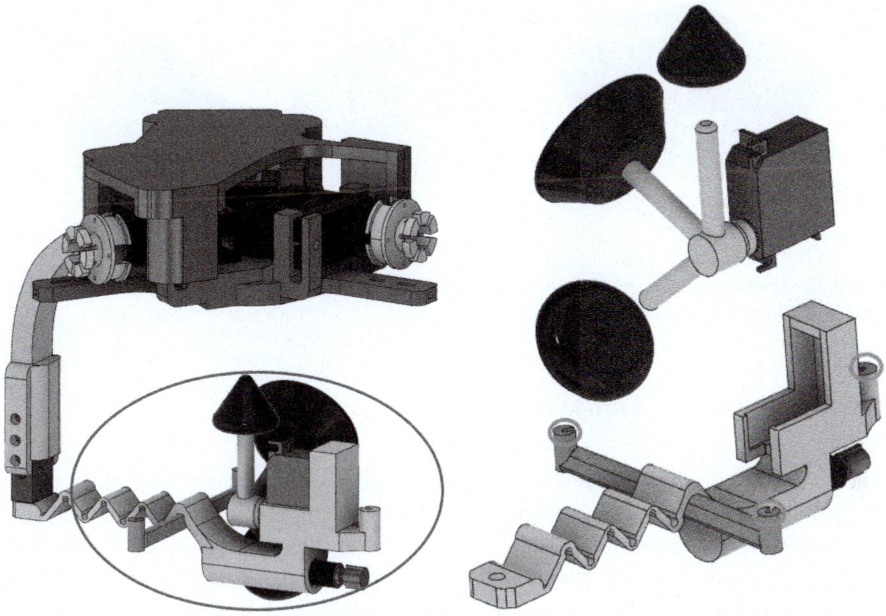

(a) (b)

Fig. 3.32 CAD model of the new HapticPalm. **a** HapticPalm CAD model. **b** New interchangeable CAD modules and new end-effector compliant structure. Copyright © 2022 Troisi et al. [86]

Interchangeability of the new modules is streamlined, as they feature a simple hole at the bottom that allows for easy assembly and disassembly without the need for tools. This maintains the HapticPalm's hallmark feature of module interchangeability (see Fig. 3.32b) while ensuring that the mobile element enables users to experience various stimuli on the palm without manual intervention. Three contact modules have been developed (see Fig. 3.33): a plane-shaped module (M1), which has been slightly modified from the previous version to better reproduce contact with edges and flat shapes; and two spherical modules (M2 and M3) with varying curvature radii, designed to simulate curved surfaces and corners, thereby providing users with different pressure cues on the palm. According to the literature, pressure combined with vibrations yields various therapeutic benefits depending on the frequency. Specifically, frequencies ranging from 50 to 400 Hz offer the following advantages: muscle relaxation at 50 Hz, inhibition of spasticity at 100 Hz, pain relief at 200 Hz, and muscle training up to 300 Hz [88]. Therefore, the HapticPalm end-effector has been designed to incorporate a vibromotor, which delivers vibrations to the palm in accordance with these clinical requirements.

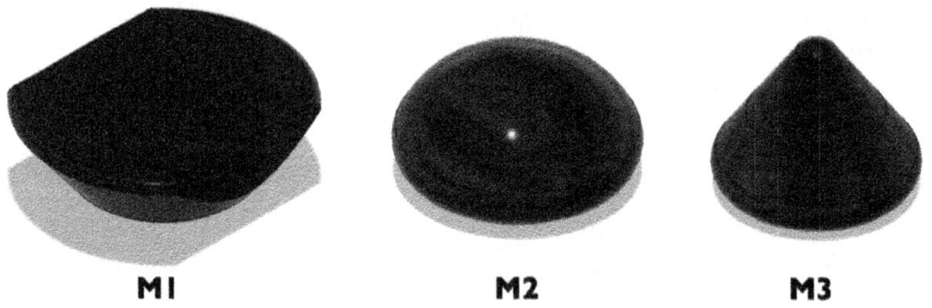

Fig. 3.33 Modules of the new HapticPalm. M1 the plane-shaped module, M2 and M3 the spherical modules. Copyright © 2022 Troisi et al. [86]

3.6.2 Structural Analyses

The design process was guided by wearability and manufacturing constraints, resulting in a structure capable of withstanding relatively high static and dynamic loads. To assess the mechanical resistance and vibration characteristics of the device's structure, a series of Finite Element Method (FEM) analyses were conducted using Fusion 360 (Autodesk Inc., US). The analysis began with a static structural evaluation, followed by an assessment of the device's response to vibrations induced by the vibromotor when vibration cues are applied.

3.6.2.1 Stationary Structural Analysis

The goal of the FEM analysis is to assess the stress response of the end-effector under various constraints and loading conditions, simulating specific pressure applications on the palm. For the static structural analysis, ABS is the material considered. Forces are applied at the three connection points of the tendons to simulate their tension on the end-effector. A constraint is imposed at the upper section of the connection site of the end-effector (lower-left part of Fig. 3.34). The following loading cases were analyzed:

- Case 1—Three forces with the same magnitude F are applied along the z-axis (Fig. 3.34a).
- Case 2—The tendon along the y-axis is exerting a force with magnitude F, while the other two with exert forces with magnitude $F/2$. This load configuration represent the case in which the device exerts a feedback force on the left/right part of the hand palm (Fig. 3.34b).
- Case 3—The tendon along the x-axis pulls the end-effector with F force, while the tensions on the other two tendons are $F/2$. This time the configuration represents the case in which I would like to move the end-effector on the upper/lower part of the hand (Fig. 3.34c).

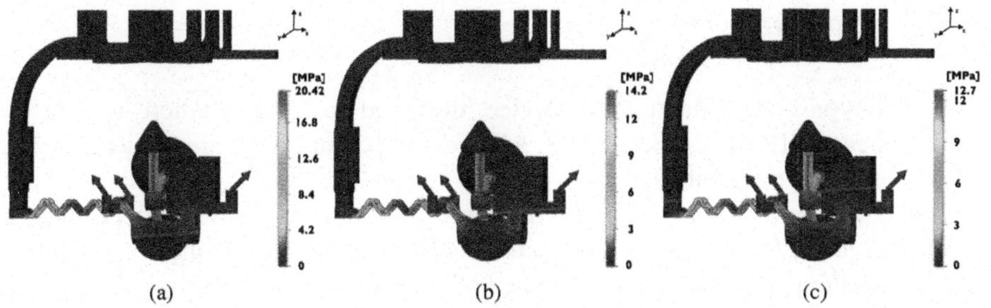

Fig. 3.34 Results of the FEM structural analysis. The blue arrows indicate the forces applied in the simulations, corresponding to tendons. Equivalent stress values obtained when **a** a pure normal force, aligned with z-axis, **b** a force with components along y and z, and **c** a force with components along x and z, are applied to the palm. Copyright © 2022 Troisi et al. [86]

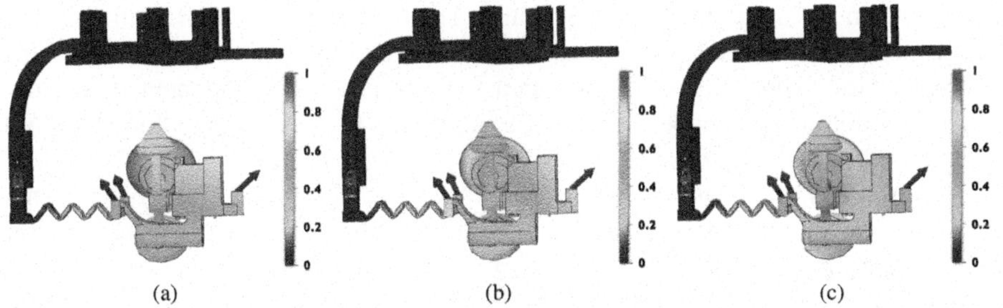

Fig. 3.35 Results of the modal analysis. **a** 110 Hz, **b** 215 Hz, **c** 375 Hz. Copyright © 2022 Troisi et al. [86]

Results relative to the numerical simulations in which $F = 1$ N are reported in Fig. 3.34. It is evident that the most stressed zone of the end-effector in each case is in correspondence of the compliant wave link.

3.6.2.2 Modal Analysis

Given that this version of the end-effector includes a vibromotor, a modal analysis was conducted to assess the vibration frequencies it can produce, focusing on those beneficial for physical therapy as previously described. The analysis targeted eight vibration modes within the frequency range of 50–400 Hz. Below, I summarize three significant results from this analysis, as illustrated in Fig. 3.35. Notably, the modes corresponding to 110 Hz and 215 Hz, shown in Fig. 3.35a and b respectively, demonstrate effective transmission of vibrations to the palm, with the 110 Hz mode being particularly effective.

3.6.3 Prototype

The prototype of the HapticPalm device, designed for rehabilitation in a virtual environment, is illustrated in Fig. 3.31. All structural components are fabricated using FDM with ABS material.

The device utilizes three MG-90S microservos powered by a 5 V battery to transmit forces to the HapticPalm end-effector, each providing a stall torque of 0.20 Nm. Control and data processing are managed by an Elegoo Nano V3+ microcontroller (ELEGOO Inc., CHN), with serial communication enabling interaction with the virtual environment, as described in Sect. 3.4.

As previously mentioned, a tendon-based parallel transmission system with three degrees of freedom (3-DoFs) generates the force applied to the palm. The cables connect the "Y-arranged" links of the end-effector to the motor pulleys located on the platform worn on the back of the hand. The minimum length of each tendon is determined by the thread length needed to link the end-effector to the platform when under tension. The pulleys are equipped with an external component that allows excess tendon to be wrapped, enabling adjustments to cable lengths for accommodating different hand sizes.

Additionally, the device is integrated into a glove designed to minimize orientation uncertainty and assist the user in positioning their hand between the tendons while wearing the device. The end-effector houses a BMS-303 micro-servo and a Micro 612 coreless vibration motor, facilitating module changes in contact with the palm and delivering vibrations in accordance with the previously mentioned clinical requirements.

Finally, the end-effector is passively supported by a 3D-printed compliant "wave"-shaped link, which allows it to detach from the palm when contact rendering is unnecessary.

3.6.3.1 VR Application

To utilize the device's various contact capabilities, a virtual reality scenario was developed using the Unity graphics engine. This scenario features interactive objects within the simulated environment, specifically designed to test the end-effector modules (see Fig. 3.36). The cube is designated for testing the M1 and M3 modules, while the sphere is used for the M2 module. When the user positions the avatar's hand over one of these objects while wearing the HapticPalm, the corresponding module is automatically selected. As the avatar's hand approaches and virtually touches the object, the user experiences the interaction through the device. Vibration can also be activated during the interaction by selecting the checkbox highlighted in Fig. 3.36. This functionality enhances navigation in the VR environment through haptic feedback on the palm and makes physiotherapy exercises more interactive, thereby improving the rehabilitation process.

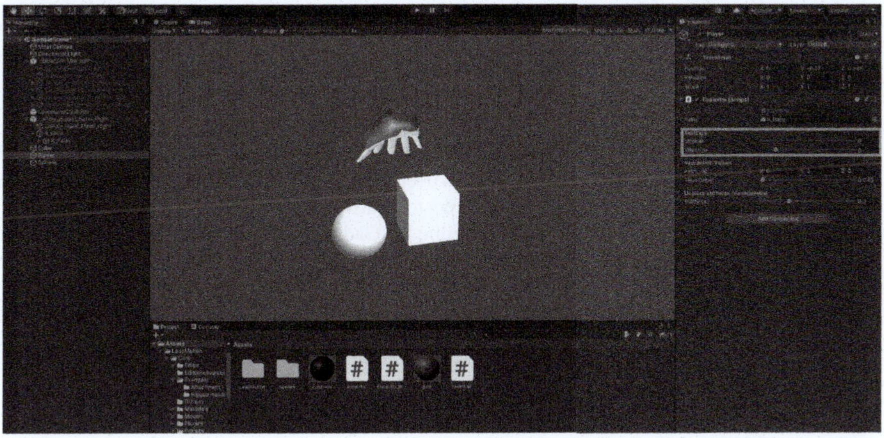

Fig. 3.36 The testing virtual scenario. It is composed by a avatar hand and two different objects. The cube allows to use M1 and M3 modules while the sphere allows to test M2 module. Copyright © 2022 Troisi et al. [86]

References

1. Abbott JJ, Marayong P, Okamura AM (2007) Haptic virtual fixtures for robot-assisted manipulation. In: Robotics research. Springer, pp 49–64
2. Battaglia PW, Kersten D, Schrater PR (2011) How haptic size sensations improve distance perception. PLoS Comput Biol 7(6):e1002080
3. Isobel S (2020) It has touched us all: commentary on the social implications of touch during the covid-19 pandemic. Soc Sci Hum Open 2(1):100051
4. Jain A, Shaikh A, Malhotra K (2020) Handshake habit amongst medical practitioners, need to abandon and embrace an alternative: analytical study in view of covid-19 pandemic. Int J Commun Med Public Health 7(6):2352
5. Cai H, Baoren T, Ma J, Chen L, Lei F, Jiang Y, Zhuang Q (2020) Psychological impact and coping strategies of frontline medical staff in Hunan between January and March 2020 during the outbreak of coronavirus disease 2019 (covid-19) in Hubei, China. Med Sci Monitor Int Med J Exp Clin Res 26:e924171-1
6. Lima CKT, de Medeiros Carvalho PM, de Araújo Silva Lima I, de Oliveira Nunes JVA, Saraiva JS, de Souza RI, da Silva CGL, Neto MLR (2020) The emotional impact of coronavirus 2019-ncov (new coronavirus disease). Psychiatry Res, 112915
7. Joshi S, Collins S, Kamino W, Gomez R, Šabanović S (2020) Social robots for socio-physical distancing. In: International conference on social robotics. Springer, pp 440–452
8. Pacchierotti C, Sinclair S, Solazzi M, Frisoli A, Hayward V, Prattichizzo D (2017) Wearable haptic systems for the fingertip and the hand: taxonomy, review, and perspectives. IEEE Trans Haptics 10(4):580–600
9. Lederman SJ, Klatzky RL (1987) Hand movements: a window into haptic object recognition. Cogn Psychol 19(3):342–368
10. Van Nierop OA, van der Helm A, Overbeeke KJ, Djajadiningrat TJP (2008) A natural human hand model. Vis Comput 24(1):31–44
11. Moss P, Sluka K, Wright A (2007) The initial effects of knee joint mobilization on osteoarthritic hyperalgesia. Manual Therapy 12(2):109–118

12. Bialosky JE, Bishop MD, Price DD, Robinson ME, George SZ (2009) The mechanisms of manual therapy in the treatment of musculoskeletal pain: a comprehensive model. Manual Therapy 14(5):531–538
13. Camarinos J, Marinko L (2009) Effectiveness of manual physical therapy for painful shoulder conditions: a systematic review. J Manual Manipulative Therapy 17(4):206–215
14. Martins DF, Bobinski F, Mazzardo-Martins L, Cidral-Filho FJ, Nascimento FP, Gadotti VM, Santos ARS (2012) Ankle joint mobilization decreases hypersensitivity by activation of peripheral opioid receptors in a mouse model of postoperative pain. Pain Med 13(8):1049–1058
15. Martins DF, Mazzardo-Martins L, Cidral-Filho FJ, Gadotti VM, Santos ARS (2013) Peripheral and spinal activation of cannabinoid receptors by joint mobilization alleviates postoperative pain in mice. Neuroscience 255:110–121
16. Salgado ASI, Stramosk J, Ludtke DD, Kuci ACC, Salm DC, Ceci LA, Petronilho F, Florentino D, Danielski LG, Gassenferth A et al (2019) Manual therapy reduces pain behavior and oxidative stress in a murine model of complex regional pain syndrome type I. Brain Sci 9(8):197
17. Beaudoin AJ, Pedneault F, Houle M, Bilodeau C, Gauvin M-P, Groleau D, Brochu P, Couture M (2021) Case study assessing the feasibility of using a wearable haptic device or humanoid robot to facilitate transitions in occupational therapy sessions for children with autism spectrum disorder. J Rehab Assistive Technol Eng 8:20556683211049041
18. Barbic F, Galli M, Vecchia LD, Canesi M, Cimolin V, Porta A, Bari V, Cerri G, Dipaola F, Bassani T et al (2014) Effects of mechanical stimulation of the feet on gait and cardiovascular autonomic control in parkinson's disease. J Appl Physiol 116(5):495–503
19. Choukou M-A, Mbabaali S, Hani JB, Cooke C (2021) Haptic-enabled hand rehabilitation in stroke patients: a scoping review. Appl Sci 11(8):3712
20. Wu H-C, Liao Y-C, Cheng Y-H, Shih P-C, Tsai C-M, Lin C-Y (2017) The potential effect of a vibrotactile glove rehabilitation system on motor recovery in chronic post-stroke hemiparesis. Technol Health Care 25(6):1183–1187
21. Brokaw EB, Murray TM, Nef T, Lum PS, Nichols D, Holley RJ (2011) Time independent functional task training: a case study on the effect of inter-joint coordination driven haptic guidance in stroke therapy. In: 2011 IEEE international conference on rehabilitation robotics. IEEE, pp 1–6
22. Timmermans AA, Lemmens RJM, Monfrance M, Geers RPJ, Bakx W, Smeets RJEM, Seelen HAM (2014) Effects of task-oriented robot training on arm function, activity, and quality of life in chronic stroke patients: a randomized controlled trial. J Neuroeng Rehab 11(1):1–12
23. Dragusanu M, Iqbal ZM, Prattichizzo MDB (2022) Exploiting a wearable extra-finger for haptic. In: Haptics: science, technology, applications: 13th international conference on human haptic sensing and touch enabled computer applications, EuroHaptics 2022, Hamburg, Germany, 22–25 May 2022, proceedings, vol 13235. Springer Nature, p 366
24. Fluet GG, Merians AS, Qiu Q, Davidow A, Adamovich SV (2014) Comparing integrated training of the hand and arm with isolated training of the same effectors in persons with stroke using haptically rendered virtual environments, a randomized clinical trial. J Neuroeng Rehab 11(1):1–11
25. Loureiro RCV, Harwin WS, Lamperd R, Collin C (2013) Evaluation of reach and grasp robot-assisted therapy suggests similar functional recovery patterns on proximal and distal arm segments in sub-acute hemiplegia. IEEE Trans Neur Syst Rehab Eng 22(3):593–602
26. Maris A, Coninx K, Seelen H, Truyens V, De Weyer T, Geers R, Lemmens M, Coolen J, Stupar S, Lamers I et al (2018) The impact of robot-mediated adaptive i-travle training on impaired upper limb function in chronic stroke and multiple sclerosis. Disab Rehab Assistive Technol 13(1):1–9
27. Broeren J, Rydmark M, Björkdahl A, Sunnerhagen KS (2007) Assessment and training in a 3-dimensional virtual environment with haptics: a report on 5 cases of motor rehabilitation in the chronic stage after stroke. Neurorehab Neur Repair 21(2):180–189
28. Huang X, Naghdy F, Naghdy G, Du H (2017) Clinical effectiveness of combined virtual reality and robot assisted fine hand motion rehabilitation in subacute stroke patients. In: 2017 International Conference on Rehabilitation Robotics (ICORR). IEEE, pp 511–515

29. Iwata H, Yano H, Nakaizumi F, Kawamura R (2001) Project feelex: adding haptic surface to graphics. In: Proceedings of the 28th annual conference on Computer graphics and interactive techniques, pp 469–476
30. Borst CW, Cavanaugh CD (2004) Haptic controller design and palm-sized vibrotactile array. Technical report
31. Bouri M, Baur C, Clavel R, Newman CJ, Zedka M (2013) "Handreha": a new hand and wrist haptic device for hemiplegic children. In: ACHI 2013, the sixth international conference on advances in computer-human interactions, pp 286–292
32. Pernalete N, Edwards S, Gottipati R, Tipple J, Kolipakam V, Dubey RV (2005) Eye-hand coordination assessment/therapy using a robotic haptic device. In: 9th international conference on rehabilitation robotics, 2005. ICORR 2005. IEEE, pp 25–28
33. Pernalete N, Gottipati R, Grantner J, Edwards S, Janiak D, Haskin J, Dubey RV (2007) Integration of an intelligent decision support system and a robotic haptic device for eye-hand coordination therapy. In: 2007 IEEE 10th international conference on rehabilitation robotics. IEEE, pp 283–291
34. Ferre M, Galiana I, Wirz R, Tuttle N (2011) Haptic device for capturing and simulating hand manipulation rehabilitation. IEEE/ASME Trans Mechatron 16(5):808–815
35. Martinez J, Griffiths D, Biscione V, Georgiou O, Carter T (2018) Touchless haptic feedback for supernatural VR experiences. In: 2018 IEEE conference on virtual reality and 3D user interfaces (VR). IEEE, pp 629–630
36. Minamizawa K, Kamuro S, Fukamachi S, Kawakami N, Tachi S (2008) Ghostglove: haptic existence of the virtual world. In: ACM SIGGRAPH 2008 new tech demos. Association for Computing Machinery
37. Minamizawa K, Kamuro S, Kawakami N, Tachi S (2008) A palm-worn haptic display for bimanual operations in virtual environments. In: International conference on human haptic sensing and touch enabled computer applications. Springer, pp 458–463
38. Achibet M, Girard A, Talvas A, Marchal M, Lécuyer A (2015) Elastic-arm: human-scale passive haptic feedback for augmenting interaction and perception in virtual environments. In: 2015 IEEE virtual reality (VR). IEEE, pp 63–68
39. Son B, Park J (2018) Haptic feedback to the palm and fingers for improved tactile perception of large objects. In: Proceedings of the 31st annual ACM symposium on user interface software and technology, pp 757–763
40. Son B, Park J (2018) Tactile sensitivity to distributed patterns in a palm. In: Proceedings of the 20th ACM international conference on multimodal interaction, pp 486–491
41. Gollner U, Bieling T, Joost G (2012) Mobile LORM glove: introducing a communication device for deaf-blind people. In: Proceedings of the sixth international conference on tangible, embedded and embodied interaction, pp 127–130
42. Martínez J, García A, Oliver M, Molina JP, González P (2014) Identifying virtual 3D geometric shapes with a vibrotactile glove. IEEE Comput Graph Appl 36(1):42–51
43. Borja EF, Lara DA, Quevedo WX, Andaluz VH (2018) Haptic stimulation glove for fine motor rehabilitation in virtual reality environments. In: International conference on augmented reality, virtual reality and computer graphics. Springer, pp 211–229
44. Kovacs R, Ofek E, Franco MG, Siu AF, Marwecki S, Holz C, Sinclair M (2020) Haptic pivot: on-demand handhelds in VR. In: Proceedings of the 33rd annual ACM symposium on user interface software and technology, pp 1046–1059
45. Kajimoto H (2012) Design of cylindrical whole-hand haptic interface using electrocutaneous display. In: International conference on human haptic sensing and touch enabled computer applications. Springer, pp 67–72
46. Zubrycki I, Granosik G (2017) Novel haptic device using jamming principle for providing kinaesthetic feedback in glove-based control interface. J Intell Robot Syst 85(3–4):413–429
47. de Tinguy X, Howard T, Pacchierotti C, Marchal M, Lécuyer A (2020) Weatavix: Wearable actuated tangibles for virtual reality experiences. In: Nisky I, Hartcher-O'Brien J, Wiertlewski M, Smeets J (eds) Haptics: science, technology, applications. Springer International Publishing, Cham, pp 262–270

48. Trinitatova D, Tsetserukou D, Fedoseev A (2019) Touchvr: a wearable haptic interface for VR aimed at delivering multi-modal stimuli at the user's palm. In: SIGGRAPH Asia 2019 XR. Association for Computing Machinery, pp 42–43
49. Trinitatova D, Tsetserukou D (2019) Deltatouch: a 3D haptic display for delivering multimodal tactile stimuli at the palm. In: 2019 IEEE world haptics conference (WHC). IEEE, pp 73–78
50. Prasad V, Stock-Homburg R, Peters J (2021) Human-robot handshaking: a review. Int J Soc Robot, pp 1–17
51. Ammi M, Demulier V, Caillou S, Gaffary Y, Tsalamlal Y, Martin J-C, Tapus A (2015) Haptic human-robot affective interaction in a handshaking social protocol. In: Proceedings of the tenth annual ACM/IEEE international conference on human-robot interaction, pp 263–270
52. Beaudoin Jonathan, Laliberté Thierry, Gosselin Clément (2019) Haptic interface for handshake emulation. IEEE Robot Autom Lett 4(4):4124–4130
53. Vigni F, Knoop E, Prattichizzo D, Malvezzi M (2019) The role of closed-loop hand control in handshaking interactions. IEEE Robot Autom Lett 4(2):878–885
54. Prattichizzo D, Chinello F, Pacchierotti C, Malvezzi M (2013) Towards wearability in fingertip haptics: a 3-dof wearable device for cutaneous force feedback. IEEE Trans Haptics 6(4):506–516
55. Chinello F, Malvezzi M, Prattichizzo D, Pacchierotti C (2019) A modular wearable finger interface for cutaneous and kinesthetic interaction: control and evaluation. IEEE Trans Ind Electron 67(1):706–716
56. Huisman G, Baldi TL, D'Aurizio N, Prattichizzo D (2021) Feedback of head gestures in audio-haptic remote communication. In: 2021 international symposium on wearable computers, pp 135–137
57. Teh JKS, Cheok AD, Peiris RL, Choi Y, Thuong V, Lai S (2008) Huggy pajama: a mobile parent and child hugging communication system. In: Proceedings of the 7th international conference on Interaction design and children, pp 250–257
58. Dragusanu M, Troisi D, Villani A, Prattichizzo D, Malvezzi M (2022) Happ: a haptic portable pad for hand disease manual treatment. In: 2022 31st IEEE international conference on robot and human interactive communication (RO-MAN), pp 345–350
59. Larson K (2016) Can you estimate modulus from durometer hardness for silicones. Dow Corning Corporation, pp 1–6
60. Pacchierotti C, Sinclair S, Solazzi M, Frisoli A, Hayward V, Prattichizzo D (2017) Wearable haptic systems for the fingertip and the hand: taxonomy, review, and perspectives. IEEE Trans Haptics 10(4):580–600
61. Dragusanu M, Villani A, Prattichizzo D, Malvezzi M (2021) Design of a wearable haptic device for hand palm cutaneous feedback. Front Robot AI 8:254
62. Dragusanu M, Iqbal Z, Villani A, D'Aurizio N, Prattichizzo D, Malvezzi M (2022) Hans: a haptic system for human-to-human remote handshake. In: 2022 9th IEEE RAS/EMBS international conference for biomedical robotics and biomechatronics (BioRob), pp 1–8
63. Meli L, Hussain I, Aurilio M, Malvezzi M, O'Malley MK, Prattichizzo D (2018) The hbracelet: a wearable haptic device for the distributed mechanotactile stimulation of the upper limb. IEEE Robot Autom Lett 3(3):2198–2205
64. Knoop E, Bächer M, Wall V, Deimel R, Brock O, Beardsley P (2017) Handshakiness: benchmarking for human-robot hand interactions. In: 2017 IEEE/RSJ international conference on intelligent robots and systems (IROS). IEEE, pp 4982–4989
65. Melnyk A, Henaff P, Khomenko V, Borysenko V (2014) Sensor network architecture to measure characteristics of a handshake between humans. In: 2014 IEEE 34th international scientific conference on electronics and nanotechnology (ELNANO). IEEE, pp 264–268
66. Pérez-González A, Vergara M, Sancho-Bru JL (2013) Stiffness map of the grasping contact areas of the human hand. J Biomech 46(15):2644–2650
67. Gao Y, Li H, Luo Y (2015) An empirical study of wearable technology acceptance in healthcare. Ind Manage Data Syst
68. Lee Y, Kozar KA, Larsen KRT (2003) The technology acceptance model: Past, present, and future. Commun Assoc Inf Syst 12(1):50

69. Hoßfeld T, Heegaard PE, Varela M, Möller S (2016) QOE beyond the MOS: an in-depth look at QOE via better metrics and their relation to MOS. Qual User Exp 1(1):1–23
70. Chinello F, Pacchierotti C, Malvezzi M, Prattichizzo D (2018) A three revolute-revolute-spherical wearable fingertip cutaneous device for stiffness rendering. IEEE Trans Haptics 11(1):39–50
71. Chinello F, Malvezzi M, Prattichizzo D, Pacchierotti C (2020) A modular wearable finger interface for cutaneous and kinesthetic interaction: control and evaluation. IEEE Trans Ind Electron 67(1):706–716
72. Swartz MH (2002) Physical diagnosis: history and examination. WB Saunders
73. Kubo K, Cheng Y-S, Zhou B, An K-N, Moran SL, Amadio PC, Zhang X, Zhao C (2018) The quantitative evaluation of the relationship between the forces applied to the palm and carpal tunnel pressure. J Biomech 66:170–174
74. Berti A, Merlet J-P, Carricato M (2013) Solving the direct geometrico-static problem of 3-3 cable-driven parallel robots by interval analysis: preliminary results. In: Cable-driven parallel robots. Springer, pp 251–268
75. Carricato M, Abbasnejad G (2013) Direct geometrico-static analysis of under-constrained cable-driven parallel robots with 4 cables. In: Cable-driven parallel robots. Springer, pp 269–285
76. Miermeister P, Kraus W, Pott A (2013) Differential kinematics for calibration, system investigation, and force based forward kinematics of cable-driven parallel robots. In: Cable-driven parallel robots. Springer, pp 319–333
77. Khosravi MA, Taghirad HD (2013) Experimental performance of robust PID controller on a planar cable robot. In: Cable-driven parallel robots. Springer, pp 337–352
78. Yao R, Li H, Zhang X (2013) A modeling method of the cable driven parallel manipulator for fast. In: Cable-driven parallel robots. Springer, pp 423–436
79. Malvezzi M, Chinello F, Prattichizzo D, Pacchierotti C (2021) Design of personalized wearable haptic interfaces to account for fingertip size and shape. IEEE Trans Haptics
80. Villani A, Dragusanu M, Prattichizzo D, Malvezzi M (2024) Validation and usability assessment of the hapticpalm, a wearable device for hand palm force feedback. In: 2024 IEEE haptics symposium (HAPTICS), pp 372–378
81. Alexander H, Cook T (1976) Variations with age in the mechanical properties of human skin in vivo. In: Bed sore biomechanics. Springer, pp 109–117
82. Kapandji A (1986) Clinical test of apposition and counter-apposition of the thumb. Annales de chirurgie de la main: organe officiel des societes de chirurgie de la main 5(1):67–73
83. Hart SG, Staveland LE (1988) Development of NASA-TLX (task load index): results of empirical and theoretical research. In: Advances in psychology, vol 52. Elsevier, pp 139–183
84. Hart SG (2006) Nasa-task load index (NASA-TLX); 20 years later. In: Proceedings of the human factors and ergonomics society annual meeting, vol 50. Sage, Los Angeles, CA, pp 904–908
85. Knight JF, Baber C (2005) A tool to assess the comfort of wearable computers. Human Factors 47(1):77–91
86. Troisi D, Dragusanu M, Villani A, Prattichizzo D, Malvezzi M (2022) Hapticpalm: a wearable robotic device for haptics and rehabilitative hand treatments. In: Cavallo F, Cabibihan J-J, Fiorini L, Sorrentino A, He H, Liu X, Matsumoto Y, Ge SS (eds) Social robotics. Springer Nature, Cham, Switzerland, pp 402–411
87. Cardinale MAJW, Wakeling J (2005) Whole body vibration exercise: are vibrations good for you? Br J Sports Med 39(9):585–589
88. Saggini R, Carmignano S, Palermo T, Bellomo R (2016) Mechanical vibration in rehabilitation: state of the art. J Novel Physiotherapies 6:314
89. Dragusanu M, Achilli GM, Valigi MC, Prattichizzo D, Malvezzi M, Salvietti G (2022) The wavejoints: a novel methodology to design soft-rigid grippers made by monolithic 3D printed fingers with adjustable joint stiffness. In: 2022 international conference on robotics and automation (ICRA), pp 6173–6179

90. Dragusanu M, Troisi D, Prattichizzo D, Malvezzi M (2023) Joint stiffness analysis and regulation for underactuated soft grippers based on monolithic structure. In: Petuya V, Quaglia G, Parikyan T, Carbone G (eds) Proceedings of I4SDG workshop 2023. Springer Nature, Cham, Switzerland,, pp 492–499

Chapter 4
Assistive Robotic Gripper Devices

Millions of people worldwide face significant limitations in their ability to reach for and manipulate objects, rendering them dependent on assistance for basic activities of daily living (ADLs). These limitations often stem from conditions affecting both the upper and lower limbs, including stroke, aging, muscular dystrophy, multiple sclerosis, and other debilitating diseases. As a result, many individuals are unable to lead fully independent lives. This highlights the urgent need for accessible and efficient assistive devices that enable users to interact safely with their environment, thereby enhancing autonomy and boosting self-esteem [1, 2]. Research consistently shows that one of the most critical challenges for individuals with temporary or permanent disabilities is the inability to grasp and handle objects, whether from a shelf or the floor. Object retrieval is a fundamental aspect of performing ADLs, and the inability to do so places a considerable burden on healthcare systems and professionals. Assistive robotic manipulators offer a promising solution for individuals with motor impairments, enabling them to perform essential tasks such as manipulating objects, assisting with personal hygiene, and even supporting nutrition. These devices can significantly improve quality of life, empowering users to regain control over their daily activities and live with greater dignity.

In addition to advancements in exoskeletons and wearable or portable devices, the research presented in this chapter focuses on the emerging field of soft robotics, specifically the development of soft robotic grippers for assistive applications. This approach holds great potential for creating versatile and user-friendly solutions in assistive robotics.

M. Dragusanu, *Design of Soft–Rigid Devices for Rehabilitative and Assistive Robotics*, Springer Theses, https://doi.org/10.1007/978-3-031-84823-0_4

4.1 State of the Art

Robotic grippers and hands are used as the primary end-effectors for robots interacting with their environment, enabling grasping and manipulation of objects. Despite the numerous robotic hands and grippers developed over the years, robotic grasping and manipulation remains a challenging, unsolved problem for researchers and engineers.

Early solutions to this problem were mostly based on rigid mechanisms, with compliance achieved through active control. These rigid approaches involved fully actuated (or hyper-actuated) hands [3, 4], composed of rigid links connected by individually controllable joints. These hands performed manipulation tasks based on models that assumed perfect knowledge of applied forces and contact points [5, 6]. While these devices offered high accuracy, they also introduced significant mechanical and computational complexity, which negatively impacted their reliability and ease of use.

In recent years, the limitations of rigid approaches in real-world applications have exposed several limitations, leading to a growing interest in a novel approach based on soft materials. Advances in new materials, technology, and the design of highly deformable structures have spurred the development of soft robotic grippers [7] and hands [8, 9]. These soft robots are inherently underactuated, meaning they have fewer actuators, i.e. degrees of actuation (DoAs), than degrees of freedom (DoFs), which results in greater robustness and reduced mechanical complexity.

The key idea behind soft manipulation is the introduction of passive compliance, allowing the hand to adapt to object uncertainties, such as unknown locations and shapes, making it particularly effective in unstructured and unpredictable environments. This compliance can be achieved through various fabrication techniques, including the use of novel deformable biomaterials [10] and advanced 3D-printing technologies [11]. Rather than requiring precise contact points or exact force application, soft grippers and hands simply enclose the object, with their intrinsic flexibility adapting to its shape [12]. Inspired by human manipulation, soft grippers can also exploit environmental constraints to compensate for the lack of controllable degrees of freedom [13, 14]. This principle has led to several practical applications, where even delicate or fragile objects can be safely grasped [15, 16]. However, when more complex manipulation tasks are required, soft hands face challenges due to their underactuation, limited ability to apply strong forces, and lack of precise modeling [17, 18].

Our research group has recently focused on the design of soft-rigid multi-fingered grippers [19, 20], which combine rigid links with deformable soft joints [21, 22]. This hybrid actuation strategy allows the gripper's rigid components to yield to external forces, reducing resistance and enhancing safety during unintended collisions.

The state of the art in assistive grippers leverages a combination of hardware underactuation through mechanical coupling of joints and deformable materials surrounding the rigid links. This approach offers a practical solution for achieving safe interactions by *embodying* part of the gripper's "intelligence" into the hardware design rather than relying solely on complex control algorithms [23]. Notable examples from our lab include the CoGripper [24], the ScoopGripper [25], and the Quad-Spatula Gripper [26]. These grippers use a tendon-driven system, with fingers constructed from 3D-printed modules featuring rigid ABS links and soft joints made from TPU [27], inspired by the design principles introduced by Dollar and Howe [28].

A key feature of these soft-rigid grippers is their ability to reproduce different finger flexion trajectories by adjusting the compliance of the soft hinges [29], enabling diverse grasping strategies that exploit environmental constraints. Joint compliance is tailored by varying the density of the material used for printing the joints. Commercial 3D printing software offers control over mechanical properties, such as infill density and pattern, while advanced techniques like multi-material 3D printing provide additional flexibility. For example, Interpenetrating Phase Composites (IPCs) allow for the design of soft grippers with customized mechanical properties using mathematically generated topologies [30].

Advanced design tools enable the synthesis of mechanisms with minimal mechanical components, ensuring desired mobility through the appropriate shaping of elements [31, 32]. These tools have been adopted in the design of compliant robotic grippers and hands [33, 34]. Building on the robust literature on flexure hinges dating back to the 1960s [35], the bending behavior of common flexure hinges has been modeled and experimentally validated to find optimal designs for fully compliant prosthetic fingers [36]. In [37], a fruit-handling gripper composed of two monolithic compliant fingers was developed using topology optimization methods. However, underactuated devices face challenges in precise motion control and the ability to resist external mechanical disturbances (e.g. , unexpected forces that may open the jaws). Furthermore, traditional control strategies [38] are not applicable to such devices due to indeterminate kinematics and difficulties in modeling compliance and its effects on transmitted forces and torques. To address these limitations, research is shifting towards more complex designs and control strategies [39]. This approach involves providing additional actuation sources, such as replicating motors, which increases the device's size and requires more sophisticated control algorithms.

In this context, the work presented in this chapter explores innovative solutions using soft-rigid grippers for assistive applications, focusing on new actuation systems and AM) technologies. First, a methodology for designing a novel robotic gripper with 3D-printed, tendon-actuated fingers is introduced. Each finger is a monolithic structure with rigid phalanges connected by flexible wave-shaped joints, referred to as WaveJoints. The characterization of these WaveJoints and the twisted-string actuation (TSA) control system used to adjust their stiffness are detailed in Sects. 4.2–4.4.

Additionally, a new tendon-driven underactuated gripper with magnetic actuation is presented in Sect. 4.5, specifically designed for safe human-robot cooperative dressing. Magnetic elements serve as additional degrees of actuation (DoAs) in specific locations of the gripper, working synergistically with the global actuation provided by motors and tendons. This approach enhances the device's capabilities for safe and efficient interactions. In following a review of the state of art in assisted dressing is presented.

4.1.1 Related Works on Robot Grippers for Assisted Dressing

Robot-assisted dressing is a highly collaborative task between humans and robots, requiring the strict adoption of the principle of "safety first". During dressing, the human and the robot operate in close proximity, often sharing the same confined space, which can lead to unintentional physical contact. In such scenarios, the robotic end-effector (EE) responsible for manipulating clothing plays a crucial role. Soft robotic grippers are particularly well-suited for these tasks due to their ability to deform upon contact, absorbing the energy from accidental collisions and ensuring safer interactions compared to rigid grippers [28].

The manipulation of garments presents a unique challenge in robotics, as clothing materials are thin, highly deformable, and difficult to control. Despite these complexities, most grippers used for garment manipulation are not specifically designed for fabric interaction [40]. Various approaches have been explored to address this challenge. For example, a versatile gripper capable of both prehensile and non-prehensile grasping is introduced in [41], while [42] proposes using needles to separate and grasp fabric layers. Rolling fingertips are employed in [43] to detect fabric corners for easier manipulation, and suction cups are explored in [44]. Multi-fingered hands provide more dexterous control over fabrics [45, 46], with the added benefit of sensorization to classify materials [47] or leverage environmental factors [48]. A jaw gripper with an integrated electromagnet, designed for manipulating garments with ferromagnetic parts, is discussed in [49]. However, none of these designs prioritize safety in human-robot interactions, as they are primarily intended for industrial applications that emphasize reliability, speed, and accuracy.

Perception of fabrics has been studied in [50, 51], and machine-learning techniques for autonomous garment manipulation have been explored in [52–54]. While these methods have shown promise, they are typically suited for scenarios where human presence is not required. In [55, 56], safety concerns and standards for physical human-robot interaction (pHRI) are addressed, and [57] outlines specific guidelines for designing collaborative grippers.

4.2 The WaveJoints

This part of the thesis introduces a methodology for designing a novel type of robotic grippers, composed of 3D-printed tendon-actuated fingers. Each finger is a monolithic structure composed of rigid segments, the phalanges, connected by flexible, wave-shaped joints known as WaveJoints.

The first key contribution of this work is the development of a procedure to define the stiffness of the flexible joints based on the specific task the gripper needs to perform. Unlike previous approaches, where the design focused primarily on achieving a predetermined closure motion for the fingers [29], this method takes into account more complex tasks that involve contact interactions with grasped objects. The proposed methodology allows for the customization of the flexible parts' characteristics-such as thickness, length, wave amplitude, and phase-enabling the tendon-driven actuation to not only produce finger flexion but also more intricate movements.

The solution presented in this section offers several advantages over existing state-of-the-art designs, particularly in its versatility, ease of manufacturing, and simplified assembly. Each finger consists of a single component made from a single material, streamlining the production process. The sinusoidal shape of the flexible components was chosen for its ability to generate a broad range of compliance values by adjusting just a few parameters.

Another major contribution is the structured synthesis procedure, broken down into distinct sub-phases, allowing designers to precisely control each phase and tailor the gripper's design to suit different tasks and objectives. The overall compliance of the flexible parts is designed in relation to the task at hand, after which the geometric parameters of the sinusoidal "wave" elements are determined to meet the desired compliance. This procedure builds on the design framework established in [29], which focused on passive joints for fingertip closure trajectories, but extends it to encompass a broader range of tasks, including grasp control and in-hand object manipulation.

To demonstrate the feasibility of this design and manufacturing methodology for soft-rigid grippers, two prototypes were developed: the WaveGripper and the Twist-WaveGripper. The WaveGripper is designed for grasping objects of various shapes, while the Twist-WaveGripper enables the in-hand rotation of a cylindrical object around an axis perpendicular to the palm surface (see Fig. 4.1).

This methodology can be further expanded and generalized to create grippers with customized finger closure trajectories tailored for specific manipulation tasks. Notably, the same tendon-driven actuation can produce different motions by simply adjusting the configuration of the wave-shaped joints, highlighting the flexibility and adaptability of this design approach.

4.2.1 Methodology

The methodology developed for the design of WaveJoints can be divided in three main steps, as summarized in Fig. 4.2.

Step 1. The primary design requirements are defined in terms of task-specific finger movements or fingertip trajectories, from which the necessary joint rotations, $\Delta\mathbf{q}$, are derived. Building on the methodology introduced in [29], these values are then used to calculate the joint stiffness. This process involves analyzing the gripper's

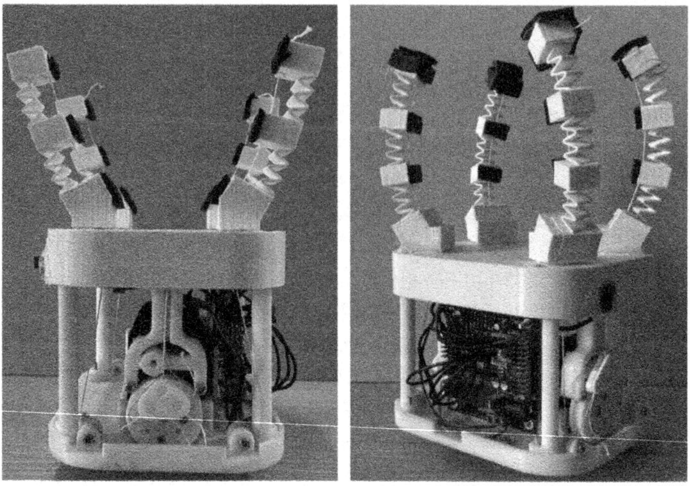

(a) (b)

Fig. 4.1 Two versions of the WaveGripper. **a** Version for power grasp. **b** Version for in hand twisting of an object

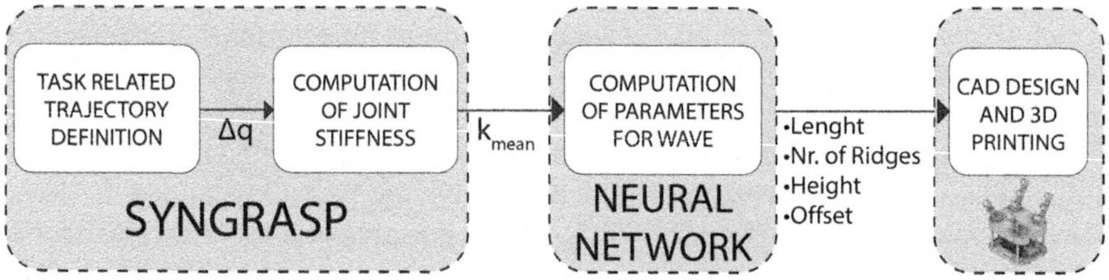

Fig. 4.2 Scheme of the procedure developed for the design of WaveGripper flexible elements. Reproduced from [58] with permission from IEEE. © IEEE 2022

kinematics and grasping capabilities. In this work, the analysis is carried out using the tools provided by SynGrasp [59].

Step 2. Definition of flexible joint geometric properties allowing to get the suitable stiffness values. A feed-forward Neural Network based procedure has been developed to solve this problem.

Step 3. The obtained parameters are sent to a parametric CAD software that generates the input for the manufacturing phase.

4.2.1.1 Parametric Definition of Gripper Elements and Joints

With respect to other solutions present in the literature, designed with a closed loop kinematic structure [31, 32, 37], the fingers presented in this section maintains a serial structure, with a sequence of rigid and flexible parts.

Gripper design parameters The design parameters regarding the whole gripper that can be selected are: (i) the number of rigid/compliant elements for each finger; (ii) the dimension and shape of the rigid parts; (iii) the number and arrangement of the fingers on the gripper palm.

Compliant element parameters Each compliant part of the finger is designed with a sinusoidal *wave* shape, chosen for several key reasons: (i) it allows parametric definition in CAD software, requiring only a few parameters for its design. This flexibility is not available with other geometries, such as the Fin Ray® effect [60], or more complex automated design methods like topology optimization [61]; (ii) compared to rectangular-section flexures, such as those discussed in [29], the sinusoidal shape is more adaptable and allows the use of the same material for both the rigid and flexible parts of the finger. Once the joint characteristics are tailored to the task, the finger's CAD model is automatically updated, simplifying manufacturing and reducing assembly complexity; (iii) by adjusting the design parameters, a broad range of stiffness values can be achieved, enabling the gripper to perform a wide variety of tasks, as will be detailed later.

The parameters defining each wave joint are: (i) joint length (l_t); (ii) number of ridges (n_r); (iii) wave height (sinusoidal amplitude) (h_c); (iv) offset (wave thickness) (t_h); (v) twist angle (α).

Table 4.1 and Fig. 4.3 provide the design parameter ranges defined in this study, enabling the creation of grippers capable of grasping and manipulating common objects. Notably, the twist angle α facilitates more complex, 3D finger movements compared to other grippers composed of soft-rigid element chains [29].

For the rigid elements, a simple rectangular design is chosen for all components, with dimensions $11 \times 15 \times 16$ mm. These elements can be modified to suit specific tasks, such as using custom shapes for handling delicate or deformable objects. Additionally, an S-shaped cavity is incorporated into the rigid links for tendon routing.

Table 4.1 Ranges of parameters for joint definition

Parameters	l_t [mm]	n_r	h_c [mm]	t_h [mm]	α [°]
Twist	15–30	3–6	8–14	0.5–0.6	0–24
Power grasp	15–30	3–6	8–14	0.5–0.6	0

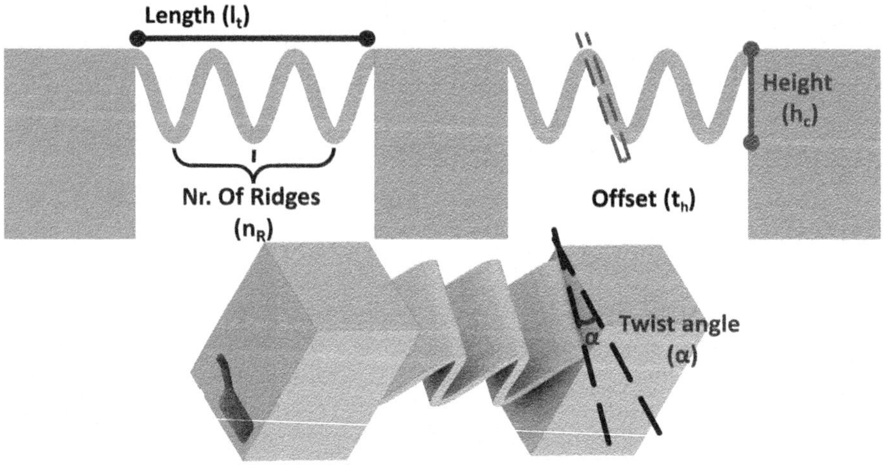

Fig. 4.3 Scheme of a single compliant element of the finger, showing the parameters that can be varied in the design process. Reproduced from [58] with permission from IEEE. © IEEE 2022

4.2.1.2 Task-Specific Joint Stiffness Evaluation

The synthesis procedure is developed based on the following key assumptions: (i) Each finger has a serial structure consisting of alternating rigid and flexible elements. (ii) Each flexible element is modeled as a 3-DoF spherical joint, meaning that tensile, compression, and shear deformations are considered negligible in comparison to bending and torsion. As shown in Fig. 4.4, the rotation angles around the local axes x, y, and z of each link are denoted by ξ, η, and ζ, respectively. (iii) A Hard-Finger contact model is assumed to describe the interaction between the fingers and the object. This model is appropriate when both the finger and the object exhibit sufficiently high contact stiffness, and the local deformation at the contact point is minimal compared to the overall problem scale. With respect to the the previous work presented in [29], where joint stiffness was computed to ensure the fingertips of a soft-rigid gripper followed a predefined closure trajectory, this new procedure introduces two main advancements.

Firstly, the full three-dimensional deformation of the flexible elements is considered, as they are modeled as 3-DoF joints. Secondly, the methodology addresses more complex finger trajectories and grasp tasks, including in-hand twisting of a grasped object. In the subsequent sections, three case studies will be presented that extend the synthesis procedure from [29]: replicating an assigned rigid-body object movement, regulating contact forces applied to the grasped object, and adjusting the overall grasp stiffness.

Assigned rigid-body object movement The first task involves defining joint stiffness values to control the motion direction of a grasped object relative to an initial equilibrium position. Specifically, this requires evaluating the joint stiffness in such

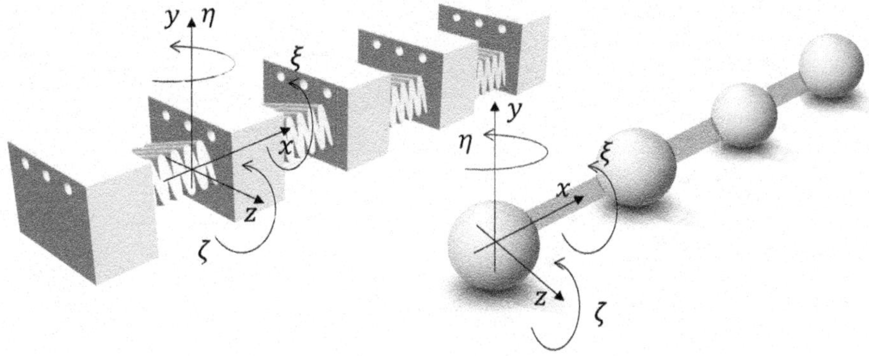

Fig. 4.4 Each flexible element is modelled as a spherical joint: reference axes and rotation angles for each flexible joint. Reproduced from [58] with permission from IEEE. © IEEE 2022

a way that, for a given grasping configuration, the object follows a predetermined motion direction when the tendons of the fingers are actuated. Additionally, it is essential that contact forces remain relatively stable throughout the motion. Such a requirement could be particularly beneficial in industrial settings, where a gripper attached to a robotic arm performs repetitive tasks on objects of similar dimensions and shapes.

Let us assume that the gripper grasps an object with its fingertips, let us indicate with n_c the number of contacts, with $\mathbf{c}_i \in \Re^3$ the position of the ith contact point with respect to a given base reference frame on the gripper support, indicated with $\mathcal{S}_0$, and with $\mathbf{v}_i \in \Re^3$ their velocities. Let us collect all the contact point coordinates in the vector $\mathbf{c}_p \in \Re^{3n_c}$ and their velocities in the vector $\mathbf{v}_p \in \Re^{3n_c}$. Let us indicate with $\mathbf{u} \in \Re^3$ the position of the origin of a reference frame $\mathcal{S}_b$ on the object with respect to $\mathcal{S}_0$ and with $\phi \in \Re^3$ its orientation, represented for instance by means of RPY angles. Let $\mathbf{v} \in \Re^3$ be the velocity of $\mathcal{S}_b$ origin and $\omega \in \Re^3$ the object angular velocity. A well-known basic definition adopted in grasp theory [62] is the so-called *Grasp Matrix* $\mathbf{G} \in \Re^{6\times 3n_c}$, whose transpose relates the object twist, $\nu = [\mathbf{v}^{\mathrm{T}}, \omega^{\mathrm{T}}]^{\mathrm{T}}$, to contact point velocities, i.e.

$$\mathbf{v}_p = \mathbf{G}^{\mathrm{T}}\nu \tag{4.1}$$

If we consider a small displacement with respect to a reference initial condition, the above relationship can be rewritten as

$$\delta\mathbf{c}_p = \mathbf{G}^{\mathrm{T}}\begin{bmatrix}\delta\mathbf{u}\\ \delta\phi\end{bmatrix} \tag{4.2}$$

It is worth noting that the motion defined in Eqs. (4.1) and (4.2) is based on rigid body assumptions, this means that contact forces are not influenced by the motion [63].

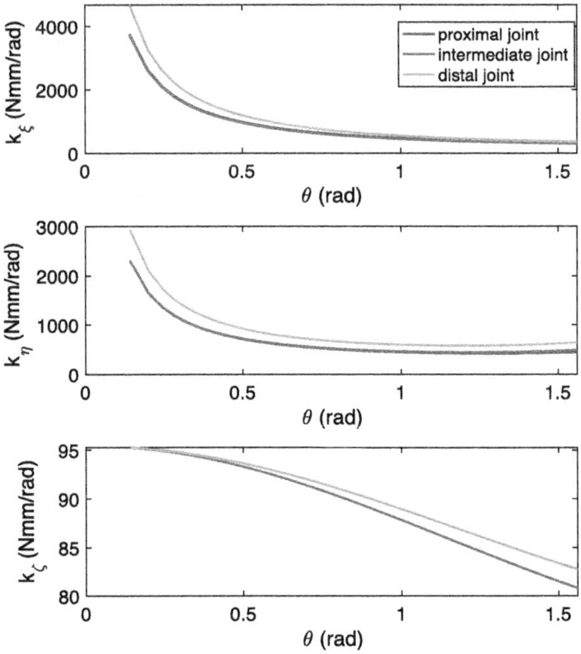

Fig. 4.5 Stiffness values for each joint of the first finger, evaluated as a function of the rotation angle $0 \le \theta \le \pi/2$ rad. Each diagram reports one of the stiffness components, i.e. k_ξ, k_η and k_ζ, in each diagram the values obtained for the three joints (i.e. proximal, intermediate and distal), are reported. Reproduced from [58] with permission from IEEE. © IEEE 2022

Let us indicate with n_i the number of flexible joints in the i-th finger. As previously introduced, each joint is represented as a 3-DoFs spherical joint, let us indicate with $\mathbf{q}_i \in \Re^{3n_i}$ a vector containing joint rotation angles corresponding to the $i-th$ finger, and with $\mathbf{q} = \left[\mathbf{q}_1^{\mathrm{T}}, \mathbf{q}_2^{\mathrm{T}} \cdots\right]^{\mathrm{T}} \in \Re^{n_q}$ the overall joint coordinate vector for the whole gripper. A standard inverse kinematics procedure can be used to evaluate joint coordinate variations $\delta\mathbf{q}$ corresponding to contact point displacement $\delta\mathbf{c}_p$ evaluated in Eq. (4.2). Let us use the procedure based on Jacobian pseudo-inverse:

$$\delta\mathbf{q} = \mathbf{J}^{+}\delta\mathbf{c}_p \tag{4.3}$$

in which $\mathbf{J} \in \Re^{3n_c \times nq}$ is the gripper *Jacobian matrix* [62] and the symbol $^+$ indicates the matrix pseudo-inverse.

Once the task specification is *translated* in a joint coordinate variation $\delta\mathbf{q}$, the procedure detailed in [29] can be adopted to evaluate the joint stiffness matrix $\mathbf{K}_q \in n_q \times n_q$. In particular, indicating with $\mathbf{Q} = \mathrm{diag}(\delta\mathbf{q}) \in \Re^{n_q \times n_q}$, with $\delta\mathbf{f} \in \Re^{n_t}$ the variation of tendon force that we apply to get the displacement described by $\delta\mathbf{q}$, and with $\mathbf{T} \in \Re^{n_t \times n_q}$ the tendon Jacobian matrix, relating joint variations to tendon displacements $\delta\mathbf{t} \in \Re^{n_t}$, i.e. $\delta\mathbf{t} = \mathbf{T}\delta\mathbf{q}$, we can evaluate the vector $\mathbf{k}_q \in \Re^{n_q}$ as:

$$\mathbf{k}_q = \mathbf{Q}^{-1}\mathbf{T}^{\mathrm{T}}\delta\mathbf{f} \tag{4.4}$$

and we can obtain the corresponding stiffness matrix as $\mathbf{K}_q = \mathrm{diag}(\mathbf{k}_q)$.

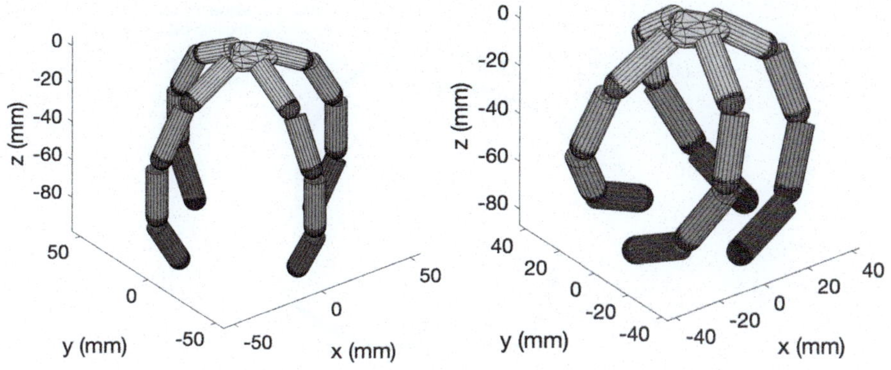

(a) (b)

Fig. 4.6 SynGrasp model of the gripper developed for realising a twist rotation of the grasped object with respect to z axis, in the initial (**a**) and final configuration (**b**). Reproduced from [58] with permission from IEEE. © IEEE 2022

Example To illustrate the process of defining joint stiffness within a grasping context, consider a gripper consisting of four fingers arranged symmetrically on its support, securely grasping a cylindrical object. Each finger comprises three rigid links connected by three flexible elements.

For this scenario, we can assume that the four contact points lie on a horizontal plane, corresponding to the xy plane of the $\mathcal{S}_r$ reference frame. Additionally, let's specify that the desired motion involves a pure rotation about the z axis.

In this case, indicating with r the cylinder radius, the Grasp matrix is:

$$\mathbf{G} = \begin{bmatrix} 1 & 0 & 0 & 1 & 0 & 0 & 1 & 0 & 0 & 1 & 0 & 0 \\ 0 & 1 & 0 & 0 & 1 & 0 & 0 & 1 & 0 & 0 & 1 & 0 \\ 0 & 0 & 1 & 0 & 0 & 1 & 0 & 0 & 1 & 0 & 0 & 1 \\ 0 & 0 & 0 & 0 & 0 & 0 & 0 & 0 & 0 & 0 & 0 & 0 \\ 0 & 0 & 0 & 0 & 0 & 0 & 0 & 0 & 0 & 0 & 0 & 0 \\ -r & 0 & 0 & 0 & r & 0 & r & 0 & 0 & 0 & -r & 0 \end{bmatrix}$$

and, by imposing a pure rotation with respect to z axis, i.e. $\delta\mathbf{u} = 0$ and $\delta\phi = [0, 0, \delta\theta]^{\mathrm{T}}$ it is straightforward to verify that

$$\delta\mathbf{c}_1 = \left[-r\delta\theta\ 0\ 0\right]^{\mathrm{T}};\ \delta\mathbf{c}_2 = \left[0\ r\delta\theta\ 0\right]^{\mathrm{T}};$$

$$\delta\mathbf{c}_3 = -\delta\mathbf{c}_1;\ \delta\mathbf{c}_4 = -\delta\mathbf{c}_2$$

Figure 4.6 illustrates the modeled gripper in both its initial and final configurations. The movement analyzed is a $\pi/2$ rad twist rotation with respect to the z axis, which is perpendicular to the reference plane of the hand palm. This specific rotation amplitude

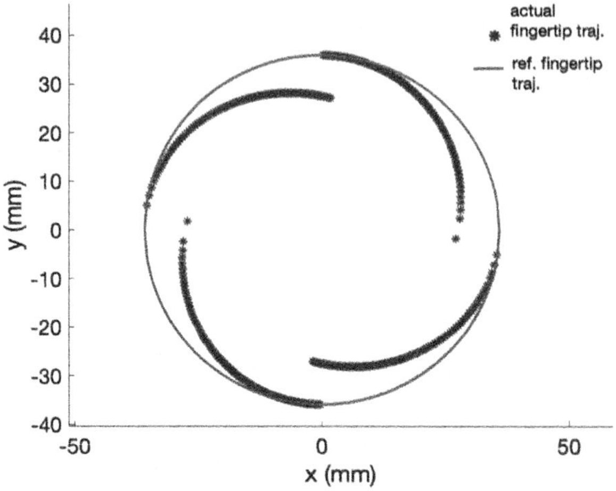

Fig. 4.7 SynGrasp simulation of the gripper developed for realising a twist rotation of the grasped object with respect to z axis: the reference fingertip trajectories (red curve) is a circumference in the xy plane, while fingertip trajectories obtained assuming constant joint stiffness values (blue curves) tends to diverge from the reference one as the rotation angle increases. Reproduced from [58] with permission from IEEE. © IEEE 2022 (color figure online)

was chosen to evaluate the gripper's performance when the fundamental assumptions used for stiffness synthesis are not met.

To achieve the overall rotation, the movement was divided into a series of 100 discrete steps, with the previously described procedure repeated for each step. For every simulation step and for each joint, three stiffness values were evaluated. Figure 4.5 presents the results obtained for one of the fingers. Analysis of the diagrams reveals that the stiffness values k_ξ and k_η show significant variations at lower rotation angles, eventually stabilizing at a sort of plateau for higher angles ($\theta > 0.7$ rad). In contrast, k_ζ alues are consistently lower and exhibit more limited variation. Additionally, it is noteworthy that the stiffness values obtained for the three joints of the finger are quite similar throughout the considered motion.

When fingers are fabricated using standard additive manufacturing processes, such as FDM, and constructed from conventional materials with approximately linear-elastic behavior, it becomes challenging to regulate joint stiffness based on deformation. As a result, only a constant stiffness value can be implemented.

To illustrate this limitation, we simulated the error that arises from assuming constant stiffness values instead of variable ones for each joint. The simulation involved a gripper with dimensions identical to those considered during the synthesis phase, with joints set to constant stiffness values calculated as the average of the curves shown in Fig. 4.5.

Figure 4.7 presents the simulation results, displaying the reference trajectory of the fingertips (a circular path in the xy plane) alongside the trajectories calculated under the assumption of constant stiffness values. While the fingertip trajectories tend to diverge from the reference path-especially at larger rotation angles-the difference is approximately 12 mm at $\theta = \pi/2$ rad. Similar discrepancies were reported in [29], where the gripper had a planar structure and a much simpler planar trajectory was considered.

4.2.1.3 Contact Force Regulation

Another critical factor in grasping tasks is contact force control, which is essential for ensuring adequate grasp robustness while also preventing excessive localized pressure that could harm the object being handled. In an underactuated compliant gripper, it is not feasible to control each contact force independently. However, by carefully selecting joint stiffness values, we can influence the directions in which contact forces increase as tendon tension is applied and determine how these forces are distributed across the various contact points.

$$\delta \mathbf{q} = \mathbf{J}^{+}\mathbf{K}_c^{-1}\left(\mathbf{I} + \mathbf{G}_K^{+}\mathbf{G}\right)^{-1}\delta \mathbf{f}_c \tag{4.5}$$

where $\mathbf{K}_c \in \Re^{3n_c \times 3n_c}$ is the contact stiffness matrix, $\mathbf{G}_K^{+} = \mathbf{K}_c\mathbf{G}^{\mathrm{T}}\left(\mathbf{G}\mathbf{K}_c\mathbf{G}^{\mathrm{T}}\right)^{-1}$ is the $\mathbf{G}$ matrix pseudo-inverse, weighted with $\mathbf{K}_c$ matrix, and $\mathbf{I}$ is the identity matrix.

Also in this case, once $\delta \mathbf{q}$ is evaluated, the procedure detailed in [29] can be adopted to find the joint stiffness matrix $\mathbf{K}_q$.

4.2.1.4 Grasp Stiffness

Grasp stiffness is a grasp property that describes how the system is able to resist to external disturbing loads applied to the object. Formally, the inverse of grasp stiffness matrix $\mathbf{K}_g \in Re^{6\times 6}$ allows to evaluate object displacement $\delta \mathbf{u}$ and rotation $\delta \phi$ to a given external wrench $\delta \mathbf{w} \in \Re^6$ applied to the object [64, 65], i.e. :

$$\begin{bmatrix} \delta \mathbf{u} \\ \delta \phi \end{bmatrix} = \mathbf{K}_g^{-1}\delta \mathbf{w} \tag{4.6}$$

According to the quasi-static model introduced in [63] and detailed in [65], grasp matrix can be evaluated as follows:

$$\mathbf{K}_g = \mathbf{G}\left(\mathbf{K}_c^{-1} + \mathbf{J}\mathbf{K}_q^{-1}\mathbf{J}^{\mathrm{T}}\right)^{-1}\mathbf{G}^{\mathrm{T}} \tag{4.7}$$

In this case, for a given grasp configuration and for a given desired value of grasp stiffness, Eq. (4.7) can be solved to find directly $\mathbf{K}_q$.

4.2.1.5 Joint Stiffness Value as a Function of Its Geometrical Characteristics and Material Properties

Analysis of a set of reference elements It is clear that the stiffness of the flexible parts depends on both its geometrical shape and dimensions, and on material properties. For instance, in a beam with a rectangular section, with cross section $w \times t$ and length l, realised with a linear elastic material with Young's modulus E, the equivalent bending rotation stiffness evaluated with standard De Saint Venant assumptions, is $k = EI/l, I = wt^3/12$. In a wave-shaped element as the one that has been chosen for realizing the fingers, De Saint Venant assumptions and results cannot be employed. A structural mechanics analysis based on FEM tools has been realized for defining the following relationship:

$$\begin{bmatrix} k_\xi \; k_\eta \; k_\zeta \end{bmatrix}^{\mathrm{T}} = \mathbf{f}(l_t, n_r, h_c, t, \alpha, E) \tag{4.8}$$

where k_ξ represent the torsional stiffness k_η is the lateral bending stiffness, and k_ζ is the longitudinal bending stiffness,

Overall 221 different configurations were generated by varying the design parameters l_t, n_r, h_c, t, and α. The material was assumed to be homogeneous and linear elastic, characterized by a Young's modulus of $E = 2.24$ GPa, Poisson's coefficient $\nu = 0.38$, and density $\rho = 1.06\,\mathrm{kg/m^3}$. The analysis was conducted using the Autodesk® Fusion 360 simulation environment, with a variable mesh defined for each simulation sample, averaging around 16,000 elements.

For each configuration, three loading scenarios were simulated: bending in the longitudinal plane, bending in the lateral plane, and torsion. The corresponding stiffness values k_ξ, k_η, and k_ζ ere then evaluated. Two examples of these simulations are illustrated in Fig. 4.8. The results for k_ζ across all simulations are summarized in Fig. 4.9, while similar diagrams were obtained for k_ξ and k_η. A comprehensive characterization from both theoretical and experimental perspectives is detailed in Sect. 4.3.

Definition of flexible joint characteristics The design process described in this part of the thesis aims to invert the relationship established in Eq. (4.8), specifically to identify the set of parameters $[l_t, n_r, h_c, t, \alpha]$ that will yield the desired stiffness values k_ξ, k_η, and k_ζ based on the specifications of the gripper. To address this challenge, various system identification techniques were explored.

The most effective solution was found to be a Pattern Recognition Neural Network, which features hidden layers comprising 45, 5, and 10 neurons, and utilizes a Scaled Conjugate Gradient training function. Two distinct Neural Networks were developed; both networks have three input parameters: k_ξ, k_η, and k_ζ. The first network outputs four parameters: l_t, n_r, h_c, and t, while the second network includes an additional output for the twist angle α. The networks were trained using data obtained from finite element method (FEM) analysis, leveraging the Deep Learning Toolbox in MATLAB. The performance of the Neural Networks, assessed using the Cross-

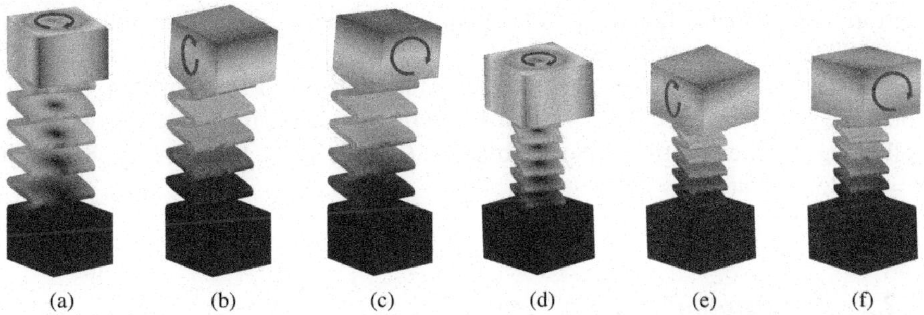

Fig. 4.8 Examples of test cases for stiffness evaluation based on FEM structural analysis. **a–c** Test case: $l_t = 30$ mm, $n_r = 5$, $h_c = 10$ mm, $t = 0.6$ mm, $\alpha = 0$. **a** Loading condition for defining k_ξ (torsion), **b** loading condition for defining k_η, **c** loading condition for defining k_ζ. **d–f** Test case: $l_t = 20$ mm, $n_r = 6$, $h_c = 10$ mm, $t = 0.5$ mm, $\alpha = 3°$. **d** Loading condition for defining k_ξ (torsion), **e** loading condition for defining k_η, **f** loading condition for defining k_ζ. Reproduced from [58] with permission from IEEE. © IEEE 2022

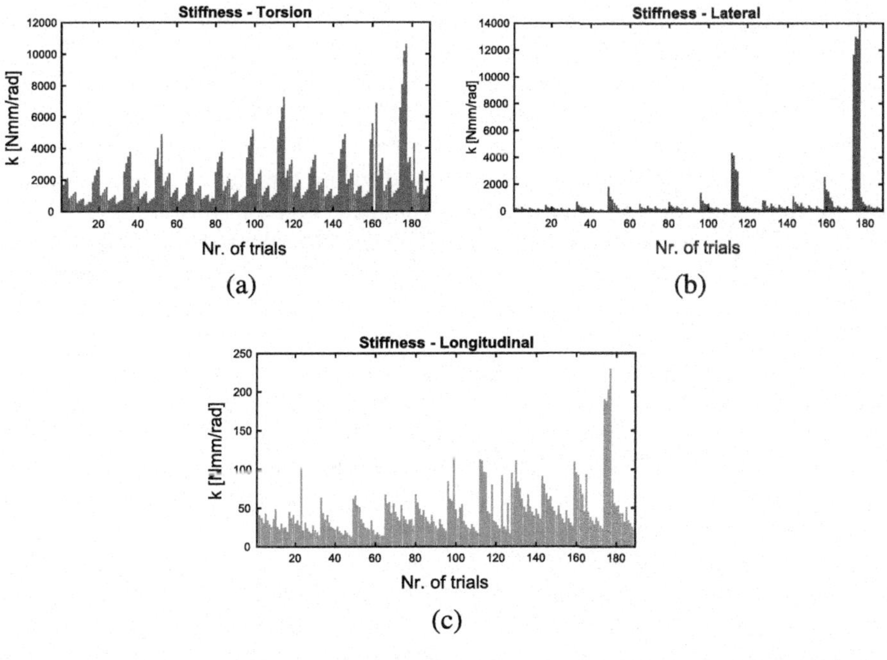

Fig. 4.9 Stiffness values obtained from FEM analysis. **a** Torsion stiffness, k_ξ. **b** Lateral flexion stiffness k_η. **c** Longitudinal flexion stiffness k_ζ

Entropy performance function, yielded values of 0.05 for the four-output network and 0.89 for the five-output network.

For instance, when the mean stiffness values calculated for achieving the twist rotation angle depicted in Figs. 4.6 and 4.7 were provided to the Neural Network, the following parameter estimates were obtained: $l_t = 19.2$ mm, $n_r = 3$, $h_c = 8.14$ mm, $t = 0.515$ mm, and $\alpha = 18°$.

4.2.2 Experiments

The methodology proposed was evaluated through the realization of two prototypes of soft-rigid grippers. The first prototype, referred to as the WaveGripper, is designed to perform power grasp tasks. The desired finger trajectories are achieved by initiating finger flexion from a straight position and allowing all joints to reach a bending angle of 30°. The corresponding joint stiffness parameters were computed, and the resulting fingers were 3D printed and connected to a palm that houses motors for tendon-driven actuation. The second prototype, known as the Twist-WaveGripper, was developed to enable twist rotation of a grasped object. This section will describe the palm and actuation system, along with the results obtained from both prototypes. The fingers of the grippers were modeled using SolidWorks (Dassault Systèmes®). An equation-driven curve tool was employed, using the values derived from the Neural Network-based procedure as input parameters for the software.

Both grippers feature four soft fingers connected to the palm via snap-fit connectors. The tendon is anchored to a differential mechanism and passes through the upper plate of the gripper. It is inserted into pre-designed slots and secured in a final module, facilitating easy finger replacement.

The entire structure, including the fingers and palm, is constructed from ABS (ABSPlus, Stratasys, USA). Actuation is provided by two Dynamixel MX-28T motors, which are capable of delivering a maximum torque of 3.1 Nm and a maximum angular speed of 684°/s. Each motor controls a pair of fingers. Additionally, a differential mechanism is integrated into the gripper palm to adapt the fingers' configurations to the shape of the grasped object.

The Arbotix-M controller (Robotis, South Korea) is used to control the Dynamixel actuators. The main technical features of the WaveGripper and its actuation system, as well as an experimental evaluation of the payload and maximum horizontal resistive force, were conducted using the same methodology outlined in [24] for the Co-Gripper. Since the results are comparable, interested readers are referred to [24] for further details. The print orientation was strategically chosen, with the WaveJoints printed on their side to ensure maximum resistance and strength.

4.2.2.1 Preliminary Tests on Two Gripper Prototypes

For both grippers, the accuracy in following the *reference* fingertip trajectory was evaluated using two metrics: the mean Euclidean distance error, $\varepsilon_{\text{mean}}$, and the maximum Euclidean distance error, ε_{MAX}. Given the two trajectories, the reference trajectory (T_{ref}) and the real trajectory (T_{real}), these values are defined as follows:

$$\varepsilon_{\text{mean}}(T_{\text{ref}}, T_{\text{real}}) = \frac{1}{N}\sum_{i=1}^{N} d(p_{\text{ref},i}, p_{\text{real},i}), \tag{4.9}$$

$$\varepsilon_{\text{MAX}}(T_{\text{ref}}, T_{\text{real}}) = \max_{i=1}^{N} d(p_{\text{ref},i}, p_{\text{real},i}), \tag{4.10}$$

where $d(p_{\text{ref},i}, p_{\text{real},i})$ represents the three-dimensional Euclidean distance. For each finger model, the mean values of $\varepsilon_{\text{mean}}$ and ε_{MAX} across ten trials were utilized to assess the tracking performance throughout the entire experiment. Real fingertip trajectories were recorded using an optical tracking system (Vicon Motion Systems, UK). The system comprised two Bonita cameras and two Vero cameras, along with the Tracker software (version 3.9.0). A single finger from each prototype was tracked during the trials. Data was collected at a sampling rate of 100 Hz, employing fourteen passive optical markers to monitor finger motion. The markers, measuring 6.35 mm in diameter, were strategically placed along the fingers and at the base to accurately determine both the position and orientation of the corresponding bodies in the workspace.

4.2.2.2 Test for Power Grasp Finger

A series of ten trials were conducted on the power grasp finger. Each trial involved flexing the finger by actuating the tendon and recording the values of the joints and fingertip positions. The reference and measured values of the fingertip trajectory from a representative trial are shown in Fig. 4.10a. It can be observed that the average $\varepsilon_{\text{mean}}$ across the ten trials in following the theoretical trajectory was 0.54 mm, while the mean ε_{MAX} was 1.74 mm.

4.2.2.3 Test for Twist Finger

The same experimental setup was applied to the twist finger. As with the power grasp finger, both theoretical and measured values of the fingertip trajectory were analyzed. The mean ε_{MAX} across the ten trials for following the theoretical trajectory was found to be 3.71 mm, while the average $\varepsilon_{\text{mean}}$ was 0.82 mm. A representative trial is presented in Fig. 4.10b.

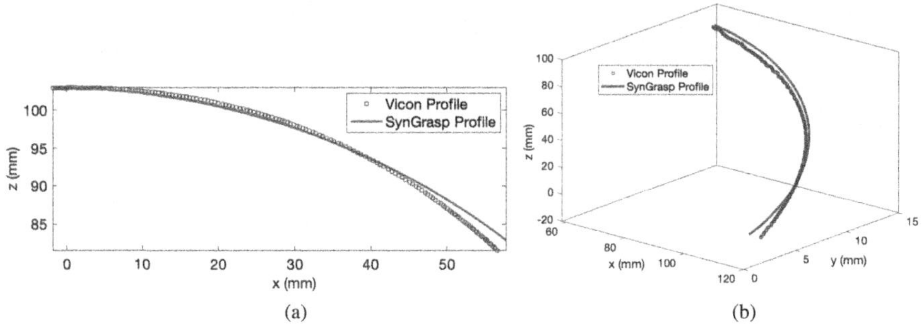

Fig. 4.10 **a** Power grasp finger test. Theoretical fingertip's trajectory and acquired vicon fingertip's trajectory during one of the trials. **b** Twist finger test. 3D-view of the theoretical fingertip's trajectory and acquired vicon fingertip's trajectory during one of the trials. Reproduced from [58] with permission from IEEE. © IEEE 2022

4.2.2.4 Grasping Object Using the WaveGripper

The WaveGripper was constructed with four fingers, each consisting of two modules, as illustrated in Fig. 4.11. Grasping trials were conducted using a variety of objects that differed in size, shape, and stiffness. Five distinct objects were selected for the experiments: a plastic bottle (approximately 1 kg), a cylindrical container, an empty rectangular box, a rigid irregularly shaped box, and a soft puppet. During the trials, the gripper was maneuvered by the experimenter via a handle attached to the base of the WaveGripper. Multiple grasping attempts were made for each object, with variations in the grasping direction. In total, 27 grasps were executed, all of which were successful, except for the soft puppet, which could not be grasped from the lateral direction due to its unique shape, and the plastic bottle, which could not be stably grasped from the top. Examples of some successful grasps are presented in Fig. 4.11.

4.2.2.5 In-Hand Rotation of an Object Using the Twist-WaveGripper

The Twist-WaveGripper is designed to perform in-hand manipulation tasks, specifically the twisting of a cylinder. The experimental setup included the prototype mounted on a robotic arm, positioned perpendicular to the working plane. A plastic cylinder with a diameter of 60 mm was placed beneath the gripper. A measurement circle was employed to assess the rotation angle, while the robot's wrist remained stationary during the manipulation task, which was executed by actuating the gripper's fingers. Figure 4.12a illustrates the initial position of the gripper and the object, while Fig. 4.12b depicts the torsion applied to the object by the gripper. Five trials were conducted, with the gripper successfully grasping the object and achieving a rota-

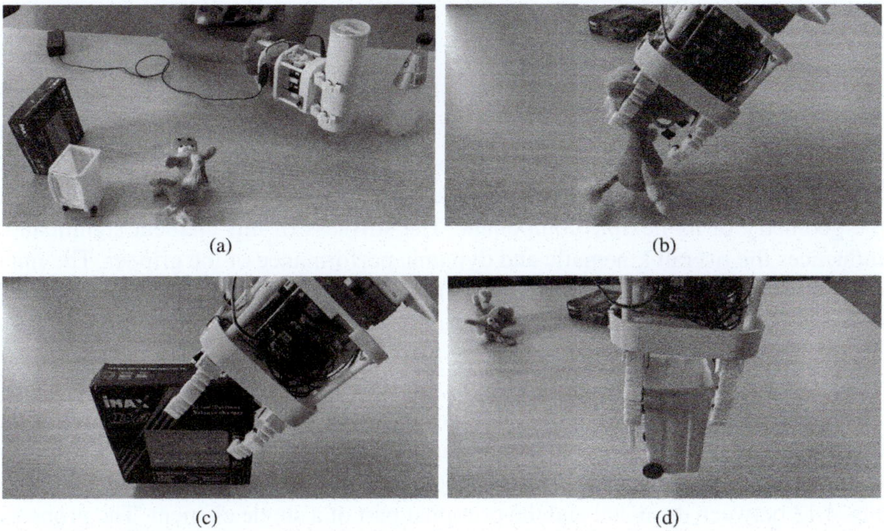

Fig. 4.11 Grasp Experiment with different objects. **a** Cylindrical box **b** Soft toy. **c** Rectangular box. **d** Irregular box

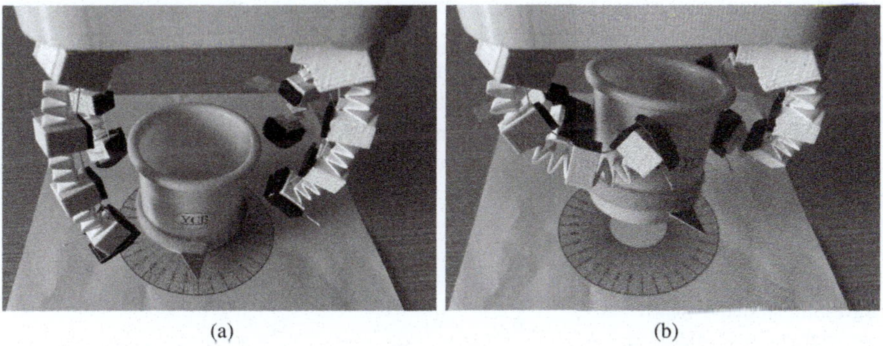

Fig. 4.12 Twist rotation experiment. **a** Initial configuration. **b** Final configuration

tion of approximately 40°. However, as the test was repeated multiple times without replacing the object, it was observed that the error tended to increase. This increase in error can be attributed to the translation of the cylinder during grasping and the smooth surface of the cylinder, which was not conducive to preventing slippage at the contact points, as well as unmodeled rolling movements.

4.3 The WaveJoint: Numerical and Experimental Characterization

This work presents the characterization of a monolithic and parametric flexible joint, referred to as the WaveJoint, which is a compliant flexible joint actuated by tendons. The primary properties of the joint are defined by geometric parameters related to the geometry of its flexible component. The stiffness of this element significantly influences the overall kinematic and dynamic performance of the gripper. The main aim of this study is to characterize the stiffness concerning its geometric parameters, utilizing both theoretical and experimental approaches, thereby providing valuable insights for the design of such elements.

The WaveJoint overcomes the need of elastic joints made of different materials by exploiting the shape of a compliant sector interposed between the two rigid modules: as a first approximation, we can represent the compliance of this part of the finger as a rotational degree of freedom allowing the rotation along the Y-axis Fig. 4.13 between the distal and the proximal part of a single element. The proposed synthesis procedure necessitates defining the properties of the flexible component as a function of its characteristics, including thickness, length, wave amplitude, and phase. The adaptability and ease of manufacturing and assembling the solution presented in this thesis offer distinct advantages compared to other designs composed of various components and materials, as noted in [67]. Each finger is constructed from a single element, utilizing a uniform material throughout.

Each compliant finger element is characterized by a sinusoidal wave shape. This shape was chosen because it is a fundamental geometric form that can be easily parametrically generated using CAD software based on a limited number of variables, as detailed in Table 4.1.

Fig. 4.13 Rotation of the WaveJoint around Y-axis. Copyright © 2022 Achilli et al. [66]

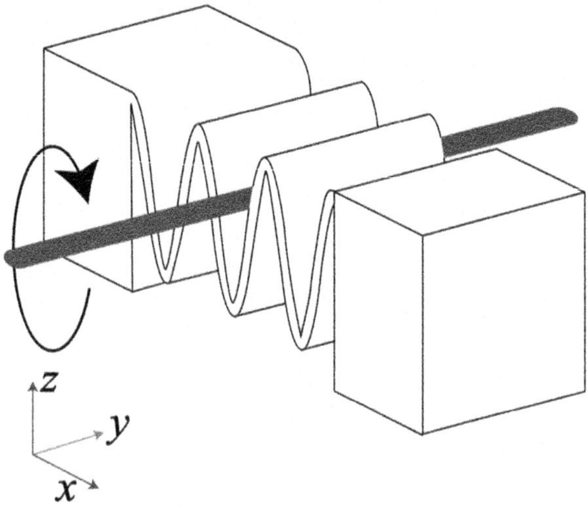

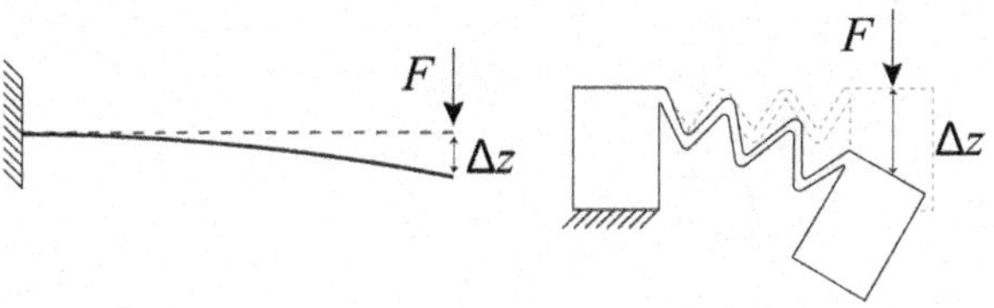

Fig. 4.14 The investigated sample. Copyright © 2022 Achilli et al. [66]

The geometric parameters serve as variables that allow for alterations in the flexibility and stiffness characteristics of the joint. These variables are incorporated into a parametric equation, which describes a cosine function characterized by amplitude, frequency, and phase. By varying the length parameter l_t, the equation takes the form $y(t) = A\cos(\omega t + \alpha)$, with t between $[0, l_t]$:

$$y(t) = -\left[\left(\frac{h_c}{2} - t_h\right) cos\left(2\pi\frac{n_r}{l_t}t\right)\right]. \tag{4.11}$$

A simple shape for the stiff joint parts is used. Indeed, in this thesis work focused on the design of flexible joints, using the same rectangular parallelepiped for all parts, with dimensions 11 × 15 × 16 mm. Further research on stiff link design may be required for specific tasks, such as grasping soft or deformable objects. All the components used for the trials were made using AM technologies.

The WaveJoint was characterized through both experimental tests and simulations. These methodologies were employed to investigate how the stiffness value k_ζ of the joint varies between the virtual and real worlds. To validate this characterization, a flexural test was performed, utilizing a sample consisting of three components: two rigid modules alternated with a flexible module, as illustrated in Fig. 4.14. In this setup, one rigid module is fixed to a support structure while the other is free to move. A vertical load is applied to the center of the upper face of the free module, allowing for a clear measurement of the joint's stiffness. Both experimental and finite element method (FEM) analyses were utilized to evaluate the joint stiffness. This characterization is essential for understanding how the WaveJoint performs within the robotic gripper's fingers. Specifically, knowing the joint stiffness of each finger is crucial for achieving a controlled grasp. Additional details on this aspect can be found in Sect. 4.2.1.2.

4.3.1 Experimental Characterization

The geometric properties of the joints were analyzed and categorized into sixteen distinct cohorts. Each cohort's sample was experimentally evaluated using the test rig depicted in Fig. 4.15a. This test rig consists of a vertical bench equipped with an IMADA ZTA-50N dynamometer and a linear encoder. The same displacement was

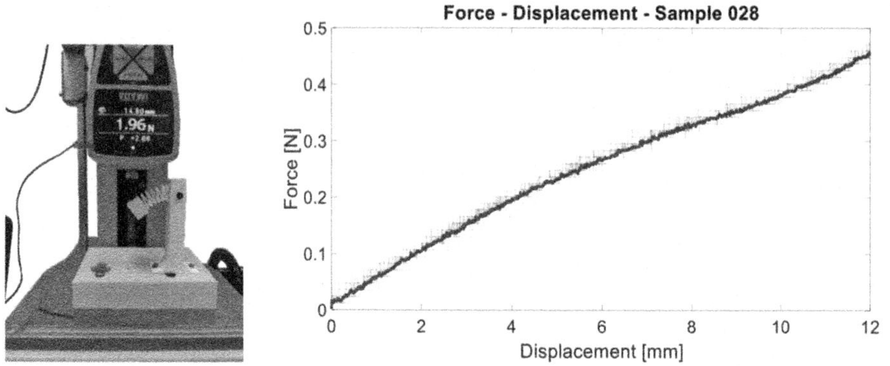

(a) (b)

Fig. 4.15 **a** Test on bench. **b** Acquired data in ten repeated tests for the cohort 28. Copyright © 2022 Achilli et al. [66]

achieved through a bending test, where the applied forces were measured alongside the corresponding deformations.

An example of the experimental results is presented in Fig. 4.15b, which illustrates the data acquired during ten repeated tests for cohort number 28. The repeatability of the results is clearly observable in this figure. On the left side, the legend indicates the mean value of the joint stiffness obtained from the tests. Additionally, Table 4.2 summarizes all the experimental results concerning stiffness for each cohort, along with their corresponding geometric characteristics.

4.3.2 Numerical Characterization

The FEM models were utilized to assess the mechanical behavior and characteristics of the samples. The simulations were performed using COMSOL Multiphysics FEM software, employing parameters that replicated the conditions of the original experiments. In the setup, the first stiff module was fully constrained, while a prescribed displacement of 12 mm along the Z-axis was applied to the second stiff module. The analysis focused on the force required to bend the WaveJoint under these constraints, along with an evaluation of how the simulation results compared to the actual test outcomes. Material parameters for the simulation were derived from the manufacturer's technical specifications. The solver for linear elastic materials necessitates inputs for Young's modulus and the Poisson's ratio of the selected material. The analysis incorporated a geometric non-linearity condition, essential for accurately examining the WaveJoint due to its unique shape, which does not conform to that of a standard beam, and its behavior, which cannot be entirely linear or elastic.

To conduct a non-linear investigation, a sweep vector p was defined, ranging from 0 to 1 in increments of 0.1. This parameter was multiplied by the prescribed

Table 4.2 Mean force applied at 12 mm of displacement

Cohorts	n_r	h_c [mm]	t_h [mm]	F_{mean} [N]	$k_{\zeta mean}$ [N/mm]
9	3	8	0.5	0.480	0.040
12	3	14	0.5	0.432	0.036
25	4	8	0.5	0.540	0.045
28	4	14	0.5	0.456	0.038
41	5	8	0.5	0.708	0.059
44	5	14	0.5	0.624	0.052
57	6	8	0.5	0.876	0.073
60	6	14	0.5	0.756	0.063
137	3	8	0.6	2.988	0.249
140	3	14	0.6	2.460	0.205
153	4	8	0.6	3.072	0.256
156	4	14	0.6	2.604	0.217
169	5	8	0.6	3.276	0.273
172	5	14	0.6	3.012	0.251
185	6	8	0.6	3.516	0.293
188	6	14	0.6	3.240	0.270

Table 4.3 Mean values of force and stiffness at 12 mm of prescribed displacement

	Cohort 12	Cohort 41	Cohort 156	Cohort 188
Force [N]	0.437	0.701	2.507	3.324
Stiffness kmean [N/mm]	0.037	0.058	0.209	0.277

displacement applied to the module. Varying the sweep parameter enabled the evaluation of the joint's behavior while minimizing the risk of unintended deformation of the solid.

Table 4.3 presents the evaluated stiffness and force values obtained at a 12 mm displacement applied to the edge of the stiff WaveJoint. Figure 4.16 displays the deformation plots, demonstrating that all samples achieved the prescribed 12 mm displacement, with all graphs maintaining a 1:1 scale factor.

4.3.3 *Results and Comparison*

The results obtained from the experimental and theoretical tests were analyzed and compared to evaluate the variation in stiffness of the WaveJoint. The experimentally

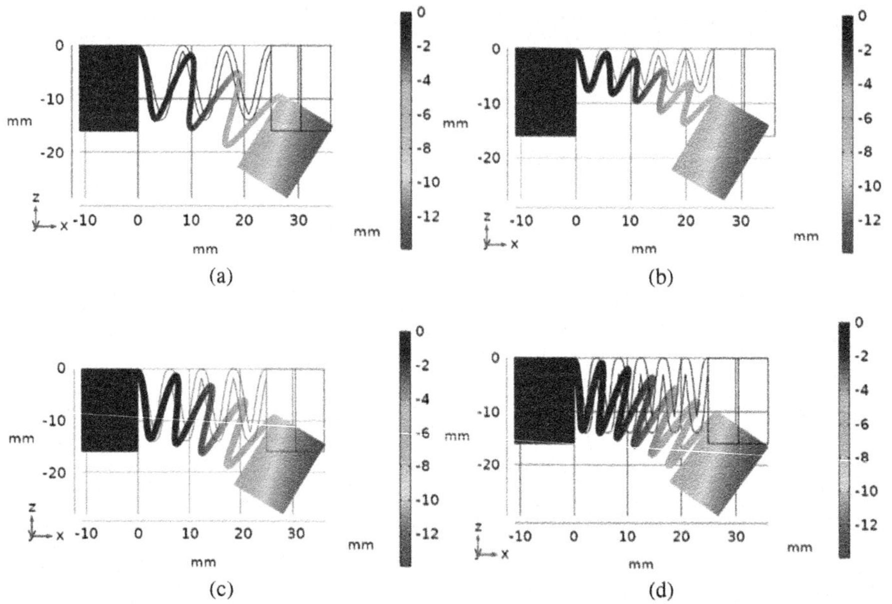

Fig. 4.16 Simulations results: **a** A sample of cohort 12. **b** A sample of cohort 41. **c** A sample of cohort 156. **d** A sample of cohort 188. Copyright © 2022 Achilli et al. [66]

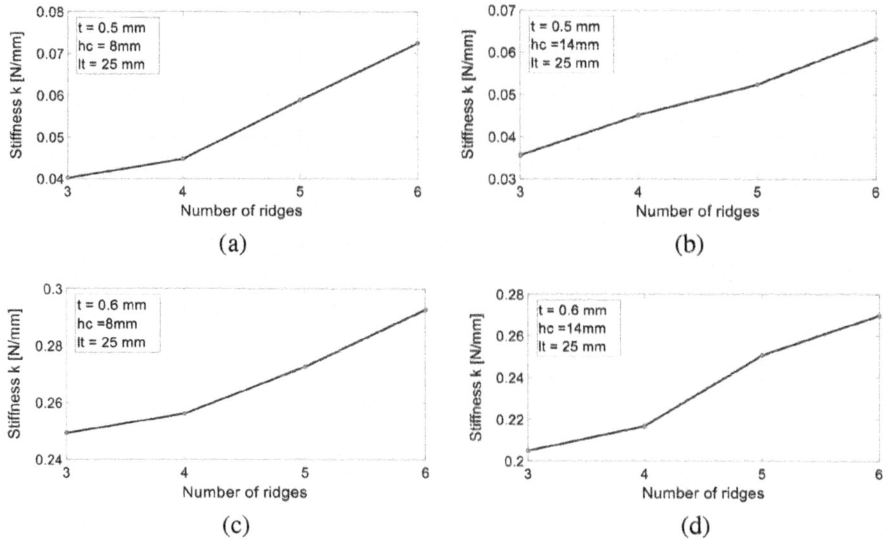

Fig. 4.17 Experimental trend of the stiffness k_ζ by varying the number of the ridges. Red dots represent the $k_{\zeta mean}$ values. Copyright © 2022 Achilli et al. [66]

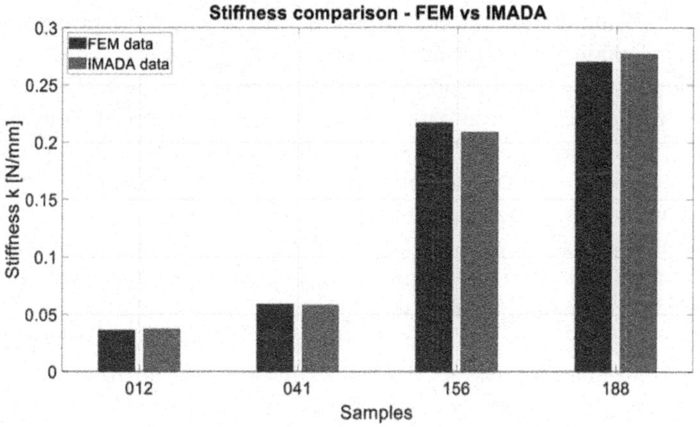

Fig. 4.18 Stiffness comparison between experimental and simulation results. Copyright © 2022 Achilli et al. [66]

evaluated stiffness for homogeneous groups of samples is presented in Fig. 4.17. The plots illustrate the trend in stiffness while maintaining fixed geometric parameters. Specifically, the analysis focuses on groups of samples with identical ridge height h_c and thickness t_h . This approach allows for a clear correlation between the joint's behavior and its geometric parameters.

All experimental tests indicate an increasing trend in stiffness that correlates with variations in geometric parameters. Across all sixteen cohorts examined, it is evident that an increase in the number of ridges n_r enhances the stiffness of the joint. Theoretical tests conducted through FEM simulations exhibited a similar behavior to the experimental results. Figure 4.18 presents a comparison between the experimental and simulation results in terms of stiffness. The discrepancies in the stiffness values k_ξ between the two sets of samples can be attributed to several factors. The 3D printing process used to fabricate the samples often leads to inhomogeneous structures. Additionally, the displacement values obtained may differ from those measured in the FEM simulations. Furthermore, the shape of the WaveJoints during the mesh generation phase can create accumulation areas around the folds, potentially altering the behavior of the deformed solid when compared to the actual samples.

4.4 The WaveJoint: Controlled Variable Stiffness Based on Twisted Strings Actuation

The methodology underlying the work presented in this section was introduced in Sect. 4.2. This prior work considered underactuated tendon-driven robotic fingers composed of rigid and compliant modular elements, evaluating the stiffness of compliant joints to achieve a specified closure motion for the finger. Elastic joints were manufactured using a soft material, allowing for regulation of stiffness during the manufacturing phase by controlling the infill density percentage. While the aforementioned studies proposed a methodology for designing passive joint stiffness according to specific requirements, these parameters become fixed once the robotic finger is manufactured and assembled. This section of the thesis aims to overcome this limitation by proposing a method to control and adapt finger joint stiffness beyond the fabrication and assembly stages, thereby enhancing the operational capabilities of the gripper throughout its lifecycle. We build upon the monolithic soft-rigid finger structure based on wave joints, introducing a novel system utilizing twisted string actuation (TSA) to regulate joint stiffness through the application of pre-compression. This pre-compression, applied via a twisted string actuator, induces a stress/deformation state in the joint that modifies its flexural stiffness. Consequently, as suggested by [69], this alteration in stiffness impacts the finger's closure motion and grasping capabilities.

This section thus combines a compliant tendon-driven finger with TSA technology to control elastic joint stiffness. We present a system for pre-compressing flexible joints through TSA, investigating the relationship between pre-compression and flexural stiffness in single wave joints. This investigation is conducted initially through FEM-based numerical simulations and subsequently through an experimental setup. To demonstrate the applicability of the proposed solution in robotic grippers and hands, we conduct a series of closure movement experiments with a tendon-actuated finger composed of three phalanges (Fig. 4.19).

4.4.1 Methodology

In this section it is introduced the variable-stiffness wave-shaped elastic joint, analyze it by means of numerical simulations and present the experimental setup realized for joint characterization.

4.4.1.1 The Wave Joints

The monolithic soft-rigid finger structure consists of compliant wave-shaped elements, known as wave joints. Each compliant finger element features a simple sinusoidal wave shape that is created and parametrically defined using CAD software, based on a limited set of parameters. This joint structure allows the use of a single material for both the flexible and rigid parts of the finger, enabling the entire finger to be fabricated as a single component and simplifying the assembly process. By varying a restricted set of parameters during the pre-processing phase of finger fabrication, i.e., including joint length, wave height, number of ridges, wave thickness, and twist angle, it is possible to achieve the desired equivalent stiffness values required for specific tasks.

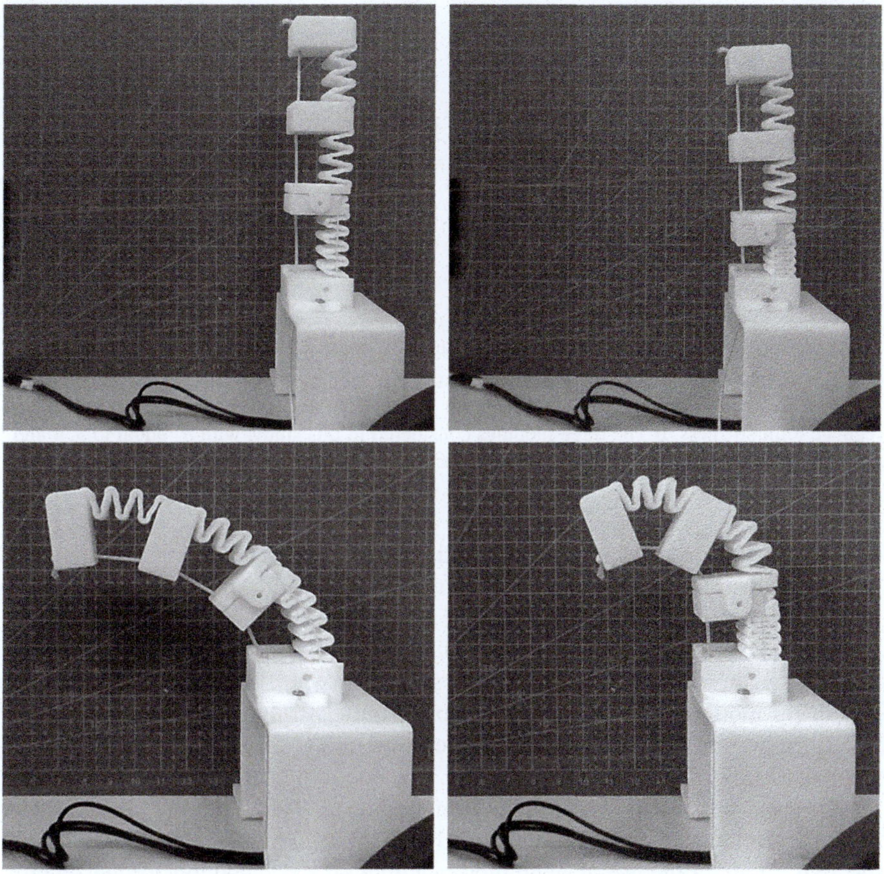

Fig. 4.19 Underactuated tendon-driven robotic finger structure based on WaveJoints, in which the proximal joint stiffness can be regulated by means of a TSA system. Top images: unactuated finger with different (softer on the left, harder on the right) stiffness values in the proximal joint. Lower images: corresponding finger closure motions. Acting on TSA actuator it's possible to regulate finger closure motion. Reproduced from [68] with permission from IEEE. © IEEE 2023

This section of the thesis introduces an additional mechanism for regulating joint stiffness: joint pre-compression produced by a twisted string actuator (TSA). This mechanism enables active and controllable changes in joint stiffness after fabrication. To illustrate the effect of the pre-compression induced by the TSA, the study initially focuses on a single joint, maintaining all parameters at their initial values (as described in Sect. 4.2), except for the number of ridges and, consequently, the joint length. With respect to Sect. 4.2, the structure of the wave joint has been slightly modified to accommodate the routing of the TSA tendons used to vary stiffness. Figure 4.20 illustrates the CAD model of the new WaveJoint module with the integrated TSA. The updated joint design features an internal pathway specifically crafted

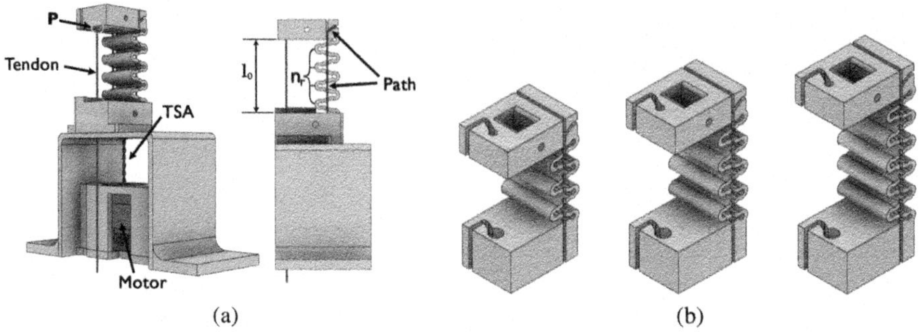

Fig. 4.20 CAD model of a wave-joint with variable stiffness. **a** The joint is actuated by a tendon connected to a motor, while Joint flexural stiffness is regulated by a TSA, that pulling the extremities of the joint, compresses the wave, increasing its stiffness. Controlling TSA stroke it's possible to regulate joint stiffness. **b** The three modules considered in this study, with n_r equal to 3, 4 and 5. Reproduced from [68] with permission from IEEE. © IEEE 2023

to route the tendons. The tendon is folded into two parts; one side is twisted, passed through a flexible tube, and fixed to the motor shaft, while the other side is routed through the compliant element following the designated path shown in Fig. 4.20.

A twisted string actuator has been utilized to apply pre-compression to the joint. The underlying principle of the TSA is straightforward: it converts rotary motion into linear motion by twisting two or more parallel strings. One end of the strings is connected to a rotary motor, while the other end is linked to a linearly moving element, such as the load to be actuated. The rotation of the electric motor causes the strings to shorten, resulting in linear motion on the load side. The kinematics and dynamics of the TSA system are detailed in [70, 71]. The unique characteristics of the TSA allow for the use of small motors with high speed and low torque, enabling the generation of significant force. This results in a cost-effective, lightweight, and compact linear transmission system [72, 73]. In this study, a polyethylene cable (Dyneema fiber, Japan) was selected for its excellent strength-to-weight ratio. The motor was positioned perpendicular to the joint tip, ensuring that the forces exerted by the twisted strings are distributed vertically along the structure.

Regarding the wave joints, the only parameter that has been altered is the number of ridges, which subsequently affects the overall length of the compliant module. Specifically, three case studies were considered, corresponding to three, four, and five ridges n_r with initial lengths l_0 of 30 mm, 36 mm, and 42 mm, respectively. This selection of values was deemed sufficiently representative and manageable for the identification procedure described in the following section, ensuring an appropriate amount of data for analysis.

Each compliant wave joint consists of a single module that is 3D-printed in ABS. Each sample comprises a rigid part, represented by cubes, and a compliant part, characterized by the wave structure. In addition to the path designed to accommodate the twisted string actuator (TSA), an additional path located on the cube edge (denoted

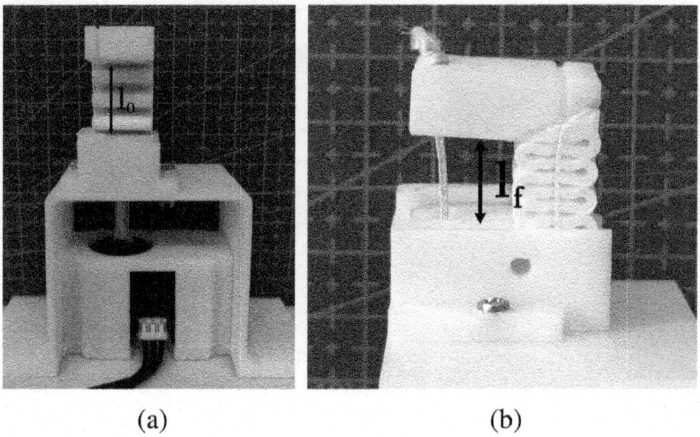

Fig. 4.21 Prototype of the wave-joint with variable stiffness for the identification of stiffness properties: **a** frontal view, where the TSA for joint stiffness regulation is evident, the joint is in its initial configuration, with length l_t equal to l_0. **b** Lateral view of the prototype with the wave-joint completely compressed, so that it's length l_t has been reduced to l_f. Reproduced from [68] with permission from IEEE. © IEEE 2023

as **P** in Fig. 4.20) facilitates the insertion of the tendon for actuating the joint's flexion. Figure 4.21 illustrates the wave joint sample with three ridges n_r and an initial length l_0 of 30 mm.

4.4.1.2 Preliminary Investigation with Numerical Simulation

A numerical structural analysis was conducted to determine whether the TSA can provide the necessary pre-compression to effectively control joint stiffness. This analysis, based on FEM, was performed using COMSOL Multiphysics® software, utilizing the previously described CAD model for structural evaluation.

A series of structural static tests were performed to preliminarily verify that the routing designed for the TSA is capable of applying pure compressive deformation. Additionally, these tests helped establish the relationship between joint pre-compression, joint deformation, and stiffness properties. Figure 4.22d presents a representative set of results from one of the three case studies. The force, indicated by the blue arrow in Fig. 4.22d, acts vertically on the wave-shaped structure to simulate the TSA, while the constrained part is represented by the cube, indicated with a white padlock. The results confirm that the applied force simulating the TSA causes compression of the joint without inducing bending or buckling effects, validating the tendon routing designed for the joint.

Further preliminary tests were conducted on all three samples to evaluate the maximum pre-compression and the force required to flex the joint under the most critical scenario, characterized by the highest joint stiffness.

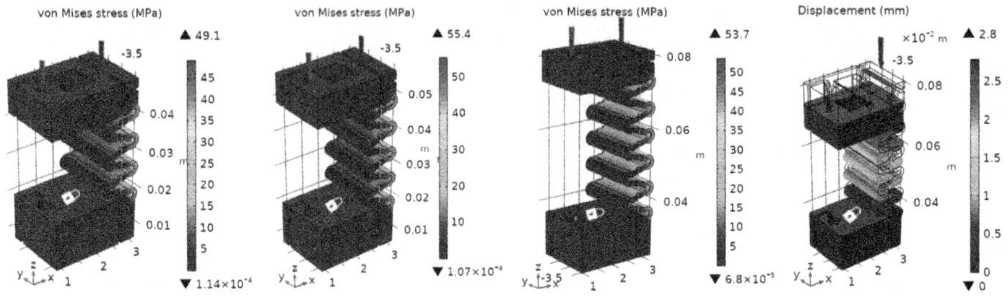

(a) (b) (c) (d)

Fig. 4.22 A subset of FEM analysis results (**a–c**). Deformation obtained by applying a force simulating the TSA to the three considered joints. **d** Results obtained by applying a joint pre-compression and an actuation force to the tendon. Reproduced from [68] with permission from IEEE. © IEEE 2023

These preliminary tests indicated that the maximum force that can be applied to the TSA is 5 N for all three samples. The maximum compression values achieved were 6 mm, 8 mm, and 12 mm for the case studies with three, four, and five ridges n_r, respectively. Figure 4.21 illustrates the preliminary test results for the maximum pre-compression.

Figure 4.22a–c display the results of the FEM analysis in terms of stress for the previously described samples. To evaluate stress, a vertical force was applied to the structure, positioned along the path created for the insertion of the cable. This force, simulating the TSA, was applied with sufficient intensity to induce displacements comparable to those observed experimentally, as indicated by the blue arrow in Fig. 4.22d. Furthermore, to simulate the tendon used to bend the finger, a force (indicated by the red arrow in Fig. 4.22d) with an intensity of 5 N was vertically applied to the cube edge corresponding to the other tendon path. The base cube of the wave-shaped joint remained constrained throughout the analysis.

It is important to note that the maximum equivalent stress that standard ABS can withstand is 60 MPa. The results demonstrate that the compliant structure is sufficiently robust to resist all simulated load cases across the different scenarios.

4.4.1.3 Joint Characterization: Experimental Setup

Regarding the characterization of the joint, the experiments aimed to evaluate the differences in wave-joint stiffness values achieved by controlling the twisted string actuator (TSA). Figure 4.23a illustrates the experimental setup, while the schematic representation is shown in Fig. 4.23b. The testing setup comprises the following components: (i) an Xsens Mi-3 inertial measurement unit (Xsens, NL), which integrates an accelerometer, gyroscope, and magnetometer within a single chip. This unit is mounted on the top of the finger to measure its orientation variation during tendon actuation, (ii) a digital dual-range Vernier dynamometer (Vernier Software & Technology, US) with an accuracy of 0.05 N, used to quantify the force applied during the

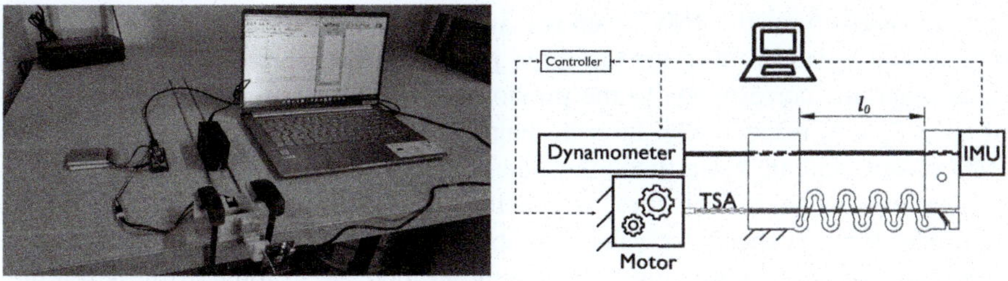

(a) (b)

Fig. 4.23 **a** Experimental setup for the wave-joint stiffness characterization. **b** Experimental setup for joint characterization, scheme. In the test, actuation force is measured by a dynamometer, while joint bending angle is measured by an IMU. For each test, the length l_0 of the joint is controlled by the TSA. Reproduced from [68] with permission from IEEE. © IEEE 2023

tests, and (iii) a microcontroller (OpenCM9.04, Robotis) for controlling the tendon, which is actuated by a Dynamixel XL330-M077-T motor, characterized by a stall torque of 0.228 Nm at 6.0 V.

The support for the twisted string actuator was fixed to the table, while a specialized path made from a brass bar was used to ensure that the tester applied a horizontal force on the compliant module in the direction of the tendon during the experiment.

Choosing to place the sample in a horizontal position, rather than vertical, allows us to mitigate the effects of gravitational force that could impact the readings of the digital dynamometer during testing. Initially, we measured the length of the compliant module, and before each test, the dynamometer was positioned to ensure the tendon was under tension.

All the samples described above were evaluated consistently and under the same conditions for ten defined twisted string actuator (TSA) motor currents (τ) during the twisting process.

Once the TSA motor reached the required τ value, the tester began to pull the tendon connected to the dynamometer, applying a force in the range of 1 to 5 N, in increments of 1 N for each torque. This created a step force function profile with a time step of 5 s. This procedure was repeated three times for each sample. Finally, when the motor reached the maximum torque τ, the corresponding final length of the joint was recorded.

4.4.2 *Results*

4.4.2.1 Results of Joint Characterization

Data from the IMU sensors were collected at a frequency of 100 Hz and subsequently processed using MATLAB. For each step of the acquired force profile, ranging from 1 to 5 N, the average force was calculated and associated with the corresponding average angle from the IMU readings. In Fig. 4.24, the results for the five most representative values of τ for the three joint samples are presented. Each of the three diagrams corresponds to the previously introduced joints with ridge counts of $n_r = 3, 4, 5$, respectively. In each diagram, the rotation angle measured by the IMU sensor is plotted as a function of the force applied to the tendon, as measured by the dynamometer. Each curve is generated by actuating the twisted string actuator (TSA) with a specific τ value. Notably, as expected, an increase in τ leads to a decrease in the bending angle, indicating an increase in joint stiffness. Furthermore, the force-to-angle behavior remains approximately constant for the first four τ values. This suggests that, at lower levels of joint pre-compression, the joint stiffness remains relatively consistent over a wide range of rotation angles. However, as the pre-compression increases, the force-to-angle curve exhibits evident non-linear behavior, likely due to significant crushing of the joint waves. Finally, a comparison of the results obtained from the three samples reveals that joint stiffness decreases as the length of the joint increases.

4.4.2.2 Feasibility Example with a Three-Phalanges Finger

In addition to the three samples of compliant joints with variable stiffness, an additive module was designed to be assembled onto these joints. This module enables the construction of a finger structure consisting of three phalanges and three joints, which could serve as a finger element for a gripper or a compliant robotic hand. As detailed in [69], passive joint stiffness plays a crucial role in tendon-driven underactuated robotic fingers by defining the closure trajectory. This prior work utilized this characteristic during the design phase and presented a procedure for synthesizing joint mechanical features based on the requirements of the gripper. In the finger design presented in this study, stiffness can be further regulated by manipulating the twisted string actuator (TSA), as previously discussed. In the second set of experiments, we analyzed how variations in fingertip trajectory, and consequently finger closure movement, can be influenced by adjusting the stiffness of the proximal joint.

In Fig. 4.20b, the hole at the top part of the rigid element is clearly visible. This feature was introduced to accommodate an interchangeable module, specifically designed for this purpose, which consists of two phalanges with $n_r = 3$. The final prototype used to evaluate the trajectories is shown in Fig. 4.25. We analyzed the closure motion of the finger under three conditions: normal stiffness (no TSA action), medium stiffness, and maximum stiffness.

To track the fingertip trajectories, we utilized Tracker, an open-source software capable of capturing the finger's position from a camera feed. The motion of the upper front edge of the rigid distal element was monitored throughout the experiments. Figures 4.25a–c display the superposition of five frames for the normal, medium, and maximum stiffness cases, respectively, during the finger's flexion motion. Additionally, Fig. 4.26 illustrates the fingertip trajectories plotted on the reference flexion plane of the finger, highlighting the changes achieved by varying the stiffness of the first compliant module.

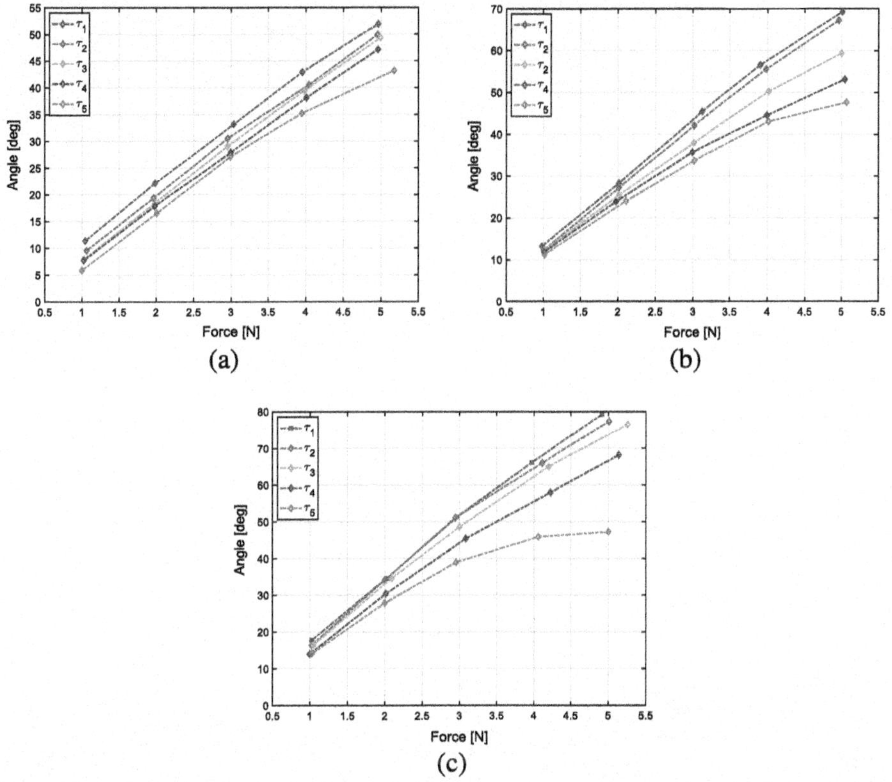

Fig. 4.24 Results of the joint characterization with $\tau_1 = 12\,\text{mA}$, $\tau_2 = 38\,\text{mA}$, $\tau_3 = 80\,\text{mA}$, $\tau_4 = 160\,\text{mA}$, $\tau_5 = 290\,\text{mA}$. **a** $n_r = 3$, $l_0 = 30\,\text{mm}$ and $l_f = 24\,\text{mm}$. **b** $n_r = 4$, $l_0 = 36\,\text{mm}$ and $l_f = 28\,\text{mm}$. **c** $n_r = 5$, $l_0 = 42\,\text{mm}$ and $l_f = 30\,\text{mm}$. Reproduced from [68] with permission from IEEE. © IEEE 2023

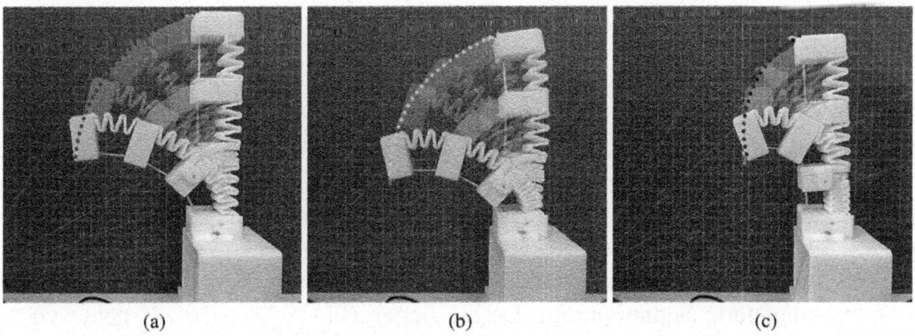

Fig. 4.25 Trajectories followed by the fingertip in the three cases: **a** normal stiffness ($\tau_{motor} = 0\,\text{mA}$); **b** medium stiffness ($\tau_{motor} = 150\,\text{mA}$); **c** maximum stiffness ($\tau_{motor} = 390\,\text{mA}$). Reproduced from [68] with permission from IEEE. © IEEE 2023

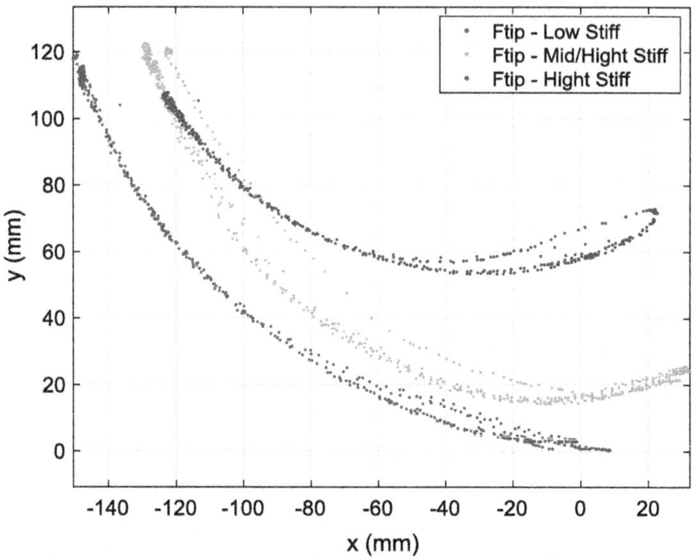

Fig. 4.26 Cloud points of the fingertip trajectories in the above mentioned cases during the finger flexion movement. Reproduced from [68] with permission from IEEE. © IEEE 2023

4.5 The DressGripper

This part of the thesis, instead, proposes a tendon-driven underactuated gripper with magnetic actuation, attained by embedding properly located magnetic elements, which can act as additional DoAs operating in specific locations of the gripper. Hence, they can act synergistically with the more global effect provided by classic actuation and transmission components (like motors and tendons), arousing a complementarity enriching of the device's capabilities. The presented gripper is specifically designed for intrinsically safe human-robot cooperative dressing [57]. By "intrinsically" safe, in this thesis framework, means that the gripper has to be capable of absorbing the impact of unexpected collisions with the human by deforming its structure, and then it has to restore its original configuration. Moreover, with "cooperation" it is means that the gripper has to enable the interaction between the robot and the human in order to achieve the common goal of dressing the human. Hence, the gripper has to ensure the grasp maintenance.

This section of the thesis introduces a tendon-driven underactuated gripper with fingertip magnetic actuation, the DressGripper (Fig. 4.27). This is achieved by embedding strategically located magnetic elements that serve as additional Degrees of Actuation (DoAs) in specific regions of the gripper. These magnetic elements work synergistically with traditional actuation and transmission components, such as motors and tendons, thereby enriching the device's capabilities through complementary functionality. The proposed gripper is specifically designed for intrinsically

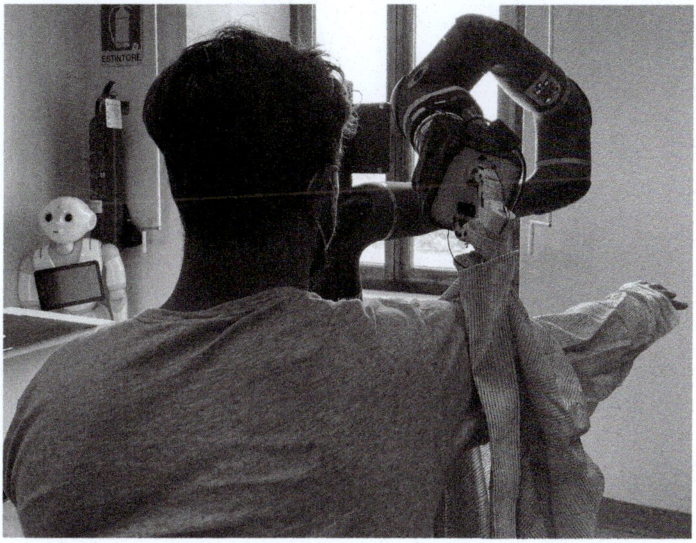

Fig. 4.27 The dressing setup, composed of a collaborative robot and the DressGripper, assisting a person in wearing a shirt

safe human-robot cooperative dressing, as outlined in [57]. In this context, "intrinsically" safe refers to the gripper's ability to absorb the impact from unexpected collisions with humans by deforming its structure, after which it can restore to its original configuration. Additionally, "cooperation" implies that the gripper must facilitate interaction between the robot and the human to achieve the shared objective of dressing the individual. Consequently, the gripper must ensure that it maintains a secure grasp throughout the operation.

4.5.1 Device Description

This subsection provides details on the design of the DressGripper, whose CAD model is illustrated in Fig. 4.28. The DressGripper is an underactuated soft-rigid gripper composed of two modular fingers connected to a base that houses all the electronic components. The design specifically aims to exploit the synergy between tendon-driven and magnetic actuation.

The fingers are actuated by tendons, which transmit force from the motor to the fingers. The fingertips are equipped with magnetic elements that facilitate magnetic actuation. While tendon-driven actuation enables flexion and extension of the fingers, magnetic actuation enhances the permanence of contact between the fingertips, thereby improving the grasping of garments.

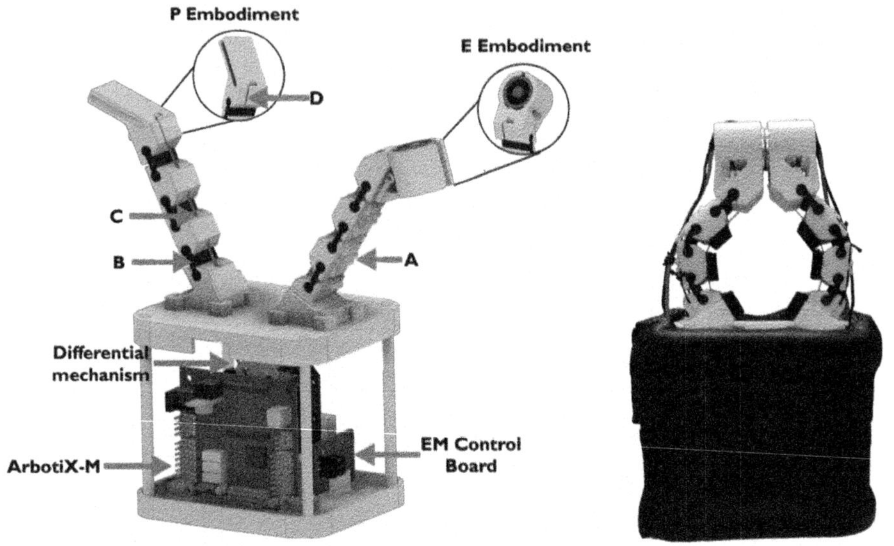

Fig. 4.28 The DressGripper: **a** CAD model, showing base, actuation mechanism, electronics, modular fingers, and fingertips embodiments ("A" rigid modules, "B" flexible joints, "C" tendon path, "E" electromagnet, "P" ferromagnetic plate). **b** EE embodiment of the DressGripper prototype, front view. Copyright © 2022 Dragusanu et al. [74]. This is an open-access article distributed under the terms of the Creative Commons Attribution License (CC BY)

Each finger of the DressGripper functions as a kinematic chain comprising two identical modules that culminate in a fingertip module. One of the fingers features a fingertip module containing an electromagnet, while the other finger can accommodate either another electromagnet or a small ferromagnetic plate (see Fig. 4.28a). This design choice depends on the specific use case. Electromagnets can exert significant grip forces but may incur considerable power consumption during prolonged use. Although higher forces are advantageous for manipulating heavy or thick garments, such power requirements necessitate a connection to a power supply.

Conversely, a fingertip that employs a single electromagnet consumes less power, making it suitable for battery operation and compatible with passive robotic arms. However, grip forces in this configuration will typically be lower than those produced by two electromagnets, making it more appropriate for thin and lightweight garments.

Each module of the two fingers consists of a rigid part 3D-printed in ABS, denoted as *A* in Fig. 4.28a, and a flexible part 3D-printed in TPU (Lulzbot, USA), indicated as *B* in Fig. 4.28a. TPU was chosen for its excellent elongation and fatigue resistance properties, allowing repeated joint movements without significant wear. Additionally, it provides a good damping ratio, which helps reduce undesired vibrations and absorb shocks [75]. Part *A* and Part *B* are connected by sliding Part *B* inside Part *A*, facilitated by appropriate grooves in Part *A*. This modular approach allows for a quick and easy assembly process. Furthermore, each module features paths (denoted as *C* in Fig. 4.28a) designed for the insertion and extraction of the tendon cable made from polyethylene (Dyneema fiber Japan).

Tendon-driven actuation is achieved through a motor and two parallel tendons, marked in red in Fig. 4.28a. Each tendon is connected at one end to the fingertip module (after passing through the intermediate modules of the fingers), while the other end connects to a differential mechanism linked to a pulley rigidly attached to a Dynamixel MX-28T motor (Robotis, South Korea). The motor boasts a maximum torque of 3.1 Nm and a maximum angular speed of 11.9 rad/s. An Arbotix-M controller (Robotis, South Korea), which includes a driver for the Dynamixel and utilizes an AVR microcontroller, is employed to control the DressGripper.

The rotational movement of the motor allows the cables to wind around a pulley with a radius of 10.5 mm (see Fig. 4.28a), facilitating finger flexion by shortening the length of the wires. Conversely, finger extension occurs through the elastic force stored in the flexible parts of the modules during previous flexion. During this release phase, the motor returns to its initial position.

Each finger connects to the base of the gripper through a dovetail joint, allowing complete rotation of the finger about its axis (perpendicular to the palm). The motor and electronic components, which are critical for robustness, are positioned under the gripper base, providing a secure location well-protected from accidental shocks and human contact.

The following sections describe the design of the two different fingertip embodiments, the trajectory design for the fingers, and the results of the stationary structural analysis of the DressGripper using FEM.

4.5.1.1 Fingertips Design

Two versions of the DressGripper fingertips have been developed, with their respective CAD models shown in Fig. 4.28a. Both modules share the same lower part, which contains an internal path designed to route and secure the tendon used for actuation.

The first design, referred to as the Electromagnet Embodiment (EE), is specifically engineered to house an electromagnet. In contrast, the second design, known as the Plate Embodiment (PE), accommodates a ferromagnetic plate. Both fingertip modules are inclined at 45 °C with respect to the intermediate modules of the fingers. This inclination aims to provide parallel surfaces after the flexion motion, making the DressGripper particularly suitable for performing pinch grasps on extremely thin objects, such as garments.

The EE module, as illustrated in Fig. 4.28a, is designed to contain an electromagnet. An ARD MAGNET-25N electromagnet, which provides a holding force of 25 N at 5 V, was selected to meet the necessary criteria regarding weight, strength, size, and ease of control. The PE module, also shown in Fig. 4.28a, features a fingertip that hosts a ferromagnetic plate. To minimize undesired interactions with ferromagnetic components potentially embedded in garments (such as buttons, zippers, and studs), a soft ferromagnetic material was chosen. This material is characterized by minimal

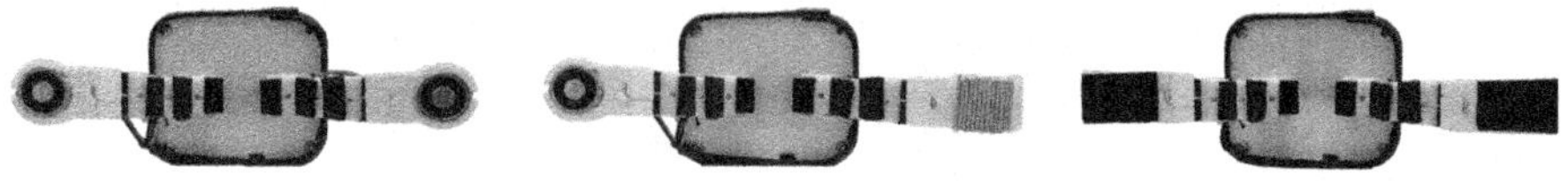

(a) (b) (c)

Fig. 4.29 The DressGripper with different fingertip embodiments: **a** EEE, two electromagnets are hosted in the fingertips, **b** EPE, an electromagnet is hosted in one tip, while the other houses a ferromagnetic plate, **c** NEPE, fingertips are simply covered with a rubber layer.

residual magnetization; it can easily magnetize when subjected to a magnetic field and demagnetize promptly when the magnetic field is removed.

More specifically, I constructed a plate measuring 22 mm× 20 mm × 3 mm, composed of adjacent steel wires held together by a thin layer of hot glue. The glue is applied at the bottom part of the plate, leaving the upper part exposed (see Fig. 4.29b). In addition, to compare the DressGripper with a simple gripper without magnetic actuation, it is considered also the NEP embodiment (No Electromagnet (nor) Plate), in which the gripper has only tendon-driven actuation, no magnetic elements are hosted in the fingertips, and the last module of the finger is similar to the intermediate ones (see Fig. 4.29c). The DressGripper prototype is shown in Fig. 4.28b.

4.5.1.2 Finger Design Trajectory

The primary objective of the hardware design was to facilitate inherently safe interactions with humans. To achieve this, a soft-rigid gripper with elastic joints has been developed. The design process for the prototype necessitated careful selection of the joints' stiffness values, which are intrinsically linked to the specific topology of the gripper. This topology defines how torque is transmitted from the motors throughout the entire finger structure. In this context, the problem was formulated with the goal of enabling effective grasping of garments. The two fingers of the DressGripper are engineered to close in a specific flexion movement that allows the fingertips to make parallel contact, thereby enabling the DressGripper to perform a pinch grasp. This closing trajectory is actuated through a tendon-driven mechanism.

Thanks to the flexible modular structure of the gripper, it was possible to tailor the closing trajectory by adjusting the stiffness of the soft joints. This approach facilitated the identification of appropriate stiffness ratios between consecutive joints, following the procedure detailed in [69]. To analyze the kinematic properties of the gripper, tools provided by SynGrasp [76] were employed. The main equations utilized for this analysis are discussed below.

Let us consider the two fingers of the DressGripper actuated by n_t tendons, where each tendon connects n_q joints. While a three-dimensional analysis of the deformation of flexible joints is presented in [77], for simplicity, we will assume that each soft joint behaves as a revolute joint, neglecting other possible deformations. Consequently, the variable q_i, which describes the displacement of the i-th joint, is interpreted as a pure rotation angle. We define the vector containing the rotations of the gripper joints as $\mathbf{q} = [q_1, \ldots, q_{n_q}]^T \in \mathbb{R}^{n_q}$, and the vector related to the displacement of the tendons, that is denoted with $\delta \in \mathbb{R}^{n_t}$. The relationship between the tendon displacement δ and the configuration of the gripper joints $\mathbf{q}$ is expressed as $\delta = \mathbf{Aq}$ where $\mathbf{A}$ is a transformation matrix determined by the size of the finger's pulley and the routing topology of the tendons [78]. Using the Principle of Virtual Work, it turns out

$$\tau = \mathbf{A}^T \mathbf{f}, \tag{4.12}$$

where τ is the vector containing the joint torques, while $\mathbf{f}$ is the vector of the tendons' pulling forces. Assuming that the gripper moves the fingers without interacting with any object or external surfaces, and that no external forces are present, the relation between the gripper configuration and the torque at the joints is described by

$$\tau + \mathbf{K}_q \Delta\mathbf{q} = 0. \tag{4.13}$$

$\mathbf{K_q} \in \mathbb{R}^{n_q \times n_q}$ is the joint stiffness matrix (symmetric and positive definite), while $\Delta\mathbf{q}$ denotes a variation of the joints configuration with respect to a reference rest position $\mathbf{q_0}$ of the gripper, i.e., $\Delta\mathbf{q} = \mathbf{q} - \mathbf{q_0}$. If the joints are independent, $\mathbf{K_q}$ is diagonal and by assuming $\mathbf{q_0} = 0$ Eq. (4.13) can be rewritten as

$$\tau + \mathbf{Qk_q} = 0, \tag{4.14}$$

where $\mathbf{Q} = diag(\mathbf{q})$ with $\mathbf{Q} \in \mathbb{R}^{n_q \times n_q}$, while $\mathbf{k_q} \in \mathbb{R}^{n_q}$ is the vector of the joint stiffness. Taking into account Eq. (4.12), the the joints stiffness can be retrieved as

$$\mathbf{k_q} = \mathbf{Q}^{-1}\mathbf{A}^{\mathbf{T}}\mathbf{f_r}. \tag{4.15}$$

Such a solution contains the stiffness values for the flexible joints of the gripper, allowing to obtain the configuration $\mathbf{q_r}$ of the joints given the force $\mathbf{f_r}$ applied by the tendons.

Moreover, to establish a basis for the subspace of possible stiffness combinations suitable for performing a desired trajectory, the vector $\mathbf{k_q}$ must be normalized. As previously noted, the shape of the finger trajectory is influenced by the stiffness ratio between two consecutive joints. To derive a complete trajectory, it is necessary to evaluate a sequence of configurations, which leads to a corresponding sequence of $\mathbf{k_q}$ values.

In [69], it is demonstrated that for various closing trajectories, similar to those required for the DressGripper, the values within $\mathbf{k_q}$exhibit slight fluctuations during the completion of finger flexion. Therefore, to effectively model the flexible joints, the average of all retrieved $\mathbf{k_q}$ values was considered, which results in an acceptable tracking error along the desired trajectory [69]. To exploit the advantages of 3D printing, flexible joints for the DressGripper were created by appropriately varying the

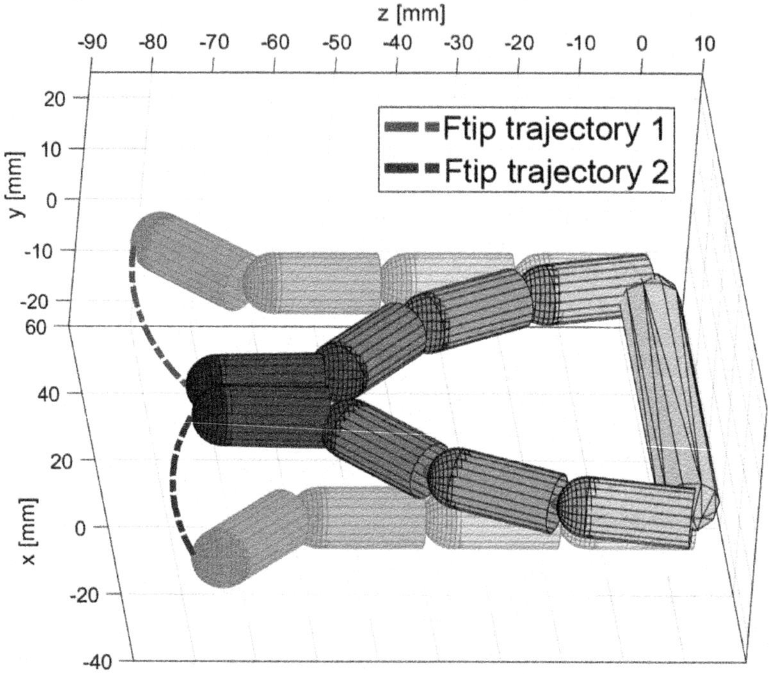

Fig. 4.30 Fingers' trajectory: initial and final configurations, simulated in SynGrasp. Copyright © 2022 Dragusanu et al. [74]. This is an open-access article distributed under the terms of the Creative Commons Attribution License (CC BY)

infill density percentage. This parameter not only alters the material's density but also modifies its mechanical properties, such as the Young's modulus. Figure 4.30 illustrates the results of the simulation conducted using SynGrasp to generate the desired trajectory.

4.5.1.3 Finite Element Analysis

This section presents the results of the structural analysis conducted in terms of stress and displacement to characterize the DressGripper under relevant conditions. The analysis encompasses the entire structure composed of the two fingers, as well as an individual finger. Both the Electromagnet Embodiment (EE) and the Plate Embodiment (PE) were considered. The resultant configurations will be denoted as "EEE" when two EE are used and as "EPE" when an EE and a PE are assembled (i.e., Electromagnet and Plate Embodiment), as illustrated in Fig. 4.29.

The Finite Element Analysis (FEA) was performed using the 3D-CAD/CAE Autodesk® Fusion 360 software, utilizing the same materials as described in Sect. 4.5.1.1. Since the base of the DressGripper is not actuated, its dynamics are neglected in the following analysis.

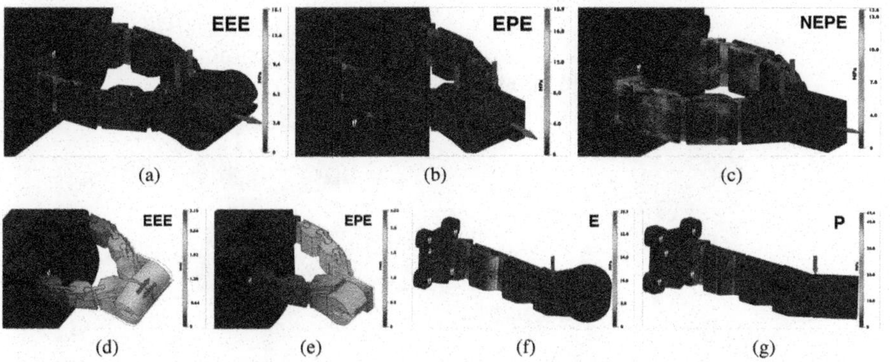

Fig. 4.31 Results of the FEM structural analysis. In **a–c** Equivalent Von Mises stress distributions when 5 N of garment weight force is applied in addition to 5 N (**a**), 2 N (**b**) and 1 N (**c**) of tangential disturbances forces, respectively. **d** and **e** report the FEM structural analyses when 1 N force at the fingertips surfaces are applied, while **f** and **g** show the Equivalent Von Mises stress distribution when 10 N force is applied. Red arrows indicate the forces applied, while the transparent wireframe CAD model shown in **d** and **e** is the reference undeformed model. The colored surface corresponds to an "actual" deformation of the DressGripper's fingers. Copyright © 2022 Dragusanu et al. [74]. This is an open-access article distributed under the terms of the Creative Commons Attribution License (CC BY) (color figure online)

Focus on Magnetic Attraction

To simulate the synergistic interaction between tendon-driven and magnetic actuation, it was assumed that the motor was activated to close the fingers until the tips were nearly in contact. Subsequently, the force required to achieve contact between the fingers was estimated. The FEM simulations applied forces at the fingertips within the range of [0.5, 1.5] N.

First, we considered the EPE configuration, where the ferromagnetic plate and the electromagnet were positioned 3 mm apart. Given that the plate is made from a soft ferromagnetic material, the magnetic field generated by the electromagnet is channeled orthogonally to the plate. Thus, a force perpendicular to its surface was simulated. The FEM analysis indicated that a force of 1 N is sufficient to bring the fingers into contact, as shown in Fig. 4.31e.

Next, we analyzed the EEE configuration. Since the magnetic attraction between two electromagnets is stronger than that between an electromagnet and a soft ferromagnetic material, a greater distance of 6 mm was allowed between the two magnetic elements. Figure 4.31d demonstrates that, similarly, a force of 1 N is adequate for establishing contact between the fingers.

These results provide the force requirements that the electromagnet must meet. Additional details regarding the validation of the electromagnet can be found in Sect. 4.5.2.

Focus on Robustness to Perturbations. To investigate the robustness of the fingertip structure, forces were applied at its tip, as this is the part of the finger most stressed

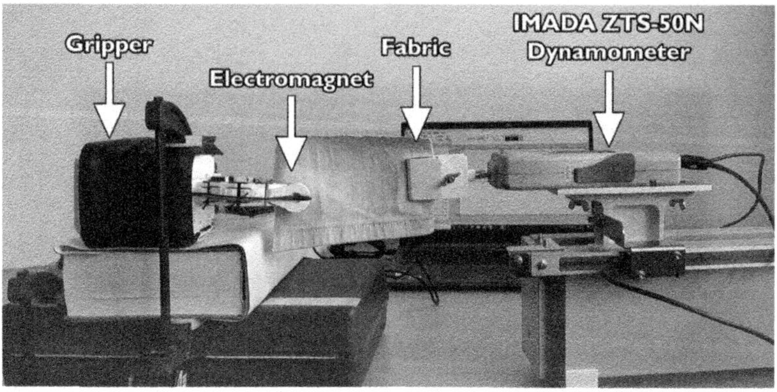

Fig. 4.32 Experimental setup for testing the DressGripper capabilities when grasping different types of fabrics. Forces needed to break the grasp have been estimated. Here it is reported the specific case where the EEE type DressGripper is tested. Copyright © 2022 Dragusanu et al. [74]. This is an open-access article distributed under the terms of the Creative Commons Attribution License (CC BY)

during the operation of the DressGripper. A force of 10 N [79] was applied in a direction perpendicular to the contact surface. This force serves as a conservative exerted by a human during garment wearing, as well as the force of attraction between the magnetic elements. The first force acts as a grasp-breaking force, while the second corresponds to an attractive force estimate of the potential (undesired) force.

Both the EE and PE were examined, and the results are presented in Fig. 4.31f and g. Notably, the maximum equivalent stress that standard ABS and TPU materials can sustain is 60 MPa and 50 MPa, respectively. The results indicate that both finger embodiments are sufficiently robust to withstand the simulated forces.

Furthermore, an investigation was conducted to evaluate the gripper's robustness when subjected to the weight force of garments and potential tangential disturbances arising from undesired collisions between the garment and the human wearing it, assisted by the robot. Such forces can lead to a grasp break due to sliding. To gain insights into these aspects, four fabrics used in Sect. 4.5.2 were selected, i.e., "Undershirt1", "Shirt1", "Fleece" and "Jeans". These fabrics were considered representative samples. By following the procedure detailed in Sect. 4.5.2, the average sliding force was conservatively estimated-the average force required to break the grasp by stretching the fabric until it slides (see Fig. 4.32).

The configurations EEE, EPE, and NEPE were investigated, yielding average forces of approximately 5 N, 2 N, and 1 N, respectively. These values were used as estimates for the aforementioned tangential disturbances. Regarding the weight force of the garment, a conservative simulation estimated a magnitude of 5 N, corresponding to a garment mass of 500 g.

Figure 4.31a–c show how the fingertip embodiment affects the stress the gripper is subjected to. In particular, in Fig. 4.31b there is a maximum Von Mises of 18.9 MPa, while in Fig. 4.31c there is a maximum Von Mises of 13.6 MPa, which is the

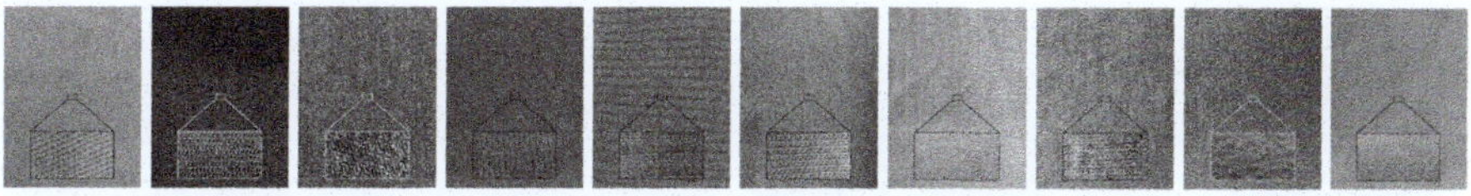

Fig. 4.33 Samples of fabrics used in the experiments on the capabilities of DressGripper. Copyright © 2022 Dragusanu et al. [74]. This is an open-access article distributed under the terms of the Creative Commons Attribution License (CC BY)

minimum stress among all of three results. However, in all the fingertip embodiments, the structure resists and has a Von Mises value lower than the maximum allowable value for the considered materials.

4.5.2 Experiments

This subsection details the experiments conducted to assess the grasping capabilities of the DressGripper.

To analytically compute the force of attraction between the electromagnets or between an electromagnet and a ferromagnetic plate, it is essential to know the specifications of the electromagnets as well as the magnetic permeability of the ferromagnetic materials involved. However, manufacturers typically do not disclose information about the internal structure of their electromagnets due to proprietary protection policies. Therefore, the setup was characterized experimentally to gather the necessary data.

Estimate of Magnetic Attraction. The DressGripper was actuated to create distances of 6 mm and 3 mm between the fingertips for the EEE and EPE configurations, respectively. These distances were measured using a caliper with a resolution of 0.1 mm.

In the setup, one electromagnet was secured using a g-clamp, while the second magnetic element (either the other electromagnet or the ferromagnetic plate) was left free to move. The non-constrained element was connected to a strain-gauge-based dynamometer (dual-range Vernier dynamometer—Vernier Software & Technology, US) with an accuracy of ±0.05 N, via a non-extensible wire (see Fig. 4.34a). The distance between the fingertips was verified again before activating the electromagnet(s). Due to the magnetic attraction, the non-constrained finger experienced an attractive force, which was measured by the dynamometer. Data were collected at a frequency of 200 Hz, and the experiment was repeated five times for each configuration. Figure 4.34b presents the force readings from the dynamometer, with average values of (0.92 ± 0.06) N for the EEE configuration and (0.75 ± 0.08) N for the EPE configuration. These results are consistent with the findings obtained from the previously reported FEM analysis.

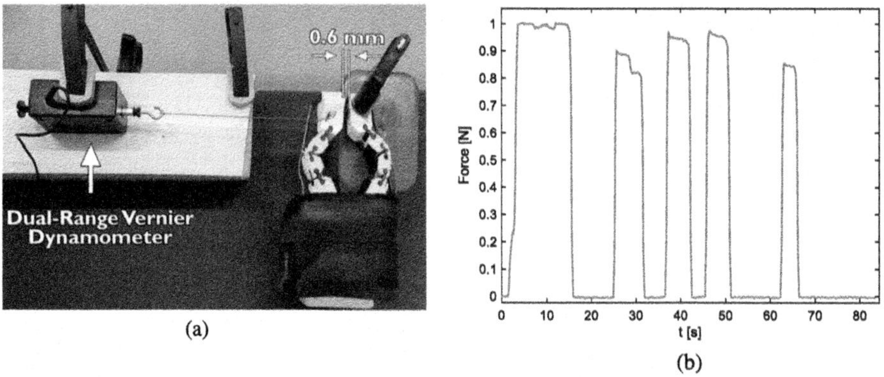

Fig. 4.34 **a** Setup for the estimate of the attractive force acting on the magnetic elements. **b** Attractive force on EE embodiment when the tips are distant 6 mm.

Table 4.4 Fabrics used for characterizing the DressGripper capabilities

Sample	W [g]	T [mm]	F_{NEPE} [N]	F_{EPE} [N]	F_{EEE} [N]
Trousers 1	6.23	0.62	0.83 ± 0.23	1.41 ± 0.16	2.19 ± 0.38
Trousers 2	7.80	0.94	0.93 ± 0.29	1.17 ± 0.13	1.74 ± 0.10
Jeans	7.07	0.72	0.97 ± 0.26	1.33 ± 0.25	3.12 ± 0.34
Undersh1	5.77	0.70	1.08 ± 0.13	1.66 ± 0.17	4.60 ± 0.57
Undersh 2	2.81	0.70	1.32 ± 0.18	2.86 ± 0.16	9.85 ± 0.48
T-Shirt	2.46	0.52	1.25 ± 0.10	2.66 ± 0.03	7.52 ± 0.68
Shirt 1	2.27	0.26	1.04 ± 0.26	1.77 ± 0.14	9.21 ± 0.25
Shirt 2	4.50	0.66	1.01 ± 0.03	1.59 ± 0.17	5.18 ± 0.41
Fleece	3.85	1.10	1.53 ± 0.13	1.61 ± 0.06	5.69 ± 0.46
Sweater	3.92	1.06	1.18 ± 0.25	1.48 ± 0.14	4.34 ± 0.13

In the last three columns, it is reported the average force required to break the grasp in the NEP, EP and EE embodiments. "W" and "T" stand for "weight" and "thickness" of the garment, respectively.

Focus on Tangential Forces breaking the grasp. To have insights on the actual performance of the DressGripper when manipulating fabrics, it was selected 10 samples of fabric commonly used for clothes (Fig. 4.33), whose weight and thickness are reported in Table 4.4 (average size of fabric sample (80 mm ± 7) mm × (240 ± 5) mm. Trousers are made of stretch cotton, with "Trouser1" more elastic than "Trouser2". "Jeans" are the less stretchy trousers. "Shirt1" is made of pure cotton, while "Shirt2" is a stretchy material containing elastane, cotton and polyester. "Fleece" is 100% polyester. "Undershirt1" is made of cotton 98%, elastane 2%, with very narrow ribs, while "Undershirt2" is made of cotton 95% and 5% elastane, and has ribs large 2 mm. "T-shirt" is made of cotton 98% and 2% elastane.

Concerning the experimental procedure, experiments were aimed at testing the DressGripper's ability to resist perturbations while pinch grasping different fabrics. A clip was attached to the fabric, and a dynamometer was attached to that clip. Forces were applied to the fabrics using an IMADA ZTS-50N dynamometer with an accuracy of ±0.01 N, which was mounted on a manual test stand HV-500N II. The test stand was equipped with a linear encoder (DMK) for displacement measurement, with an accuracy of ±0.03 mm. Once the fingers were closed, the fabrics were trapped between the fingertips. Tractions were exerted on the fabric until the sample began to slide. The procedure was repeated ten times, and the forces were averaged. The results for the EEE, EPE, and NEPE configurations are reported in Table 4.4. It can be observed that the force required to break the grasp in the NEPE configuration is the lowest among the fingertip embodiments, and this force is relatively independent of the fabric type. This observation suggests a correlation with the underactuated structure of the gripper. Among the different embodiments, the EE configuration provides the strongest forces, while the EP configuration yields intermediate results, highlighting the dependency on the magnetic permeability of the selected plate.

Regarding garment types, trousers (Figs. 4.33a–c) exhibited the most sliding. This can be attributed to their dense and combed fabric weave. The sweater (Fig. 4.33j), made of microfiber, also has some friction; however, its dense weave leads to intermediate results in terms of F_{EEE} and F_{EPE}. The fleece (Fig. 4.33i), while made of lighter fabric, has a dense but looser weave than the aforementioned materials. The small protrusions and slippery nature of polyester reduce the fabric's adherence to the fingertips, resulting in intermediate performance. The other garments, which perform better, are primarily made of cotton, featuring a looser weave and thinner construction (Figs. 4.33d, f, g).

Additional considerations regarding the EE embodiment can be noted. Figure 4.35 illustrates how the fabric material influences the traction applied by the HV-500N. As the HV-500N wheel rotates, the force applied to the fabric increases until sliding occurs, reaching a plateau associated with dynamic friction.

As seen in Fig. 4.35, non-stretchy samples slide earlier. This trend is evident for Jeans, Trousers2, Shirt1, and Sweater. The more pronounced (Undershirt2, see Fig. 4.33e) and sharper (Undershirt1, Undershirt2) the ribbed pattern, the sooner the grasp breaks. Conversely, the flatter and more homogeneous the pattern (T-Shirt and Shirt1), the higher the breaking force. Under similar patterns, the stretchiness of the fabric affects the breaking force (e.g. , T-Shirt vs. Shirt1).

Fleece, Undershirt1, and Shirt2 (Fig. 4.33h) exhibit similar behavior, although the fleece starts sliding earlier. All three fabrics are somewhat stretchy; however, the fleece has a highly inhomogeneous pattern. Among these fabrics, the fleece experiences the highest breaking forces due to its low thickness, which allows for stronger attraction between the electromagnets. However, it breaks earlier due to the relatively low stretch of the material.

The experiments reveal that thickness is not the sole parameter to consider for understanding the force required to break the grasp. Relevant characteristics include: (i) fabric slip, (ii) pattern orientation in the vertical direction, and (iii) fiber density. Regarding (i), a higher presence of synthetic fibers leads to a more slippery fabric

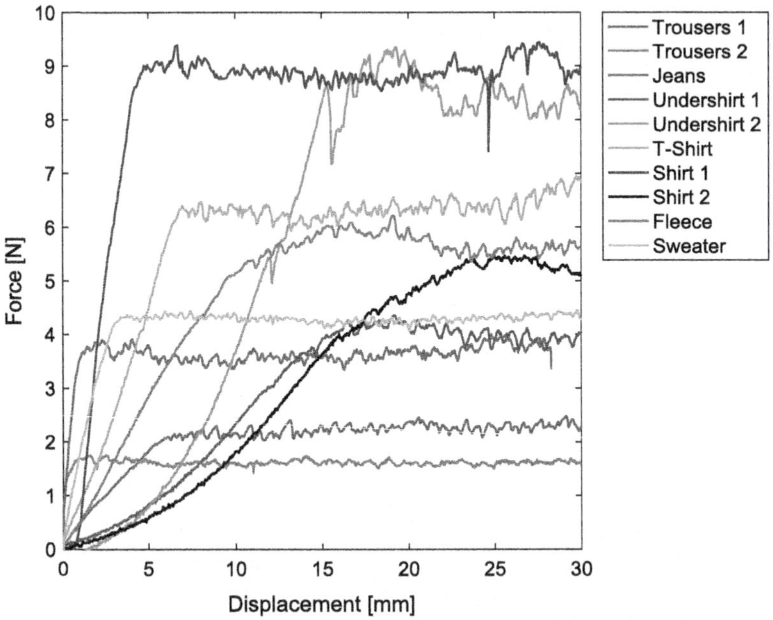

Fig. 4.35 Forces exterted on different fabrics while performing tractions aimed at retrieving insights on the DressGripper capabilities. Copyright © 2022 Dragusanu et al. [74]. This is an open-access article distributed under the terms of the Creative Commons Attribution License (CC BY)

(as noted through tactile feedback). In terms of (ii), a more irregular arrangement of full and empty spaces in the vertical direction (as seen in fleece) facilitates grasp breakage. Concerning (iii), the denser the fabric is in both the horizontal and vertical directions, the stronger the magnetic force must be to maintain a secure grasp.

To gain insights into the DressGripper's capabilities during robot-assisted dressing, a human-robot cooperative scenario was implemented, utilizing the collaborative 7-DoF Sawyer robotic arm (Rethink Robotics). Given that a non-passive robot was employed, the EEE DressGripper configuration was chosen, which has proven to exhibit greater resistance compared to the EPE configuration.

Through kinesthetic teaching, we recorded a trajectory for the robotic arm to assist a human in wearing the sleeve of a shirt. For this test, a different shirt was utilized compared to those in the previous subsections. The human was positioned with one arm almost straight in front, while the robot grasped the shirt near the neck and gently moved it toward the human, successfully fitting the sleeve onto the human arm.

References

1. Tiboni M, Borboni A, Vérité F, Bregoli C, Amici C (2022) Sensors and actuation technologies in exoskeletons: a review. Sensors 22(3):884
2. Hussain I, Salvietti G, Spagnoletti G, Prattichizzo D (July2016) The soft-sixthfinger: a wearable EMG controlled robotic extra-finger for grasp compensation in chronic stroke patients. IEEE Robot Autom Lett 1(2):1000–1006
3. Bae J-H, Park S-W, Park J-H, Baeg M-H, Kim D, Oh S-R (2012) Development of a low cost anthropomorphic robot hand with high capability. In: 2012 IEEE/RSJ international conference on intelligent robots and systems. IEEE, pp 4776–4782
4. Grebenstein M (2012) Approaching human performance. Ph.D. thesis, Springer
5. Bicchi A (2000) Hands for dextrous manipulation and robust grasping: a difficult road towards simplicity. IEEE Trans Robot Autom 16(6):652–662
6. Prattichizzo D, Trinkle J (2008) Grasping. In: Siciliano B, Kathib O (eds) Handbook on robotics. Springer, pp 671–700
7. Shintake J, Cacucciolo V, Floreano D, Shea H (2018) Soft robotic grippers. Adv Mater 30(29):1707035
8. Santina CD, Catalano MG, Bicchi A, Ang M, Khatib O, Siciliano B (2020) Soft robots. In: Encyclopedia of robotics, vol 489
9. Deimel R, Brock O (2016) A novel type of compliant and underactuated robotic hand for dexterous grasping. Int J Robot Res 35(1–3):161–185
10. Jones TJ, Jambon-Puillet E, Marthelot J, Brun P-T (2021) Bubble casting soft robotics. Nature 599(7884):229–233
11. Hussain I, Al-Ketan O, Renda F, Malvezzi M, Prattichizzo D, Seneviratne L, Abu Al-Rub RK, Gan D (2020) Design and prototyping soft-rigid tendon-driven modular grippers using interpenetrating phase composites materials. Int J Robot Res 39(14):1635–1646
12. Pozzi M, Marullo S, Salvietti G, Bimbo J, Malvezzi M, Prattichizzo D (2020) Hand closure model for planning top grasps with soft robotic hands. Int J Robot Res 39(14):1706–1723
13. Deimel R, Brock O (2015) Soft hands for reliable grasping strategies. In: Soft robotics. Springer, pp 211–221
14. Pozzi M, Marullo S, Salvietti G, Bimbo J, Malvezzi M, Prattichizzo D (2020) Hand closure model for planning top grasps with soft robotic hands. Int J Robot Res 39(14):1706–1723
15. Deimel R, Brock O (2015) A novel type of compliant and underactuated robotic hand for dexterous grasping. Int J Robot Res
16. Sotiropoulos P, Roa MA, Martins MF, Fried W, Mnyusiwalla H, Triantafyllou P, Deacon G (2018) A benchmarking framework for systematic evaluation of compliant under-actuated soft end effectors in an industrial context. In: 2018 IEEE-RAS 18th international conference on humanoid robots (humanoids), pp 280–283
17. Santina CD, Piazza C, Grioli G, Catalano MG, Bicchi A (2018) Toward dexterous manipulation with augmented adaptive synergies: the Pisa/IIT SoftHand 2. IEEE Trans Robot 34(5):1141–1156
18. Pozzi M, Salvietti G, Bimbo J, Malvezzi M, Prattichizzo D (2018) The closure signature: A functional approach to model underactuated compliant robotic hands. IEEE Robot Autom Lett 3(3):2206–2213
19. Catalano MG, Grioli G, Farnioli E, Serio A, Piazza C, Bicchi A (2014) Adaptive synergies for the design and control of the Pisa/IIT Softhand. Int J Robot Res 33(5):768–782
20. Hussain I, Salvietti G, Spagnoletti G, Prattichizzo D (2016) The soft-sixthfinger: a wearable EMG controlled robotic extra-finger for grasp compensation in chronic stroke patients. IEEE Robot Autom Lett 1(2):1000–1006
21. Guo X-Y, Li W-B, Gao Q-H, Yan H, Fei Y-Q, Zhang W-M (2020) Self-locking mechanism for variable stiffness rigid-soft gripper. Smart Mater Struct 29(3):035033
22. Cheng P, Jia J, Ye Y, Wu C (2021) Modeling of a soft-rigid gripper actuated by a linear-extension soft pneumatic actuator. Sensors 21(2):493

23. Achilli GM, Valigi MC, Salvietti G, Malvezzi M (2020) Design of soft grippers with modular actuated embedded constraints. Robotics 9(4):105
24. Salvietti G, Iqbal Z, Hussain I, Prattichizzo M, Malvezzi D (2018) The co-gripper: a wireless cooperative gripper for safe human robot interaction. In Proceedings of the IEEE/RSJ international conference on intelligent robots and systems, Madrid, Spain
25. Salvietti G, Iqbal Z, Malvezzi M, Eslami T, Prattichizzo D (2019) Soft hands with embodied constraints: the soft scoopgripper. In: Proceedings of the IEEE international conference on robotics and automation, pp 2758–2764, Montreal, Canada
26. Gafer A, Heymans D, Prattichizzo D, Salvietti G (2020) The quad-spatula gripper: a novel soft-rigid gripper for food handling. In: Proceedings of the IEEE international conference on soft robotics (RoboSoft), New Haeven, USA, pp 39–45
27. Malvezzi M, Iqbal Z, Valigi MC, Pozzi M, Prattichizzo D, Salvietti G (2019) Design of multiple wearable robotic extra fingers for human hand augmentation. Robotics 8(4):102
28. Dollar AM, Howe RD (2010) The highly adaptive SDM hand: design and performance evaluation. Int J Robot Res 29(5):585–597
29. Salvietti G, Hussain I, Malvezzi M, Prattichizzo D (2017) Design of the passive joints of underactuated modular soft hands for fingertip trajectory tracking. IEEE Robot Autom Lett 2(4):2008–2015
30. Hussain I, Iqbal Z, Malvezzi M, Prattichizzo D, Salvietti G (2020) How to 3D-print compliant joints with a selected stiffness for cooperative underactuated soft grippers. In: Ferraguti F, Villani V, Sabattini L, Bonfé M (eds) Human-friendly robotics 2019, vol 12. HFR 2019. Springer, Cham, pp 139–153
31. Xu H, Knoop E, Coros S, Bächer M (2018) Bend-it: design and fabrication of kinetic wire characters. ACM Trans Graph (TOG) 37(6):1–15
32. Megaro V, Zehnder J, Bächer M, Coros S, Gross M, Thomaszewski B (2017) A computational design tool for compliant mechanisms. ACM Trans Graph (TOG) 36(4):1–12
33. Mutlu R, Tawk C, Alici G, Sariyildiz E (2017) A 3D printed monolithic soft gripper with adjustable stiffness. In: IECON 2017-43rd annual conference of the IEEE industrial electronics society. IEEE, pp 6235–6240
34. Tawk C, Gao Y, Mutlu R, Alici G (2019) Fully 3D printed monolithic soft gripper with high conformal grasping capability. In: 2019 IEEE/ASME international conference on advanced intelligent mechatronics (AIM), pp 1139–1144
35. Weisbord L, Paros JM (1965) How to design flexure hinges. Mach Des 27(3):151–157
36. Mutlu R, Alici G, in het Panhuis M, Spinks G (2015) Effect of flexure hinge type on a 3D printed fully compliant prosthetic finger. In: 2015 IEEE international conference on advanced intelligent mechatronics (AIM). IEEE, pp 790–795
37. Liu C-H, Chiu C-H, Chen T-L, Pai T-Y, Chen Y, Hsu M-C (2018) A soft robotic gripper module with 3D printed compliant fingers for grasping fruits. In: 2018 IEEE/ASME international conference on advanced intelligent mechatronics (AIM). IEEE, pp 736–741
38. Bicchi A, Kumar V (2000) Robotic grasping and contact: a review. In: Proceedings 2000 ICRA. Millennium conference. IEEE international conference on robotics and automation. Symposia proceedings (Cat. No.00CH37065), vol 1, pp 348–353
39. Bhatt A, Sieler A, Puhlmann S, Brock O (2021) Surprisingly robust in-hand manipulation: an empirical study. Science and Systems XVII, Robotics
40. Borràs J, Alenyà G, Torras C (2020) A grasping-centered analysis for cloth manipulation. IEEE Trans Robot 36(3):924–936
41. Donaire S, Borras J, Alenya G, Torras Carme (2020) A versatile gripper for cloth manipulation. IEEE Robot Autom Lett 5(4):6520–6527
42. Kondratas A (2005) Robotic gripping device for garment handling operations and its adaptive control. Fibres Text East Eur 13(4):84
43. Sahari KSM, Seki H, Kamiya Y, Hikizu M (2010) Clothes manipulation by robot grippers with roller fingertips. Adv Robot 24(1–2):139–158
44. Cubric G, Cubric IS (2019) Study of grippers in automatic handling of nonwoven material. J Inst Eng (India): Ser E 100(2):167–173

45. Ramisa A, Alenyà G, Moreno-Noguer F, Torras C (2012) Using depth and appearance features for informed robot grasping of highly wrinkled clothes. In: 2012 IEEE international conference on robotics and automation, pp 1703–1708
46. Twardon L, Ritter H (2015) Interaction skills for a coat-check robot: identifying and handling the boundary components of clothes. In: 2015 IEEE international conference on robotics and automation (ICRA), pp 3682–3688
47. Le T-H-L, Jilich M, Landini A, Zoppi M, Zlatanov D, Molfino R (2013) On the development of a specialized flexible gripper for garment handling. J Autom Control Eng 1(3)
48. Eppner C, Deimel R, Ruiz J, Maertens M, Brock O (2015) Exploitation of environmental constraints in human and robotic grasping. Int J Rob Res 34(7):1021–1038
49. Marullo S, Bartoccini S, Salvietti G, Iqbal MZ, Prattichizzo D (2020) The mag-gripper: a soft-rigid gripper augmented with an electromagnet to precisely handle clothes. IEEE Robot Autom Lett 5(4):6591–6598
50. Jiménez P, Torras C (2020) Perception of cloth in assistive robotic manipulation tasks. Nat Comput 19(2):409–431
51. Kaltsas PI, Koustoumpardis PN, Nikolakopoulos PG (2022) A review of sensors used on fabric-handling robots. Machines 10(2)
52. Yang P, Sasaki K, Suzuki K, Kase K, Sugano S, Ogata T (2017) Repeatable folding task by humanoid robot worker using deep learning. IEEE Robot Autom Lett 2(2):397–403
53. Tsurumine Y, Cui Y, Uchibe E, Matsubara T (2019) Deep reinforcement learning with smooth policy update: application to robotic cloth manipulation. Robot Auton Syst 112:72–83
54. Colomé A, Torras C (2018) Dimensionality reduction for dynamic movement primitives and application to bimanual manipulation of clothes. IEEE Trans Robot 34:602–615
55. Colgate E, Bicchi A, Peshkin MA, Colgate JE (2008) Safety for physical human-robot interaction. In: Springer handbook of robotics, pp 1335–1348
56. Bellamy DD, Chance G, Caleb-Solly P, Dogramadzi S (2021) Safety assessment review of a dressing assistance robot. Front Robot AI 8:161
57. Salvietti G, Iqbal Z, Hussain I, Prattichizzo D, Malvezzi M (2018) The co-gripper: a wireless cooperative gripper for safe human robot interaction. In: 2018 IEEE/RSJ international conference on intelligent robots and systems (IROS). IEEE, pp 4576–4581
58. Dragusanu M, Achilli GM,Valigi MC, Prattichizzo D, Malvezzi M, Salvietti G (2022) The wavejoints: a novel methodology to design soft-rigid grippers made by monolithic 3D printed fingers with adjustable joint stiffness. In: 2022 international conference on robotics and automation (ICRA), pp 6173–6179
59. Malvezzi M, Gioioso G, Salvietti G, Prattichizzo D (2015) Syngrasp: a matlab toolbox for underactuated and compliant hands. Robotics Autom Mag IEEE 22(4):52–68
60. Crooks W, Vukasin G, O'Sullivan M, Messner W, Rogers C (2016) Fin Ray® effect inspired soft robotic gripper: from the robosoft grand challenge toward optimization. Front Robot AI 3:70
61. Zhang H, Wang MY, Chen F, Wang Y, Senthil Kumar A, Fuh JYH (2017) Design and development of a soft gripper with topology optimization. In: 2017 IEEE/RSJ international conference on intelligent robots and systems (IROS). IEEE, pp 6239–6244
62. Prattichizzo D, Pozzi M, Malvezzi M (2020) Dexterous manipulation. In: Ang HM, Khatib O, Siciliano B (eds) Encyclopedia of robotics. Springer, Berlin, Heidelberg
63. Prattichizzo D, Malvezzi M, Gabiccini M, Bicchi A (2013) On motion and force controllability of precision grasps with hands actuated by soft synergies. IEEE Trans Robot 29(6):1440–1456
64. Kao I, Ngo C (1999) Properties of the grasp stiffness matrix and conservative control strategies. Int J Robot Res 18(2):159–167
65. Malvezzi M, Prattichizzo D (2013) Evaluation of grasp stiffness in underactuated compliant hands. In: 2013 IEEE international conference on robotics and automation. IEEE, pp 2074–2079
66. Achilli GM, Logozzo S, Valigi MC, Dragusanu M, Malvezzi M (2022) Theoretical and experimental characterization of a new robotic gripper's joint. In: Niola V, Gasparetto A, Quaglia G, Carbone G (eds) Advances in Italian mechanism science. Springer International Publishing, Cham, pp 738–745

67. Malvezzi M, Valigi MC, Salvietti G, Iqbal Z, Hussain I, Prattichizzo D (2018) Design criteria for wearable robotic extra–fingers with underactuated modular structure. In: The international conference of IFToMM ITALY. Springer, pp 509–517
68. Dragusanu M, Troisi D, Prattichizzo D, Malvezzi M (2023) Compliant finger joint with controlled variable stiffness based on twisted strings actuation. In: 2023 IEEE international conference on robotics and automation (ICRA), pp 7378–7384
69. Salvietti G, Hussain I, Malvezzi M, Prattichizzo D (2017) Design of the passive joints of underactuated modular soft hands for fingertip trajectory tracking. IEEE Robot Autom Lett 2(4):2008–2015
70. Palli G, Natale C, May C, Melchiorri C, Wurtz T (2012) Modeling and control of the twisted string actuation system. IEEE/ASME Trans Mechatron 18(2):664–673
71. Würtz T, May C, Holz B, Natale C, Palli G, Melchiorri C (2010) The twisted string actuation system: Modeling and control. In: 2010 IEEE/ASME international conference on advanced intelligent mechatronics. IEEE, pp 1215–1220
72. Tsabedze T, Hartman E, Abrego E, Brennan C, Zhang. Tsa-brag: a twisted string actuator-powered biomimetic robotic assistive glove. In: 2020 international symposium on medical robotics (ISMR). IEEE, pp 159–165
73. Lee D, Kim DH, Che CH, In JB, Shin D (2019) Highly durable bidirectional joint with twisted string actuators and variable radius pulley. IEEE/ASME Trans Mechatron 25(1):360–370
74. Dragusanu M, Marullo S, Malvezzi M, Achilli GM, Valigi MC, Prattichizzo D, Salvietti G (2022) The dressgripper: a collaborative gripper with electromagnetic fingertips for dressing assistance. IEEE Robot Autom Lett 7(3):7479–7486
75. Xu T, Shen W, Lin X, Xie YM (2020) Mechanical properties of additively manufactured thermoplastic polyurethane (TPU) material affected by various processing parameters. Polymers 12(12):3010
76. Malvezzi M, Gioioso G, Salvietti G, Prattichizzo D (2015) Syngrasp: a matlab toolbox for underactuated and compliant hands. IEEE Robot Autom Mag 22(4):52–68
77. Hussain I, Renda F, Iqbal Z, Malvezzi M, Salvietti G, Seneviratne L, Gan D, Prattichizzo D (2018) Modeling and prototyping of an underactuated gripper exploiting joint compliance and modularity. IEEE Robot Autom Lett 3(4):2854–2861
78. Birglen L, Lalibertè L, Gosselin C (2008) Underactuated robotic hands, vol 40. Springer tracts in advanced robotics. Springer
79. Li M, He B, Liang Z, Zhao C-G, Chen J, Zhuo Y, Xu G, Xie J, Althoefer K (2019) An attention-controlled hand exoskeleton for the rehabilitation of finger extension and flexion using a rigid-soft combined mechanism. Front Neurorobot, 34

Chapter 5
Conclusions

This thesis presents the outcomes of research on rehabilitative and assistive robotics, with a focus on a rapidly growing and highly impactful area within the scientific community, i.e., human-robot interaction. In this context, three key domains of robotics are explored: exoskeletons, haptics, and robotic grippers. The research focuses on the design strategies for assistive and rehabilitative devices, beginning with an analysis of state-of-the-art solutions and leading to the development of novel robotic systems that advance the current technological frontier. The increasing demand for rehabilitation and assistance among individuals with disabilities suggests that assistive and rehabilitative robotics will play a pivotal role in the coming years. Today, research on the use of robotic systems in healthcare-related fields is widespread, and the literature offers numerous promising solutions. Robots are now recognized as sophisticated therapeutic tools, though in most applications, human therapists are still essential for guidance. However, advancements in artificial intelligence hold the potential to enable more autonomous and intelligent processes in neurorehabilitation. Such advancements could enhance the effectiveness of rehabilitation by increasing the frequency of exercises and reducing costs for both patients and the broader healthcare system. Nevertheless, barriers remain to the widespread adoption of robotic systems in everyday life due to their complexity and cost, representing a significant engineering challenge. The primary focus of this research, particularly in the exoskeleton field, is not only to present designs for rehabilitation and assistive systems but also to propose new user-centered, patient-driven strategies for wearable robotics. By employing topological optimization and tailoring all aspects of development to the needs of the individual, the devices are designed with constant feedback from the user, ensuring that they are fully adapted to each person's specific requirements.

M. Dragusanu, *Design of Soft–Rigid Devices for Rehabilitative and Assistive Robotics*, Springer Theses, https://doi.org/10.1007/978-3-031-84823-0_5

Chapter 1 provides an introduction to assistive and rehabilitative robotics, with a particular emphasis on human-robot interaction and the specific areas explored in this research. It also outlines the organization and main contributions of the thesis, offering a brief overview of the works detailed in the following chapters.

Chapter 2 focuses on exoskeletal systems for the upper limbs, particularly the hand and wrist. Initially, a prototype of a tendon-actuated exoskeleton designed for wrist rehabilitation is presented. This device utilizes a tendon-driven transmission system to replicate human wrist movements. By using such an actuation mechanism, the exoskeleton remains unconstrained by rigid mechanical structures. A tracking system, consisting of two IMUs, enables the capture and estimation of wrist motions. Additionally, the user interface allows patients to comfortably perform and monitor their rehabilitation exercises at home.

The chapter then shifts to hand exoskeletons, discussing several proposed solutions. These exoskeletons are designed for use in rehabilitation, assistance, training, and haptic applications. Designing a hand exoskeleton poses significant engineering challenges, as it requires balancing conflicting requirements. Ideally, the device should be lightweight, minimally restrictive, and capable of applying suitable forces and torques for the intended application. Three different solutions are proposed in the thesis, each driven by a single motor per finger, taking a modular approach. The third solution demonstrates the best results in terms of wearability, lightweight design, strength, and versatility.

Furthermore, the hand and wrist modules are combined into an integrated exoskeletal system aimed at assisting and rehabilitating both the hand and wrist. This device was designed to enhance user independence during rehabilitation and training, reducing the need for constant specialist supervision. The main objective is to develop a modular device that is easy to wear, even independently, for patients with temporary or permanent conditions such as limb-girdle muscular dystrophy. This design philosophy guided the development of an automatic locking mechanism that fastens the wrist support to the patient's forearm and the wireless communication with a PC. A key feature of the system is its ability to record therapist-guided exercises using the device's sensors, allowing the patient to replay them in future sessions. Each session can be recorded to track the patient's progress over time. The system is modular, enabling users to customize it according to their specific needs. Although the thesis presents the integrated hand-wrist system, the wrist and hand modules can be used together or independently, based on user preferences. The graphical user interface (GUI) manages single or multiple modules, and even allows the user to operate at the finger level. Depending on the user's needs, they can activate individual fingers, the entire hand, the wrist, or the complete hand-wrist system. The proposed device is especially valuable in the context of telerehabilitation, which has become increasingly important in recent years. The ability to create and upload customized exercises, and to record and replay sessions guided by a physiotherapist, reduces the need for direct physical interaction between patients and specialists. This, in turn, reduces both the fatigue and costs associated with rehabilitation, facilitating a more effective and sustainable recovery process. In addition, the thesis demonstrates rehabilitation exercises for the wrist, individual fingers, and the entire hand. These exercises are programmed using specific mathematical functions or are recorded through demonstrations conducted by a physiotherapist, enabling patients to perform them independently.

Finally, towards the end of Chap. 2, an innovative actuation system is introduced, in which the movements of two adjacent fingers are coupled through a differential mechanism. This differential gear system evenly distributes the actuator force while maintaining independent finger motion. If one finger encounters an obstacle and is blocked, the other finger remains free to move. The reduction in the number of actuators, driven by user feedback regarding device weight, represents a significant advancement in the design of the hand exoskeleton. The new system results in a lighter, more energy-efficient, and less complex device. Moreover, the updated transmission system achieves a range of motion for the phalanges that is approximately 10% greater than the previous version, all while maintaining the same actuator stroke. Additionally, the device was tested for compatibility with simple, widely-used, low-cost tracking systems such as the Leap Motion Controller. This test demonstrated that the latest version of the hand exoskeleton is not only capable of performing physiotherapy tasks but can also record and remotely monitor those tasks. This compatibility expands rehabilitation opportunities for patients, doctors, and physiotherapists by allowing for remote therapy management. Compatibility with widely-used tracking systems also improves patient engagement by enabling interaction with virtual environments, making therapy more interactive, enjoyable, and potentially competitive, either against digital avatars or artificial intelligence systems.

This chapter highlights how the rapid growth of additive manufacturing (AM) technologies, combined with topological optimization and advanced materials, has allowed for novel configurations that reduce device weight while maintaining functionality and structural integrity. The ultimate goal is to enhance portability and wearability by reducing mass while ensuring adequate strength and resistance. This phase of the project demonstrates how topological optimization and advanced materials are invaluable tools in the design and realization of patient-centered devices.

It is worth underlining that that throughout this project, the end users, i.e., patients with upper limb disabilities and motor limitations, were actively involved at every stage, from the initial design phase to the development and testing of the prototypes.

The complete hand/wrist exoskeleton system presented in this thesis has achieved a Technology Readiness Level (TRL) of 4. Its hardware structure will undergo further optimization in the near future. In the next phase of development, the design will be refined based on feedback from users and physiotherapists. In particular, the finger modules will be further miniaturized, and a dedicated app for smartphones and tablets will be developed to enhance user accessibility.

Moreover, the hardware structure will be improved with the aim of allowing patients with limited arm and hand mobility to independently assemble, disassemble, and wear the modules. An additional goal is to develop a thumb exoskeleton capable of controlling all thumb movements, a challenging engineering task that remains a high priority. Furthermore, new scenarios have opened, thanks to preliminary studies on compliant structures explored in grippers. This research is paving the way for new types of exoskeletons, such as the "suit-glove" hand exoskeleton, which employs twisted string actuators (TSA) and compliant structures to perform hand movements. The next steps in this research will involve extending this approach to the elbow, and eventually to the shoulder.

Chapter 3 introduces devices developed for haptic robotics, specifically tailored for rehabilitation and assistance, with a focus on the hand. The chapter distinguishes between grounded and wearable haptic devices. Among the grounded devices is HAPP, a portable haptic device designed for preclinical investigation of the mechanical therapy effects for hand pathologies, such as Complex Regional Pain Syndrome Type-I and stroke. It also allows systematic and remote control of manual therapy exercises via a graphical user interface. HAPP features a 3-DoF parallel structure that can orient its end-effector beneath the patient's palm, delivering local force stimulation. The end-effector is interchangeable, and in this work, a solution was presented to exert targeted forces in predefined areas of the palm. Future work will explore the integration and control of vibratory stimuli in specific areas of the hand. The graphical user interface already includes a feature for adjusting vibration intensity. In addition, a PID controller is planned to precisely control the end-effector, employing a novel system that accounts for the real-time position of the hand on the device.

In this chapter, the wearable devices developed for assistance and rehabilitation are presented. Among these, the first device introduced is *HANS*, a novel system designed for both rehabilitative and assistive purposes. Specifically, HANS is showcased as a wearable haptic device capable of facilitating remote human-to-home handshakes. Despite handshakes being widely regarded as a significant social gesture, there has been no wearable technology designed to measure and convey this interaction remotely.

Throughout this thesis, both the sensing and actuation components of HANS are detailed, with their design driven by the specific characteristics of a handshake. The experimental results demonstrate that HANS effectively enables users to perceive and transmit a handshake experience that closely mimics a natural human handshake, even while using everyday objects. Remarkably, the device also allows individuals with mobility impairments to participate in this fundamental social ritual. For example, a user with reduced upper limb mobility was invited to test HANS and responded enthusiastically, appreciating how the device enabled a handshake without discomfort or tension.

Looking ahead, future work will focus on integrating HANS with common social platforms, enabling users to combine tactile interaction with visual and auditory cues during a remote handshake. Although current limitations include the absence of the shaking motion and temperature exchange associated with a real handshake, future developments aim to address these aspects.

Additionally, this chapter introduces the *HapticPalm*, a wearable tactile device designed for cutaneous stimulation of the hand palm, particularly in virtual reality environments. The HapticPalm is engineered to render the forces generated during palm-to-environment interactions. The design employs a tendon transmission system with a passive element that disengages the end-effector from the palm when no force is required. The core mechanism involves a parallel tendon arrangement, driven by three motors positioned on the back of the hand. These motors drive the tendons, which symmetrically transmit forces from a "Y-shaped" platform to an end-effector arranged in a similar "Y-configuration."

To enhance functionality, several interchangeable modules have been 3D-printed, enabling the reproduction of a wide range of surface sensations. These modules are designed for quick attachment and detachment using a "T-shaped" socket and magnetic clip system, making the device adaptable for different tasks. The HapticPalm was thoroughly tested to validate its performance and assess usability in both rehabilitation and virtual reality contexts.

Following user feedback from preliminary tests, a new and improved version of the HapticPalm was developed. The end-effector was slightly modified based on user suggestions to enhance wearability and ease of use. Additionally, the introduction of new interchangeable modules and the replacement of the spring with a wave-joint shaped link-based on a compliant structure-has further improved its usability. A vibromotor was also incorporated, providing a more immersive virtual reality experience and potentially serving as a distraction from hand pain during rehabilitation.

In the initial stages of this work, theoretical and maximum normal forces that the HapticPalm could apply to a typical human hand were calculated under static conditions. These theoretical values were experimentally validated through testing.

As for future developments, the primary focus will be on enhancing the transmission system. A fully tendon-driven design is planned, with antagonistic tendons replacing the current spring or compliant structures. This update will eliminate the force reduction caused by the current design, which currently limits the force and torque generated by the motor to under 50%.

In Chap. 4, just before concluding the thesis, the focus shifts to the topic of assistance in human-robot interaction (HRI), specifically through the use of robotic grippers. The first work introduces a novel methodology for designing soft-rigid grippers, utilizing additive manufacturing (AM) technologies and compliant structures. AM technologies are continually evolving and offer interesting possibilities in the design and production of robotic and mechatronic devices.

The grippers developed through this method can execute various finger flexion trajectories using the same tendon-driven actuation system. The central idea is to create joints with predefined stiffness by modifying a few parameters of a design function. This approach enables the 3D printing of a monolithic finger with specific joint stiffness, which can then be easily attached to a palm base containing the actuation mechanism. The study details the characterization of the wave-shaped joints, reporting both numerical and experimental results on flexible joints based on compliant structures. Specifically, the relationship between the bending stiffness and the geometric characteristics of the joints is explored. While the study did not reveal any significant issues regarding parameter convergence, a formal analysis of optimization parameter convergence properties will be a topic for future investigations.

Additionally, a potential solution for controlling the flexural joint stiffness in underactuated tendon-driven robotic grippers is presented, which involves applying precompression to the joints using a twisted string actuator (TSA). This approach allows for active adjustment of the joint stiffness, thereby modifying the finger's overall closing movement and grasping properties. Stiffness regulation is achieved by integrating an active system into the joint, which applies controlled precompression to the gripper's elastic joints. The TSA actuator is compact enough to be embedded within the rigid parts of the finger modules, maintaining the modular structure of the gripper. Depending on the application, certain joints can have variable stiffness, while others maintain constant stiffness, reducing the number of actuators required.

Continuing the focus on assistance, particularly in the context of personal care, the latter part of Chap. 4 introduces the *DressGripper*, a collaborative robotic gripper specifically designed for assistance in dressing. Robotic dressing assistance is a particular type of collaborative robotic activity, as the robot's end-effector often comes into direct contact with the user's body. Therefore, the gripper cannot be rigid, and intrinsically safe solutions, such as soft forceps, are required. The *DressGripper* is an underactuated device that exploits a synergy between tendon-driven and magnetic actuation, with magnetic elements embedded in the fingertips.

Future developments in this field will focus on creating a new type of gripper that integrates compliant structures, magnetic and tendon actuation synergy, and TSA-based actuation, combining the best features of these technologies to enhance robotic assistance capabilities.

Author Biography

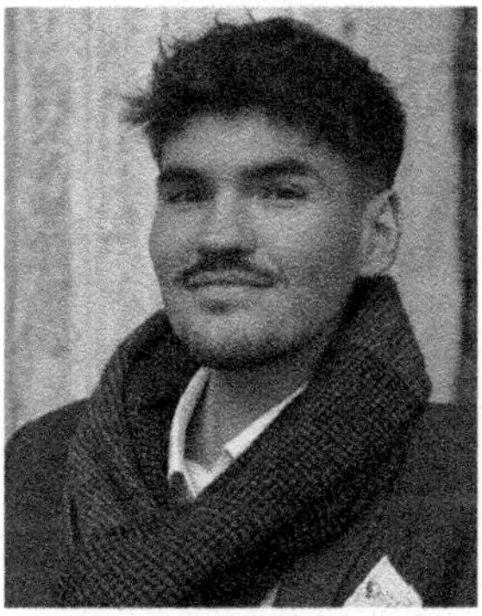

Dr. Mihai Dragusanu is currently an Assistant Professor of mechanics and mechanism theory with the Department of Information Engineering and Mathematics, University of Siena, Italy. He is also a researcher and carries out his research activities at SIRSLab (Robotics and Systems Lab) at the University of Siena, coordinated by Prof. Domenico Prattichizzo. His research interests include robotics and haptics focusing on exoskeletons, rehabilitation and medical robotics, and assistive soft rigid gripper.

Dr. Dragusanu received his Bachelor's Degree in Computer and Information Engineering in 2016, his M.Sc. in Computer and Automation Engineering in 2019, and his Ph.D. in Information Engineering and Science, specializing in applied mechanics, in 2023. All '*cum laude*' from the University of Siena.

He is currently Associate Editor for the International Conference on Robotics and Automation (ICRA), and he is one of the mentors at the University of Siena for diversity, equity, and inclusion.

Dr. Dragusanu has been honored with several awards throughout his young career. He was awarded with the *Best Student in Computer Science and Information Engineering* by the University of Siena. In 2022, he was finalist for the *RSJ Pioneering Research Award in Robot and Human Interactive Communication* at IEEE Ro-Man 2022 conference and in 2023 he received the *IEEE Fabrizio Flacco, Young Author Best Paper Award 2023, Chapter Italy—IEEE Robotics and Automation Society*. Most recently, he was honored with the prestigious award *Most Promising Researcher in Robotics and AI* by Fondazione Mondo Digitale, at RomeCup 2024, recognizing him as the top emerging researcher in Italy in the field of robotics and artificial intelligence.

Mihai's full CV and list of publications are available at https://www3.diism.unisi.it/~dragusanu/.

M. Dragusanu, *Design of Soft–Rigid Devices for Rehabilitative and Assistive Robotics*, Springer Theses, https://doi.org/10.1007/978-3-031-84823-0

The manufacturer's authorised representative in the EU is Springer Nature Customer Service Centre GmbH, Europaplatz 3, 69115 Heidelberg, Germany. If you have any concerns regarding our products, please contact ProductSafety@springernature.com

Printed and bound by CPI Group (UK) Ltd, Croydon, CR0 4YY
30/09/2026
02225500-0003